Homeopathy
as Energy Medicine

"Richard Grossinger is the Joseph Campbell of our time. The scope and depth of his knowledge of planetary medical systems are unparalleled. *Homeopathy as Energy Medicine* guides the reader to a place of self-discovery on their healing journey, offering insight into interpreting pain and suffering with wisdom. This profound book charts new territory in understanding the recovery of the human body, its sovereignty, and interconnected complexities, catering to both professionals and laypeople alike. Medicine is preexisting in our own bodily being and environment, waiting to be recognized by a knowledgeable therapist. This book places homeopathy in the rarified pantheon of correct evolutionary medicine. Brilliant!"

MICHAEL J. SHEA, PH.D., AUTHOR OF
THE BIODYNAMICS OF THE IMMUNE SYSTEM

"*Homeopathy as Energy Medicine* plumbs the historical depths of homeopathy and the various ancient principles from which it draws and then explores the last half-century of developments in the science and art of homeopathy, with a healthy nod to its futuristic concepts and applications. Grossinger was originally trained as an anthropologist, and this training is clearly evident as he describes with elegance and eloquence this amazing, compelling, and somewhat strange system of healing."

DANA ULLMAN, MPH, CCH, AUTHOR OF 10 BOOKS
INCLUDING *THE HOMEOPATHIC REVOLUTION*

Homeopathy as Energy Medicine

INFORMATION
IN THE NANODOSE

Richard Grossinger

Healing Arts Press
Rochester, Vermont

Healing Arts Press
One Park Street
Rochester, Vermont 05767
www.HealingArtsPress.com

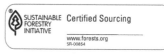

SUSTAINABLE Certified Sourcing
FORESTRY
INITIATIVE
www.forests.org
SR-00854

Text stock is SFI certified

Healing Arts Press is a division of Inner Traditions International

Portions of this text were originally published as part of *Planet Medicine: From Stone Age Shamanism to Post-Industrial Healing* by Anchor Press in 1980, Shambhala Publications in 1982, and North Atlantic Books in 1990.
Edited and expanded version published in 1993 as *Homeopathy: An Introduction for Skeptics and Beginners* by North Atlantic Books.
Revised and updated version published in 1998 as *Homeopathy: The Great Riddle* by North Atlantic Books.

Note to the reader: *This book is intended to be an informational guide. The remedies, approaches, and techniques described herein are meant to supplement, and not to be a substitute for, professional medical care or treatment. They should not be used to treat a serious ailment without prior consultation with a qualified health care professional.*

Cataloging-in-Publication Data for this title is available from the Library of Congress

ISBN 978-1-64411-966-2 (print)
ISBN 978-1-64411-967-9 (ebook)

Printed and bound in the United States by Lake Book Manufacturing, LLC
The text stock is SFI certified. The Sustainable Forestry Initiative® program promotes sustainable forest management.

10 9 8 7 6 5 4 3 2 1

Text design by Debbie Glogover and layout by Priscilla Baker
This book was typeset in Garamond Premier Pro with Legacy Sans, Plantin, and Quasimoda used as display typefaces

To send correspondence to the author of this book, mail a first-class letter to the author c/o Inner Traditions • Bear & Company, One Park Street, Rochester, VT 05767, and we will forward the communication, or contact the author directly at **richardgrossinger.com**.

Scan the QR code and save 25% at InnerTraditions.com. Browse over 2,000 titles on spirituality, the occult, ancient mysteries, new science, holistic health, and natural medicine.

For MDs and other mainstream physicians
searching for the true medicine:
Stefan Andren, Chiara Battelli, Steve Curtin,
Michael Heniser, Caitlin Kaufman, Brian Keroac,
Sirish Maddali, Gordon Murphy, Jessica Radway,
Marcey Shapiro, and Peter Then.

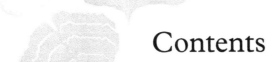

Contents

Foreword

Ever since Samuel Hahnemann, a German medical doctor, linguist, and researcher, discovered homeopathy and published the very first edition of *The Organon of Rational Medicine* in 1810, people have asked, "What is homeopathy?" This question is being asked even today, more than two hundred years after the birth of homeopathy, and this is the reason why you are drawn to reading Richard Grossinger's book *Homeopathy as Energy Medicine: Information in the Nanodose.*

This question has not stopped people from using homeopathy for the past two centuries, and presently, despite the heroic efforts by health authorities to eradicate homeopathy, it has survived successfully on every continent of the world, and in many countries it is supported and approved by the government as a valid healing modality. Homeopathy could survive against all odds, even while facing questions about what it is, only on the basis of the clinical results it gives, both historically and to this day. People, now more aware, informed, and literate than in the past few centuries, see the results for themselves. They see that homeopathy does not cause dependency, addiction, suppression of the immune system, or noxious side effects. They see that the oft-repeated phrase "The treatment is worse than the disease" does *not* apply when they use homeopathy for their acute and chronic health complaints. Encouraged and emboldened, they continue to use homeopathy for pregnant women, for newborn babies and the elderly, for their pets and farm animals, and even for their plants and gardens. Nevertheless, its popularity, based purely on clinical results, does not stop the curious folks from asking, "What is homeopathy, and how does it work?" Fair enough.

Richard Grossinger has attempted to answer this eternal question in his book *Homeopathy as Energy Medicine: Information in the Nanodose.* Richard has more than fifty years of intimate experience with homeopathy. As a university professor, he taught courses on homeopathy; as a consumer, he used it successfully for himself and his precious family; he has written books and papers about it; and he regularly refers his peers, friends, and relations to various homeopaths. Over and above all, he is a deep thinker, philosopher, and prolific writer, habituated to sinking deep into a subject and coming out of that deep dive with a unique, brilliant, and in-depth understanding of the intricacies of otherwise complicated matters. Richard has done the same magic this time, and he has devoted ample time (several decades) to scrutinize, study, understand, make sense of, and imbibe the truth contained in homeopathy into his psychic being and his vast intellect. This book, *Homeopathy as Energy Medicine: Information in the Nanodose,* born out of such heart- and intellect-based scholarship, will enable you to see homeopathy with fresh insight and understanding.

As you read this book, you will come to appreciate the fact that Dr. Hahnemann used the most sophisticated terminology and concepts available to him in his day to explain the philosophy, research, methodology, experimentations, and findings in *The Organon* more than two hundred years ago. As a medical doctor at the cutting edge of his field, Samuel Hahnemann revised his *Organon* six times, and this book became the bible of homeopaths. It was translated from German into English and carried to every corner of the world by his students. Since Hahnemann's time, there has been a prolific explosion in understanding the mind-body-psyche axis. Many other healing modalities have come to light that have based themselves on this holistic view of the human organism, just as homeopathy has since its birth. Richard Grossinger has studied this bible of homeopaths and synthesized his own thinking, interpretation, observation, and understanding of homeopathy using the sensibilities of the twenty-first century. Alongside that work, he has studied other healing modalities as well to see how homeopathy compares with and differs from them. He uses the latest scientific paradigms to examine homeopathy and lays out the intricacies of this healing art and science in terms and concepts that resonate with the modern reader. He helps us make sense of heart, soul, meaning, and purpose of homeopathy.

After reading *Homeopathy as Energy Medicine: Information in the Nanodose,* you will certainly know more and better about what homeopathy is. You will also understand that homeopathy is undoubtably the medicine of a utopian time when the human organism will be seen as a holistic entity that engages and interacts with the visible and invisible energies of the universe, and the mind-body-psyche of humans will be seen as a part of the cosmic web of energies, of which homeopathy itself is a part.

VATSALA SPERLING, M.S., PH.D., PDHOM, CCH, RSHOM

VATSALA SPERLING, M.S., Ph.D., PDHom, CCH, RSHom, is a classical homeopath who grew up in India and earned her doctorate in clinical microbiology. Before moving to the United States in the 1990s, she was the chief of clinical microbiology at the Childs Trust Hospital in Chennai, India, where she published extensively and conducted research with the World Health Organization. A founding member of Hacienda Rio Cote, a reforestation project in Costa Rica, she runs her own homeopathy practice in both Vermont and Costa Rica. She lives in Rochester, Vermont.

Homeopathy:
The Great Riddle

There are many books about the practice of homeopathic medicine, including self-help manuals, primers for patients and parents, and applications for cats, dogs, horses, fish, even hedgehogs. These texts depict its principles, remedies, and character types. This book, *Homeopathy as Energy Medicine: Information in the Nanodose*, explores what homeopathy is and attempts to place it in a larger framework of energy medicine and microdose effects.

By *energy medicine*, I mean healing—cures or beneficial changes in organisms—through stimulating or enhancing their immune systems, vital force, and natural resilience—reestablishing their homeostasis and mind-body-spirit field, as opposed to ridding them of symptoms. Energy medicines are holistic, constitutional, psychosomatic, and morphogenetic; they are synergized through mitochondria and other organelles and cells and their networks of organized tissues. The roster of energy modalities is broad and diverse: acupuncture, homeopathy, cranial osteopathy, shamanic rituals and ceremonies, Reiki, prayer, crystals, mineral baths, and treating by sound, color, scent, and taste. The effects of energy medicines are usually unquantifiable, but when they "take," they are deep and cascade outward.

While homeopathy is holistic and dynamic in the way that many

Indigenous medicines are, it is not for the same reasons. Homeopathy is clinical and objective, not totemic or ceremonial. At a "Global Healers Conference," homeopaths and shamans would head to opposite sides of the hall.

By *nanodose*, I mean the chemistry of trace, micro, nano, and/or quantum-entangled substances and those substances' imprints in water and other mediums and their radiation into living systems. In particular, I cite the assimilation, activation, catalysis, and synergization by tiny potentized molecules in homeopathic pharmacy. Though I use the word *nanodose* in this book's title, I more commonly use the word *microdose* in the text. That is because microdose is the accepted homeopathic term—the entire "nano" world was unknown at the time of the origin and development of homeopathic medicine, but it is a more accurate description of the scale at which homeopathic medicines are prepared and transfer information.

Homeopathy may also work by focused and "intentioned" thoughtforms, hence the possibility of placebo effects and other telekinetic thoughtforms.

Homeopathy also activates the *life code*. By that I mean RNA and DNA—amino acid helices in spiral strands that store and transfer biological information in cell nuclei. DNA may also form interdimensional helices such that they become *nadis* that transfer life codes from the Etheric realm into matter. Throughout this book, I will allude to the Etheric as well as the material basis of health. You can take the Etheric plane as a metaphor for energy medicine or as an actual transdimensional field. Etheric and Astral energy and information may be the main features underlying health, as they flow from the subtle body into embodiment as tissue layers. They may explain homeopathy's seeming placebo effect.

Defining homeopathy is next to impossible, as you may already suspect. For one, by modern experimental standards the system has no physical, biochemical, or anatomical explanation. Originating at the close of the eighteenth century, when modern sciences were emerging, it has rested almost solely since on its apparent success in curing sick people, particularly those with chronic diseases—a success that its detractors, if they acknowledge homeopathy at all, attribute to placebo or by doing nothing, hence causing no iatrogenic harm—physician- or treatment-instigated diseases.

Three things stand against this appraisal: (1) homeopathy's cure rates exceed ordinary placebo effects; (2) placebo is unjustly denigrated, for if the mind—as thoughtforms—can cure pathologies, it is one of the most powerful forces in nature; and (3) homeopathy's cures arise from discrete protocols rather than nebulous suggestibility around pill-taking.

In chapter 2, "The Origins of Homeopathic Medicine," I discuss medical and pharmaceutical forerunners of homeopathy. Homeopathy borrowed many of its principles and methods from earlier medicines and recombined them in a new system.

The core of this book is chapter 3, "The Tenets and Rubrics of Homeopathic Medicine." It is a brief immersion in homeopathic philosophy and practice. Followers explain homeopathy by a medley of archaic and futuristic paradigms ranging from alchemy and voodoo to quantum physics and chaos theory.

In chapter 4, "Homeopathy and Modern Medicine," I examine the relationship between homeopathy and the general practice of medicine as a clash of principles.

Chapter 5 follows the discovery and development of homeopathy by Samuel Hahnemann and explains how a doctor and medical scholar codified ancient and unorthodox healing methods while converting them into the most advanced medical system of his time.

Chapter 6 describes homeopathy's brief renaissance in nineteenth-century North America, followed by its almost total abandonment in the 1920s and then its revival in the counterculture of the 1970s.

Chapter 7 discusses three broader applications of homeopathic philosophy: pill-less pharmacy, the microdose basis of astrology, and psychic and dream homeopathy.

Appendices include a case study, a comparison of homeopathy to other alternative and mainstream modalities, and a short resource guide.

A briefer version of *Homeopathy as Energy Medicine* appeared as four chapters in *Planet Medicine: From Stone Age Shamanism to Post-Industrial Healing* (1980). After being edited and expanded, these chapters were published in their own volume as *Homeopathy: An Introduction for Skeptics and Beginners* (1993). I revised and updated this volume when I renamed it *Homeopathy: The Great Riddle* (1998). The book in your hands represents the most recent full revision and the most extensive one, expanded to cover energy medicine and nano-science in general.

1

What Is Homeopathy?

Homeopathy was developed by German physician Samuel Hahnemann (1755–1843) at the turn of the nineteenth century and soon became a popular medical modality in much of the Western world. Its ascent was swiftest in North America, cresting during the decade from 1880 to 1890. Its decline was swiftest there too. When laboratory science took over medicine, homeopathy was undermined by its own internal contradictions and absence of biophysical and biochemical evidence. It lost its independent identity as part of a general recompartmentalization of medical education.

So, what *is* homeopathy? In a 1992 article in the *New York Times Magazine*, journalist James Gorman noted confusions fostered by homeopathy's revival within a cornucopia of alternative medicines. He acknowledged that it is not a botanical or New Age pharmacy, remarking, "Few people who buy the new over-the-counter homeopathic remedies realize that homeopathy is not herbal or Chinese medicine. It is not naturopathy, osteopathy or acupuncture, not bodywork, shiatsu or chiropractic."[1]

That excludes the usual suspects, so what is left?

Homeopathy is first, and perhaps foremost, an extension of empirical and vitalistic traditions in Western medicine. Its paradigms and philosophy arise from direct observation and treatment of

1

sick people, and its claims are based on results, not theory. You can practice homeopathy without understanding or even believing in it, and you can be cured by its medicines while presuming that they are something other than what they are.

By today's reductionist requirements homeopathy is *not* a science; it doesn't check any of the boxes: peer review, universal repeatability, evidence-based cause and effect. While many of its supporters proffer that it is "another scientific medicine," I would more accurately call it "the medicine of an unknown science." The quantum leap that its principles require is decades or centuries ahead of its clinical practice. It shares that status loosely with Lamarckian evolution of acquired traits, paranormal phenomena (psi effects and UFOs), Carl Jung's theory of synchronicity, Wilhelm Reich's orgone biology, and "spooky influence at a distance" in quantum mechanics.

Homeopathy also combines elements of alchemy, hermeticism, and early pharmacology reconceived as a single method.

In another sense, homeopathy is the single branch of hermetic and vitalistic science that earned professional standing in a secularized world. That alone is an accomplishment for a nineteenth-century system once relegated to a historical memento.

Homeopathy is based theoretically on the responsiveness of an organism's defense mechanism and general homeostasis. These attributes are not associated with any organ, protein, enzyme, or biochemical network, though they are integrated within the molecular processes of the immune system. Their operation is intrinsic to the integrity of the organism, whether that is understood as a morphic field, a biomolecular cohesion, or the interplay of chi (often anglicized as *qi*) and yin and yang.

The organism's defense mechanism, when homeopathically activated rather than (in baseball parlance) "pinch-hit for" by pharmaceuticals or surgery, has the capacity to respond dynamically to any disease. In that state, it is a direct heir to the vital force of Greek and medieval medicine and a descendant of the alchemical botany of Paracelsus and Jan Baptista van Helmont. In all vitalistic systems, disease is an "invasive idea" imposed on a self-healing matrix at the core of every life form. That matrix is the vital force's epigenetic driver without which it could not exist. Whether its prototype arises vibrationally in Etheric, Astral, or other subtle planes is a metaphysical question that can be ignored in matters of homeopathic medical efficacy, though it will always be a part of existential inquiries around homeopathy.

Homeopathy is based on three central principles: the Law of Similars, attunement of tiny bits of information (micro- or nano-doses) in biological systems, and potentization with specification. Separately, each is scientifically accepted—the Law of Similars in vaccinations; microdose transmission in the biochemistry of enzymes and trace minerals, exoplanet exploration, and telecommunications; and potentization in applications ranging from music, applied algebra, and biotech to data storage and bartending—crickets, pipes, and crystals each attune at specified frequencies.

Combined in homeopathy, these precepts do not receive the same scientific pass.

The Law of Similars

The idea that a disease can be treated with a remedy whose effects mimic those of the disease being treated is known historically as the Law of Similars. Treatment by Similars uses substances that cause symptoms resembling those caused by an ailment in order to cure that ailment, matching medicinal and disease frequencies even if the match means initially increasing symptomology.

The Law of Similars challenges modernity's prime medical dictate: the "Law of Contraries" or antidoting pathological responses almost exclusively by drugs or surgery. Whether you treat symptoms as healing responses that a doctor should enhance or as diseases a doctor needs to eliminate is a fundamental medical dichotomy in both model and practice.

In action, the Law of Similars "tells" a physician to stimulate the body's natural immunity, vital energy, and internal coction (metabolism) instead of imposing an external intervention. If, for argument's sake, we consider homeopathic pills to be drugs, which they are and aren't, then following the Law of Similars means prescribing activating and aggravating rather than sedating and enervating ones.

Isopathy, healing by injecting or ingesting a form of the disease-causing substance *itself* (most notably in immunization), resembles healing by Similars but isn't. *Homeo* ("like," meaning "*not* the same") is different from *iso* ("equal," meaning, "yes, the same"). Likeness makes use of natural substances' vitality, whereas sameness requires deadened proxies: disease products, depotentized viruses, or genetically modified codes. A corollary of the Law of Similars is that isopathic substances, even when refined for vaccines or allergy shots, do not provide the differential leverage needed for an organism to "recognize" its own disease state.

In pre-Hahnemannian medicine, the use of Similars as remedies was liberally mixed with the use of Contraries, and most doctors treated maladies on a circumstantial basis. By basing homeopathy *solely* on the Law of Similars, Hahnemann formalized the distinction between a medicine that encourages symptoms *and all other medicines*. While homeopaths define their systems as treatment by Similars—*homeopathy* (from the Greek for "like treatment"), distinguishing it from *allopathy* (from the Greek for "other treatment")—*allo* does not mean healing by Contraries; it means all medicines that are not homeopathic (not chosen according to the Law of Similars). Hahnemann included in allopathy common treatments based on the Law of Contraries, plus any other medicines prioritizing individual symptoms over disease wholes or by abstract categories of pathology rather than ailments in actual patients.

Today, allopathy has become synonymous with the medical establishment, its name used pejoratively by homeopaths and proudly by allopaths who happen to know the word. Yet these same "allopaths" paradoxically use isopathy—vaccines—to prevent diseases and antidote allergies. Isopathy has immunological benefits but (again) does not treat according to whole constitutions and disease complexes or by differentiations of tiers of energy. "Treatment by like" is not energy medicine. Contemporary homeopathic author Dana Ullman highlights the key distinctions between homeopathy and isopathy:

> Some conventional medical treatments are ultimately [also] based on the Law of Similars, though they should not be considered homeopathic medicines for two basic reasons: 1) each medicine is not prepared in the pharmacological procedure of dilution and succussion common to homeopathic medicines; 2) each medicine is not individually prescribed in the sufficient detail common to homeopathic medicines.
>
> A homeopathic medicine is not prescribed for a specific disease *per se,* but for the pattern of symptoms that the original medicinal substance in crude form is known to cause in overdose when given to healthy people. The concept of a pattern or syndrome of symptoms is an integral part of homeopathic care. This is simply a systems concept of looking at symptoms in context with the whole. The challenge to the person prescribing homeopathic medicines then is this individualization of drug prescription.[2]

In order to understand the Law of Similars, we have to recognize that it is not only discrete but parabolic. Though based on treating like with like, it goes past simple stimulation of the immune response toward a ricochet effect at the source of life, health, disease, and healing. On the spectrum of energy medicines including homeopathy but also (as noted) traditional Chinese and ayurvedic pharmacies and other shamanic and psychic modalities, each arrives at its own non-linear application of Similars, reactivation of the defense mechanism, and homeostasis.

A homeopathic remedy resembles—mirrors—an illness, sometimes to a T, but it is *not* the illness, so in effect it fools the organism into both recognizing and then curing the disease. The vibration of the Similar, resonating through the nucleic codes of the body, provides a safe, biologically compatible context for clearing a pathological predisposition, much as it likely cleared away impediments in the embryonic development of the organism. The underlying pathology is relieved by a matching "nonpathology." Without that intercession, the distortion will continue to blossom into new symptom-bearing diseases.

Homeopathy (again, if you accept its premises) uses individual diseases themselves to boost and reinforce health, and that is secondary to removing their symptoms forthwith (or not). We might also say a homeopathic medicine elicits what was *constitutionally* lacking so that its deficiency is no longer expressed pathologically. A minute dose of a Similar shocks the system into action, causing it to supply the missing ingredients itself.

Most diseases (by homeopathic rationale) are themselves the *precisely* correct response of the organism to a mind-body lesion, but a sick organism can get stuck in its own stalled homeostasis. It engages with its pathology in systemic folly, even to death.

But energy must be *individually* "energized" rather than mimicked or replicated—the definition of a Similar. Otherwise, the patient's resistances and systemic torpor may snub or wrongfoot the cure—so-called side effects. It is as if the organism needs a good show to acknowledge how complex and suspenseful or vivid its situation is. It needs to be *seen*. Potentized Similars are a total outrage, the organismic equivalent of a good joke or prank, or a molecular expression of Carl Jung's trickster archetype. Lay homeopath Theodore Enslin put the matter this way:

> [The Similar] is a parallel. It is a recognition of the fact that the unwanted manifestations can only be braked by producing other unwanted manifestations which are similar. And there's a great difference between similar and the same. There's a popular conception: if the guy gets gas from eating cabbage, you give him a high dilution of cabbage, and that's going to cure him. That's not what's done at all. Actually, the medicines are not medicines at all. The process is an outrage of the system itself. A diseased system is an apathetic one: it just doesn't give a damn. But in many—most cases, unless the thing has gone too far—that apathy can be overcome by introducing a parallel. When that parallel becomes apparent to the organism, it's outraged—and cures itself. The medicine actually has very little to do with it.[3]

An organism that responds to Contraries or medicalized isopaths is still basically sluggish. To avoid relapse, it must ultimately be treated, or treat itself, homeopathically.

Disease is a natural expression of misdirects or obstacles in nature. It can't be manipulated or uprooted by material interventions, nor can it be effaced directly. If it goes away, it will return, probably in another form. One might as well, like Ahab in Herman Melville's *Moby Dick*, attack the sun. The only rival to a disease is the life essence of the organism. If that life essence can be provoked into dialogue with the pathology, then even the most severe ailment can, in principle, be healed. Conversely, an allopathic attempt to alter a disease's course may end up being as much an attack upon the organism as it is upon the illness.

Of course, Contraries are used effectively within the framework of an individual's time-bound biology. Every treatment can't be a total "cure" or an ultimate medicine; some alleviate symptoms by bringing relief and buying time for the organism to reorganize and heal. There is a place for allopathy and a reason why it has become a universal medicine. Yet the purist position gives a sense of how Similars are meant to work and how, if you accept homeopathy's premise, they can sometimes spark miracle cures. The best healing is an abbreviated re-embryogenesis (or reboot) drawing on the first one occurring at conception.

Microdoses

Homeopathy's microdose imperative establishes the use of very small, in fact increasingly smaller, doses of substances for paradoxically more powerful effects. Using information-transmitting microdoses rather than kinesis-assigning substances means stimulating the organism's innate healing capacity at subtrace and subenzymatic levels. Homeopathic microdoses do not just convey biochemical signals; they turn elemental properties into vital patterns with apparent tipping-point effects—what I call the information in the microdose.

Discovery of the microdose effect came *after* the Law of Similars was established and then fused with it in a novel fashion. As we shall see, Hahnemann was initially only trying to treat diseases with Similars—prescribing remedies that cause rather than suppress symptoms. His goal was to stimulate a healing response by an artificial, nonpathological surrogate. Because he was using some toxins and poisons, he kept reducing his dosages in order to arrive at the minimum suspension of molecules that retained a medicinal virtue.

However, the degree of dilution at which a solution would forfeit every molecule of its original basis (soon to be specified as Avogadro's constant) was still uncalculated, so Hahnemann shot right past it, and in fact continued diluting his medicines hundreds and thousands of times more, beyond the point at which any molecules of its pharmaceutical substrate statistically remain. Yet he found that the greater the dilution with succussion (heavy shaking), the more powerful and deep-acting as well as less toxic the "pill." He had stumbled upon an energetic dose as well as an unknown biochemical principle.

In the absence of a recognized pharmaceutical explanation, modern homeopathy falls back on speculative nanopharmacy and metaphors from subatomic physics, but these are props or alibis for something happening at a moleculo-cellular level.

Potentization

According to the homeopathic rule of empowerment, the smaller the dose, the more potentized its effects and the deeper its activation, as long as the active property is succussed and signified. Succussion is crucial. The explanation for medicinal activity must include the sequence and method of preparation as well as the raw potency of the molecular substances of the original solute. Otherwise, all microdoses and molecules in the world—the air we breathe, the water we drink, the particles of food we swallow—would be causing willy-nilly, conflicting nanodose effects. Succussions activate the vital force.

Potentizing means reifying molecular suspensions during succussion—forceful shaking at each phase of dilution. This has a music-like effect, setting them in a cohesive scale that stands out from environmental white noise. While repertorizing by Similars specifies the type of substance, microdosing raises and transduces the energy, and potentization apparently sets its frequency.

Homeopathy potentizes its ingredients by diluting and shaking in decimal or other algebraic sequences. Indigenous medicines employ a potpourri of techniques for dynamic activation: brushing, tapping, blowing, breathing on, Kirlian touch, modulated sound, and drumming. In some Indigenous systems, hot springs or ice caves and ice bathing play activating roles. Each of these processes, if performed properly, has somatic as well as emotional effects. These could either occur inside cells or be transmitted across extracellular matrices—membranes, fascia, and tissues—or both.

Why is the homeopathic remedy so much more noticeable to the organism than everything else in the environment? One, it is precisely specified (a true Similar), and, two, it is potentized on a dynamic plane at the same frequency as the disease.

Beyond the Law of Similars, microdosing, and potentization, the following homeopathic precepts are also definitive: diagnosis by holistic patterns of mind, body, and spirit rather than by isolated symptoms or disease categories; treating sick individuals rather than abstract diseases; choosing treatment on the basis of prior medicinal provings rather than intellectual explanations of pathological processes; regarding the body as an energetic field rather than a chemico-molecular machine; and diagnosing diseases as representatives of layers of evolutionary and civilizational latencies and suppressed maladies as opposed to chance entropic occurrences by virilization and other accidents under random thermodynamics.

Homeopathy, as we know it, was a singular achievement by Samuel Hahnemann. Many streams fed its watershed, but his discovery launched a branch of metaphysical science as summarily as the laws of Isaac Newton and Charles Darwin define physics and biology. Although individual aspects of homeopathic thought were widespread centuries before Hahnemann, the system itself arose as abruptly from his synthesis as Mormonism did from the golden tablets of Joseph Smith. Before Hahnemann, there was no homeopathy; since the birth of Hahnemannian philosophy, homeopathy has changed less than biology and physics over the same duration. That is usually a system's death knell, but it can also be the mark of a paradigm ahead of its time.

Homeopathy did not begin as an unorthodox or alternative system. During Hahnemann's lifetime, professional medicine was still in a formative phase, barely removed from the gallimaufry of the Middle Ages. Few theories or facts were firm. Practice relied on procedures that today would be considered primitive, dangerous, and ineffective. Even a hundred years after Hahnemann, by acknowledgment of medical historians, physicians stood as much a chance of harming as helping a patient.

Nor was Hahnemann a reformer or maverick by temperament or intent—he intended only an expurgation of sloppy methods of diagnosis, inconsistent treatments, and poor hygiene, modest contributions to the practices of his time. As the "first homeopath," he thought instead that he had clarified and systematized universal laws of cure that doctors had been applying for centuries, and that mainstream science would eventually corroborate him.

The initial responses to Hahnemann's work were not out of keeping with his expectation. Though he wasn't received with open arms, homeopathy wasn't rejected. Peer doctors didn't know whether its principles were reasonable inductions or errors of observation and logic. Thus, homeopathy had conditional support at a time of competing paradigms. There was also no regulatory body, medical or legal, to adjudicate, nor did any generally agreed-upon principles of physics or chemistry then either vindicate or challenge homeopathy— or *any* medical system—in its claim of being scientific. Hahnemann was another candidate seeking a constituency and verdict.

It was not until the early twentieth century that homeopathy was rejected by mainstream medicine, and then only because science established general *non*vitalistic guidelines and scientists presumed they had discovered laws of science that disproved microdose potentization per se, thereby invalidating homeopathy.

Hahnemann did not even recognize the revolutionary nature of his own work. He followed a labyrinth of experimental successes to a minotaur of medical meanings without understanding their consequences. His nonmaterial "cures" had implications so radical and far-reaching that, in truth, they could never be included in prevailing medical or scientific thought—not then, not now. While in its early years until a century or so later, homeopathy had provisional status as legitimate medicine, that cachet evaporated almost entirely with the anointment of Avogadro's number. Suddenly people said, "The emperor's got no clothes. He's treating patients with infusions of Nothing."

Many homeopaths *still* hope to see homeopathy validated within general medical science, but without a revolutionary change at the roots of molecular science, homeopathy cannot gain standing among anatomy, chemistry, and biology. It passes muster in Europe, India, and Asia for some of the same reasons that other "folk" medicines do. These cultures are not as dominated by technocracy and its regulating agencies and are more tolerant of Indigenous beliefs and inexplicable mechanisms; thus they can sanction opposing or unofficial practices.

In India today, homeopathy is rated over and above folk medicine, on equal footing with conventional allopathic medicine. More than a hundred government-approved and government-funded medical schools graduate thousands of students annually with a bachelor's degree in homeopathic medicine. They leave resolution of the system's causal basis (Similars and microdosing) to future experimentation. Outside the West, where materialism is not worshipped as the only agency, the homeopathic enigma can be left in abeyance.

Most modern practicing homeopaths also adhere to real-world standards. They don't eschew blood tests, scans, and ultrasounds. Tissue and cell etiologies are useful as long as information is distinguished from treatment. Homeopathic medical programs include courses in laboratory science, biochemistry, anatomy, psychology, infectious diseases, and surgery. To get a degree, one learns to do a thorough physical examination that includes pulse taking, temperature measurement, and assessment of the eyes, nose, ears, teeth, mouth, glands, abdomen, face, hair, nails, and feet. Students are trained to use a stethoscope and to examine urine and feces. They learn the physiology and pathology of the disease process in much the way that allopathic doctors do. Homeopathy serves as a different philosophy of disease and cure—sickness and health—not as a dissident anatomy and biology. Where homeopaths have not been marginalized, they are functionally comparable to other alternative and integrative physicians.

When clinical homeopathy could not be verified in the twentieth century's high-tech laboratories, it seemed to indicate, prematurely, that scientific testing had dismissed *all* of its claims. Numerous homeopaths refuted this, citing an array of experiments in the molecular chemistry of enzymes, colloids, crystals, even fractals, though none of these addressed homeopathic claims specifically. In the twenty-first century, novel research has tilted in homeopathy's favor, and many older experiments that seemingly invalidated Hahnemann's system have been reinterpreted at the level of nanomatter, homeopathy's home turf. But it still boils down to isolated events without controlled retesting or deference to the consensus of medical science, nor (again) does any of the research test the exact claims of homeopathy.

If we were to side with orthodoxy here on the basis of the impossibility of homeopathic cure beyond placebo, we would still be left with two significant events: one, the repeated therapeutic success of hundreds of thousands of homeopathic physicians in all parts of the world for, by now, two centuries of practice, and two, a homeopathic critique of mainstream medicine and materialistic science that does not require acceptance of homeopathy for validation.

The development of homeopathy has also been marked by internal disagreements as to what its ground rules are. While these have contributed to critiques of homeopathy as a consistent science and led to multiple interpretations of homeopathic principles in conflict with one another, they also point to the complexity and uncertainty states of microdose potentization itself (per chaos theory and quantum physics). The biggest split is between self-declared Hahnemannian purists and later, more pragmatic adaptors. The purists insist on following their interpretations of Hahnemann's rules scripturally to the exclusion of all other applications. The pragmatists, on the other hand, continue to reinvent and modernize Hahnemann's principles and terms as realms of science, medicine, physics, and cosmology evolve.

The issues on which homeopaths differ raise a number of medical and ontological paradoxes and lead to discrepancies between treatments and philosophy. In fact, in homeopathy, it is difficult to distinguish between ontological and practical rubrics. Controversies include whether homeopathy must be practiced immaculately or whether it can be combined with allopathy and/or other vitalistic modalities; whether homeopathic cures must be delivered as a single dose of the correct remedy, the Simillimum, or whether remedies can be more or just as effectively combined; whether to prioritize low-potency doses (less diluted, less succussed, and more resembling conventional allopathic pharmacy) or high-potency doses (more diluted, more succussed, and more "energetic"); whether "wrong" remedies, especially in high potencies, are dangerous (because they are powerful) or ineffective and harmless (because they have no pharmaceutical substance and are attuned "off frequency"); whether remedies, once assimilated, continue to be effective and must *not* be repeated in order to retain their integrity or, the other way around, whether they must be periodically boosted and can be antidoted and reversed by coffee, alcohol, dental drills, radiation, and a variety of other culprits; whether homeopathy has a conventional biophysical explanation that can be experimentally codified or represents a paraphysical force that needs to be applied by precedent without understanding its mechanism; and whether homeopathic cures require microdose pharmacy or can be transferred without a pill in psychic, spiritual, clairvoyant, or radionic forms.

Ironically, Hahnemann was a Hahnemannian only insofar as he proposed axioms that later purists adopted. Over his lifetime, he repeatedly broke his own rules, replacing old orthodoxies with new ones. In addition, his pursuits encompassed a number of realms outside pristine homeopathy. Hahnemannian medicine in its era was not even initially "homeopathy," let alone *Hahnemannian* homeopathy. It was public health and hygiene too. As noted, Hahnemann did not consider himself the inventor of a new system; he regarded his work as general medicine, to which he made numerous contributions, of which homeopathy was merely one.

Yet in his era and continuing through most of the nineteenth century, the full body of thought summarized in Hahnemann's 1810 textbook, *The Organon of Rational Medicine*, was considered "homeopathy." Much of its lexicon, however, dealt with diet, sanitation, immunization, the preparation of medicines, and even germ theory and techniques of surgery. These protocols were adopted almost in total by the establishment and remain a crucial aspect of allopathy, so much so that twentieth-century allopathic medical facilities were named after Hahnemann. Only his homeopathic precepts were "invalidated" and dropped from general practice.

Homeopathy is neither the first nor will it be the last attempt to develop a vitalistic scientific medicine. Alchemists, animists, Rosicrucians, odylists, and radionic "electricians" worked for prior centuries toward a cure based on the individual life force and primal energies in nature. Johan Wolfgang von Goethe, Rudolf Steiner, Carl Jung, and Wilhelm Reich followed Hahnemann in a German vitalist tradition. Homeopathy is most notable for its unlikely combination of elements and its time of birth. There seems no reason why it should have arisen when it did, at the turn of the nineteenth century when hermetic and magical sciences were in decline and the scientific revolution was well on its way toward a crescendo we live so deeply within that we don't recognize that it even has a context. Surely, if there were a microdose phenomenon, ancient Egyptians or Greeks would have happened upon it, or Paracelsus would have incorporated it in his hermetic corpus. In a way they all did; they applied nanophysics subconsciously before the present reign of quantity and before relationships among quantum, micro, macro, and vital effects—qualities and quantities—had been sorted. Still, why should a *new* hermetic science address ancient esoteric riddles during a broader demise of occult research? Hahnemann was unknowingly rowing against a rip tide.

Conversely, it would seem that if homeopathy had not been discovered in the Middle Ages or Renaissance, it would have skipped a few more centuries toward the quantum and nanosciences of the future. Yet it appeared, no doubt justifiably—by the rubric "things happen for a reason"—at a hiatus in magical inquiry in which hermetic erudition hadn't entirely dissipated and its scientific replacements hadn't yet been fully vested. Then it persisted as a clinical discipline through the nineteenth and early twentieth centuries before the advent of organized paraphysical studies. It stands today as a singularly tantalizing clue to how we might address polluted seas, a hydrocarbonized atmosphere, and future plagues. If curative energy is stored in the atomic structure and dimensional basis of matter and can heal acute and chronic diseases with potentized microdoses, then might not diseased ecosystems—contaminated rivers, dying forests and coral reefs, overheated water and air—be restored by potentized gases, fluids, and soils as part of an epic paradigm shift? Nanoscience would be far more efficient as well as less dangerous than dumping metallic particles into the atmosphere and other manipulations of geoenginering and synthetic biology.

Yet in a gap between practice and paradigm, nothing in homeopathy is objective enough to reapply ecologically, let alone at oceanic and atmospheric scales.

These conundrums all reflect an overriding paradox that led me to name the previous edition of this book *Homeopathy: The Great Riddle*. Still, no matter which camp a practitioner belongs to or believes, so long as their remedies are chosen on the basis of the Law of Similars, they seem to work. Homeopathy may, in fact, be overdetermined, with multiple pathways to healing. If so, it is a matter of not which form of homeopathy is correct but which brings the most optimal outcomes. Moment by moment, living systems change and adjust, and potentized microdoses are only one contributor to that process. If a microdose doesn't put a pool ball in a corner pocket, it still realigns the table with new probabilities. The system adjusts and reoptimizes.

Another way to phrase the relationship between the homeopathic Law of Similars and innate overdetermination in nature is to note that a potentized remedy interacts on a vital or energetic level with the vital force itself. In practice, this may not be as doctrinaire as a potentized Similar healing symptoms opposite those of its unpotentized source material, nor is it simplistically mechanical or merely the transfer of a biological, mental, or spiritual vibration across planes with a curative outcome by an antithetical effect. The Law of Similars is usually or approximately a healing by a potentized substance such that it has a therapeutic rather than a pathological repercussion, but it isn't *only* that. It is more correctly healing by inducing the vital aspect of a substance to interact energetically with the vital force of the living organism. Because vital-force medicine was rediscovered *in the context of Similars* after it was peremptorily rejected by materialistic science, it gained fresh legitimacy, but Similars never transcended vital-force interaction, and some successful homeopathic interactions may be partial opposites or induce entirely unpredictable results that are neither literally Similars nor Contraries but rather new information altogether. That then becomes the basis of healing.

In conversation with me, acupuncturist Robert Johns described a similar situation with traditional Chinese medicine's "needle and meridian" classics. Some of the oldest, most thoroughly tested means of balancing energy in meridians are transmitted in metaphors—sutras and songs—because of ancestral masters' incremental guiding to the right arrangements and the subtlety of application itself. Even when characters are mistranslated—Johns cites the instance of *shu* points as valleys or receptables rather than as transport positions—the reading can have a positive effect. That's overdetermination! Johns portrays some practitioners as riding two horses sidesaddle, the horses representing five-element theory and yin-yang energy transfer. His view is that the historical evidence indicates that yin/yang theory is the more accurate interpretation, but that doesn't preclude alternate healing concordances.

In 1977, as part of my research, I sat in (with patient permission) on cases during two afternoons at the Hering Clinic in Berkeley, California. I watched as pills and epistemologies collided, putting the ambiguity of the "cure" at *at least* three levels—pharmaceutical, psychiatric, and cultural. No wonder practitioners disagree with one another. There is no way around homeopathy's basic enigma: succussed microdoses are a *transmutation* of matter. Yet ordinary Americans marched in and out of Hering, oblivious to subtext, and got well as if the pills were "real." Even the doctors seemed unaware that they were practicing one (or more) of three forbidden arts: placebo, telekinesis, and magic.

Decades later, before prescribing a remedy for me, Vatsala Sperling remarked: "My teacher, Misha Norland, has said, if homeopathy does not work for you, just try a different homeopath. He was not joking. And, by the way, I am *with* you in considering homeopathy as magic."

2

The Origins of
Homeopathic Medicine

Homeopathy and Isopathy

Although Samuel Hahnemann invented the system we call "homeopathy," most of its rubrics had been in existence beforehand. Of particular note, the practice of using Similars—of giving a medicine that initially heightens symptomology or feeds the symptoms—was a mainstay of Hippocratic medicine. The power of Similars was likely discovered by herbalists, witches, and shamans many times over during tens of thousands of Stone Age years before medicines were committed to written record-keeping.

Homeopathic and isopathic principles are built into nature and lie close to the molecular threshold between inanimate and animate forms of organization. Isopathy was critical in natural selection, for no protoplasm-based biont would have survived without coevolution of an immune system. Isopaths are artificial, speeded-up serologies insofar as vaccines replicate the origin of species in high-microbe environments. We have since developed artificial prophylaxes against predators that are viral (nucleic), bacterial (protist), and parasitological (insect and worm) and would otherwise have consumed our species beyond the direst imaginings of Stephen King and Ridley Scott.

Small hunters are ubiquitous and travel with winds, tides, tourists, cargo, and conquistadores—ask the First Nations of the Americas and Australia.

Empirical immunology has been documented from 1000 BCE in China, where blow tubes were crafted to shoot dried-up lightly infected scabs of smallpox up the nostrils of healthy people, conferring immunity to deadlier diseases. The technology traveled via Mongolia to Turkey to central Europe.

In the late eighteenth century, "inoculation" reached England. Edward Jenner discovered that patients who had been exposed to less virulent cowpox were immune to smallpox. He took an additional step. Two months after inoculating a boy with a cowpox vesicle, he jabbed him (immodestly) with smallpox. The boy stayed healthy, with no pox or worrisome symptoms. That's a quick "birth of isopathy" précis.

Empiricism, Rationalism, and Vitalism

In order to understand Hahnemann's homeopathic heritage, we must also disinter an age-old rivalry between two medical lineages: pragmatic theoreticians (the so-called rationalists) and more empirical nurse-practitioners. The rationalist view, originating in Paleolithic times, evolved into guilds of bonesetters, surgeons, and pharmacists. Their tools and knowledge were passed down by clans and sodalities into early civilizations in the form of medical customs. They marked the origin of medicine as an occupation. Through medieval times, rationalist healers allied with barbers and smiths.

Their rivals were shamans, street healers, barefoot doctors, herbalists, and medical intuitives. As shamans, they made spiritualized potions and called on supernatural forces. As doctor-priests, they developed herbalism and witchcraft. As lay physicians, they were humankind's original medics and EMTs (emergency medical technicians). They treated patients by pragmatic methods, always setting the goals of cure, safety, and "urgent care" above rationalist theories. In prehistory and early recorded history, they were indistinguishable from doctors; in fact, they *were* the doctors.

A shaman could be both a spiritual healer and a surgeon (or pharmaceutical herbalist). Personae could switch with alternating "hats" or totem masks. Even when they were not fused in the personality of a single "medicine man" (or "medicine woman"), they were in balance and accord tribally. It was only gradually, as objectified science imposed itself, that healers as a class were ostracized by a credentialed medicine guild.

As academic training and formal philosophy became prerequisites for practice, doctors divorced themselves from manually skilled practitioners of massage and palpation as well as from the general lay practice of healing. By the twentieth century, rationalists had taken over the medical profession, achieving full status as an intellectual guild and trade union.

Homeopathy was one expression of the dialectic between these two traditions.

In his four-volume chronicle of healing appropriately named *Divided Legacy*, historian Harris Coulter defined a distinct "empirical tradition" based on diagnosing from observation, interpreting symptoms as signs of deeper holistic changes, and developing a compendium of remedies from the treatment of the sick. From the days of early civilization, pure empiricism was countered by rationalism, which was based on the use of precedent and logic to develop universally applicable etiologies of disease and cure and a general theory to explain diverse elements and actions that are successful in individual treatments: for example, the laws at work behind cures. Taxonomy of disease forms later gave rise to a science of pathology. The methods of modern orthodox medicine, refined over centuries, are, in essence, applications of cause and effect from rationalist models of biomechanical action.

Empirical medicine, by contrast, bypassed such laws as mirages or intellectual abstractions. Empiricists go from case to case, developing an intuitive art, trying to cure each sick individual. They place less value on medical knowledge because they regard each new patient as an irreducible whole. For empiricists, there are no categories of disease, only people who are ill. The empirical art of medicine as categorized by Coulter is different from the equally empirical search for rationalist categories, a discrepancy that pervades modern medicine beneath its rigorous empirical exterior.

Where rationalists may jump on a symptom, such as bloody stools and its likely cause, empiricists see a message with a variety of possible interpretations, some of them antipodes of each other. They look at a symptom's placement and stage in a sequence. One of the authors of the ancient Greek library summarized as the Hippocratic Corpus expounded the terms of empirical diagnosis in the fifth century BCE:

> Men are not feverish merely through heat . . . the truth being that one and the same thing is both bitter and hot, or acid and hot, or salt and hot, with numerous other combinations, and cold again combines with other *dynameis*.* It is these things which cause the harm. Heat, too, is present, but merely as a concomitant, having the strength of the directing factor which is aggravated and increases with the other factor.[1]

Since coction is constitutional and performed as part of the body's intrinsic capacity for healing, the doctor's task is to recognize and foster its actions. Insofar as a symptom is dynamic, an activation

---

Dynameis is a transliteration of the Greek δυνάμεις, which means "powers." Here it suggests both the vital force and metabolic and other physiological processes.

of the organism's immune response and reorganization, neutralizing it in a misguided endeavor to reduce its damage will stifle or oppose coction's natural healing.

Medicines chosen empirically according to the Law of Similars bolster cures by providing an extra jolt in the disease's own direction: empirical mirroring as opposed to empirical typology.

Because rationalist laws of cure tend to oversimplify sequences of cause and effect, physicians relying on them often miss far-reaching secondary and holistic effects of a remedy; thus they inadvertently foment new diseases that are caused by the treatments themselves, especially when the treatments obstruct the immune response as if *it* were the disease. In effect, they transform older known diseases into a new class of iatrogenic ailments that are difficult to unravel or cure.

The illusion that one can limit an attack to selected symptoms has reached a reductio ad absurdum in the modern rationalist's spectrum of antibiotics that inculcate long-term side effects and create toxic environments that breed resistant bacteria—superbugs—and antivirals that spawn new viruses as well as foster their mutations and recombinations under natural selection.

Hahnemann scoffed at the idea that a medicine could be instructed to do only benign healing when in the body. One might as well, he wrote, instruct the carbon, nitrogen, and hydrogen in a meal of cabbage, roast beef, and wheat cakes, telling them what part of the body to nourish and what part to stay out of. Yet this has been pretty much the lone game in town. Homeopathy extricated itself from this dilemma by substituting for medicines nonmedicines—that is, substances that affect the system not by digestion or assimilation but by the nonlinear information they provide to resilient, nonlinearly responsive homeostases.

Whenever their prehistoric origin, Similars were formalized in classical Greek and then Roman times to constitute a "homeopathic" branch of healing. Their rules of observation and practice were incorporated in a paradigm that Hahnemann followed without deeming it more than tradition and medical common sense.

A doctor had to choose not only the right Similar but the moment of fruition in the progression of a disease; otherwise, the "cure" may not activate coction, the body's natural conversion and cure by its own metabolic heat. The same historic physician also distinguished between primary disease, which comes from the healthy reaction of the vital force (and *can* be treated by Similars), and secondary disease, which is a sign of the capitulation of the patient's healing capacity.

According to principles of balancing humors in early Hippocratic medicine, hemorrhages, hemorrhoids, nosebleed, diarrhea, and headaches were all signs that a disease was trying to work its way out and were encouraged. For an enlarged spleen, dysentery was considered progress. Diarrhea was usually interpreted as a ripening of white phlegm. Pain in the joints indicated that a fever was beginning to disperse. Varicose veins and hemorrhoids in an insane person were desirable consequences of the reentry of disease into the watery earthen body from the mental sphere where it was incurable.

On the other hand, angina followed by lung disease was a sign not of healthy coction but of rawness taking over. Rashes were considered a sign of healthy pepsis, for they marked the progression of a disease outward from the core, but not if one should disappear abruptly without some other corresponding improvement elsewhere. However, if skin eruptions were not accompanied by general systemic improvement, they were an indication that the underlying pathology had abandoned a safer outlet and deepened. In this case a new course of treatment was recommended.

Diarrhea, nosebleed, and expectoration were presumed to provoke a crisis, with overall improvement following or else the disorder was thought to have settled deeper, with a weakening of the vital force. Most of these observations passed into homeopathy and underlay

Hahnemann's use of Similars. It was never just a matter of like curing like. It was an art of reading indications and matching progressions sequentially.

Though rationalism and empiricism go hand-in-hand today, they took separate paths in the development of Western medicine, and empiricism was at least as often affiliated with vitalism. Not all empiricists are vitalists, and even those who are do not share interpretations of the vital force. The spirits and voodoo powers of shamans are as much foolishness to many acupuncturists and homeopaths as they are to surgeons. Not all vitalists are empiricists either. Nonempirical vitalists propose spiritualized energies and even draw esoteric anatomies in textbooks of physiology, adding sheaths of Etheric and Astral bodies to bones and nerve nets.

Homeopathy is unique in being *both* empirical and vitalistic, a quality it shares with ayurveda, cranial osteopathy, anthroposophical medicine, and many other systems (see appendix II).

Whereas empirical interpretations and methods were favored in the Hippocratic Corpus (representing pre-fifth-century BCE medicine), rationalism appears to have flourished among a slightly later group of physicians associated historically with the Cnidians (Cnidus being a cosmopolitan Ionian free city in western Anatolia). They presumed drugs and herbs to work on a piecemeal counterhumoral basis without a priority of holism or recognition of a vital force.

Their treatments by opposites are still familiar to us: A fever must be lowered to get the patient out of danger from heat itself. In the cases of diarrhea, the physician should attack the dissipating cause in the gut. Pus in the lungs should be drained.

Early rationalists were innately preoccupied with figuring out how the body functions, with an emphasis on its chemical and mechanical properties. Diseases gradually came to be seen as absolute entities rather than fluid patterns marked by shifting patterns of symptoms. By the time of Aristotle (384–322 BCE), abstract classifications were starting to invent their own realities. Coulter pointed out "the 'fallacy of misplaced concreteness,' of [the physician] thinking he knows something about the organism when he has given names to its imaginary components."[2] Today, for example, cancer, Lou Gehrig's disease (ALS), Parkinson's, Alzheimer's, AIDS, arthritis, tuberculosis, and other disease and autoimmune narratives take precedent over the treatments of unique sick individuals with their individual symptom complexes and potentials for cure. It might be hard to reinstate "beginner's mind" on this matter, for disease categories have become as embedded as species of plants and animals, but not everyone gets sick in the same fashion or has the same potential for decline or cure.

As taxonomy became more sophisticated, only those symptoms viewed as contributing directly to a particular pathology were assigned value; the rest were ignored or deemphasized. A disease gradually became a discrete entity with its own nature, tracked according to precedent, hence the durability of labels for processes rather than processes as such. Secondary or sporadic effects were minimized and often forgotten. Numerous ancient allopathic disease names are now common names for diseases, and as taxonomic brands, they are half of every explanation as well as half of diagnosis and treatment: packets of memes in place of individualized diagnoses and treatments. While the same disease names may be used in homeopathy, they are not considered *actual* diseases but distribution paths of symptoms.

The "human body" of the Alexandrian physician Erasistratus (born around 300 BCE) was a precocious robot, a porous machine processing food and air as corpuscles. The stomach and colon ground up matter and supplied organs much in the manner of a grain mill. Basing their remedies on chemico-mechanical precedents, Cnidian physicians prescribed "scientifically," giving their chemical potions to neutralize toxicity, arouse sluggish organs, and dissolve congestions, respectively. When they found pus in the lungs, kidneys, or elsewhere, they aborted therapeutic coction in order to eliminate a source pathogen. Later in history, with sharper knives, they excised the diseased tissue itself.

Empirical remedies were, conversely, almost always administered with a goal of assisting coction and evacuation. According to Coulter, "The aim of therapy is to assist the organism to combat the disease along the lines already selected by the organism; the medicines and techniques employed to this end may be described as operating on the basis of 'similarity' in that they stimulate the organism to continue along the path which it has already chosen."[3] Thus, herbs promoting heat were given in a fever, and cold baths prescribed for a chill. Though this does not seem "modern" at first glance, Bikram yoga (aka "hot yoga," practiced at 105 degrees Fahrenheit), sweat lodges, cryotherapy, and ice bathing have made twenty-first-century comebacks.

Tracking the paths and stages of symptoms was a required skill set of empirical doctors. In Coulter's account: "Diseases cure themselves from the inside to the outside, the process of cure involves the appearance of new symptoms. . . . [The empiricists sought] cure through spontaneous evacuation of the *materies morbi*, fever and sweating [considered] as favorable prognostic signs [with] the general idea that disease is resolved through an eruption or evacuation, with consequent suppuration or empyema if the evacuation is not complete."[4]

Since it was important to assist the exiting of a disease—and the coction that catalyzed it—the empiricist's prime directive was, in the words of Hippocrates (460–377 BCE), "Do not disturb a patient either during or just after a crisis, and try no experiments, neither with purges nor with other irritants, but leave him alone."[5] In other words, first do no harm.

The empiricist physician waited patiently and observed, sticking to the notion of a unique, unnameable disease complex corresponding to a single force of action or coction. The appearance of multiple sequential "diseases" or symptoms was thought to represent variability of either coction or a particular constitution. Hippocrates developed the notion of individual constitutions: "Cheese does not harm all men alike; some eat their fill of it without the slightest hurt, nay, those it agrees with are wonderfully strengthened thereby. Others come off badly. So the *physies* of these men differ, and the difference lies in the constituent of the body which is hostile to cheese, and is aroused and stirred to action under its influence. . . . But if cheese were bad for the human *physis* [nature or cause of being] without exception, it would have hurt all."[6]

Both perspectives of the body have survived into modernity: the mechanical robot and the nonlinear field. Yet each had to go through the cauldron of the Middle Ages to launch a scientific revolution. Greek and Roman medicine may have sparkled with analytic gems, but it lacked shadows of creative tumult from deeper catacombs. The Dark Ages with their occult signifiers added something that classical scientists missed: the implicate depth of the world's complexity. Heraclitus needed Augustine to incubate Alfred North Whitehead. Democritus's atom could only get to Ernest Rutherford's atom by way of the gargoyle and castle. It took tens of thousands of masses, murals, and icons to cross a bridge the Greeks built but never saw. But it ultimately led to chaos theory, complexity, qubits, and nonequilibrium dynamics.

The most innovative empirical physician of the Alexandrian era was Herophilos of Chalcedon, who, among other things, charted the courses of diseases through a connection he discerned between cycles of natural *physis* (physicality) and rhythms of the pulse. Coulter summarized his art: "[Herophilos] developed a body of pulse doctrine in which pulse rates were classified according to size, speed, strength, rhythm, order, disorder, and irregularity. To make this knowledge graphic he based it on analogies with musical rhythms. He also compared various pulses to the movements of the gazelle, the ant, and the worm."[7]

Pulse-based diagnosis is a mainstay of empirical medicines like ayurveda and traditional Chinese medicine and was eventually incorporated into the homeopathic medical curriculum.

As Roman science enveloped the Hippocratic Corpus, rationalists became even more mechanistic, demoting coction itself to an abstraction. Conversion by bodily heat was cumbersome to conceive mechanically, indefinable, and—if it existed at all—indecisive about which direction it might be going (toward health or morbidity), and the same could be said about what doctors could do to aid or steer it. Furthermore, a medicine of Similars was circuitous by comparison with a medicine of Contraries by which a doctor could administer a neutralizing agent and produce a quick heroic cure.

A new mode of thinking favored intellectual shortcuts and quick results over individualized diagnoses and stratified treatments. Medicine became less an art and more a rule-bound ideology with sequential fads dominating treatment modes. Through the scientific resolution into modernity, doctors lost a sense of whether their treatments actually cured diseases, caring more about whether they fit established categories, a predicament characterized by George Bernard Shaw in the preface to his 1906 play *The Doctor's Dilemma*—better the patient die than be cured against the rules of the medical guild. This happens more than politicians, doctors, or administrators admit. Nowadays medicine treats mostly by precedent and reactions to pharmaceuticals. Disease categories have replaced individual sick people, and generics have superseded metabolisms, immunities, and coction.

Ultimately rationalist practitioners adopted a version of Erasistratus's anatomy: an animated corpse operating by solely mechanical laws, translating food and air into flesh and movement by the breakdown and rearrangement of raw materials—forerunners of molecular particles. Coction was still invoked—it became the ghost behind the machine—but the predilection was to resolve it in terms of the dynamics of heat, moisture, and dissolution, which was considered a refinement, not a reduction, of its original meaning.

In its most extreme form, rationalism became methodism, with all organic activity, including that of the mind, viewed as the result of chance interactions of atoms—essentially the current belief system, in which identity itself is seen as a neurochemical hallucination of a series of mirages. The Roman methodist school of the Greek physicians Themison and Thessalus proposed that the body was a porous pipe through which fluids circulated, too quickly if the pipe was overrelaxed, and too slowly if it was too restricted. Sweating and bloodletting were favored for a restricted flow, whereas darkness, quiet, and a diet of thick porridge and soft-boiled eggs were used to remedy agitated flow.

The gap between the concrete mechanism and a ghostlike vital force widened. Even as rationalists heralded vivisection and dissection as the ultimate tools in pinning down the proximate causes of illnesses, empiricists rejected the possibility of learning *anything* about health and disease from analysis of corpses or laboratory experiments. As the first-century Roman physician Aulus Cornelius Celsus (25 BCE–50 CE) concluded: "All that is possible to come to know in the living, the actual treatment exhibits."[8] The science of anatomy was headed in a direction from which Hahnemann would have to backtrack all the way to Celsus, who wrote: "Nor is anything more foolish . . . than to suppose that whatever the condition of the part of a man's body in life, it will also be the same when he is dying, nay, when he is already dead . . . it is only when the man is dead that the chest and any of the viscera come into the view of the medical murderer, and they are necessarily those of a dead, not of a living man."[9] By then, the notion that anything vital animated the machine had been dismissed or disregarded in the mainstream. A biochemical residue had replaced the life force.

Coulter cited some of Celsus's proto-homeopathic interpretations:

Madness is relieved by the formation of varicose veins, by dysentery, or by bleeding hemorrhoids. The cause of epileptic fits can be discharged through the stools. Watering of the eyes is benefited by diarrhoea. Shoulder pains spreading to the shoulder blades or hands are relieved by a vomit of black bile. Prolonged diarrhoeas are suppressed by vomiting. . . . Dysentery benefits enlarged spleen. . . . Round worms in the stool at the disease crisis are a good sign. If bleeding hemorrhoids are suppressed, a sudden and serious disease is liable to supervene.[10]

Celsus was also loyal to the healing power of Similars. Coulter elucidates:

He calls for black hellebore in disease where black bile is present, white hellebore in disease with white phlegm, and ox spleen as a remedy for enlarged spleen. Embedded splinters are drawn to the surface by a poultice made of pole-reed because [Celsus proposes] "of splinters the pole-reed is the worst because it is rough. . . ." Likewise [in Celsus's translated words], "the scorpion is the best remedy against itself. Some pound up the scorpion and swallow it in wine; some pound it up in the same way and put it upon the wound; some put it upon a brazier and fumigate the wound with it. . . ."[11]

The remedy for an earache with maggots is oil in which maggots have been boiled. Hydrophobia was sometimes treated by throwing the patient into a pond.

It is not only homeopathy that is portended here but also modern sympathetic medicine: the unwindings of osteopathy, the participatory traumas of gestalt psychotherapy, and the biochemical discharges of ayahuasca, kambo, and iboga.

Galenic Medicine

Renowned second-century Roman physician Galen (129–216 CE) was a vintage rationalist. Scion of a wealthy family in Pergamon (Asia Minor), he was superbly trained for his time, studying as a teenager with Aristotelians, Platonics, Stoics, and Epicureans. At the age of twenty he moved to Alexandria, where he lived for eight years and completed his education. After serving four years as physician to the gladiators of Pergamon—EMT at its most challenging—he set out for Rome at the age of thirty-two. He distinguished himself there for both his superior knowledge and his arrogance, as he was indisputably the dominant medical mind of his epoch.

Galen's work summarized the entire body of knowledge that preceded him. His thirty or so volumes of writings (twenty surviving) provided the main archive for the subsequent development of medicine in the West. In the absence of any general theory of therapeutics, they served as a surrogate authority, partly by sheer mass of their scholarship and partly because they had no rival.

While Galen did not favor methodism, he supported the rational approach and made it the bellwether medical compass for the next *fourteen hundred* years. At the same time, he attempted to meld the many different techniques and philosophies—coction, physis, and assorted laws of cure—into one basic logos. In so doing, he inadvertently endowed the organs with categorical expressions, assigning to them powers in the form of *dynameis* (crossover vital and organismic forces). For the stomach, it was digestive power; for the heart, pulsation; for veins, blood making. Additionally, each of the organs encompassed four primal *dynameis*: attraction, retention, alteration, and expulsion.

Despite his acknowledgment of a vital force, Galen separated organs from their organismic wholeness by partitioning them into heterogeneous capacities. Coction was defined as the dynamic interplay of the four elements under the law of Contraries: "Bodies act upon and are acted upon by each other in virtue of the Hot, Cold, Moist, and Dry. And if one is speaking of any activity, whether it be exercised by the veins, liver, arteries, heart, alimentary canal, or any part, one will be inevitably compelled to acknowledge that this activity depends upon the way in which the four qualities are blended."[12]

Galenic medicine, along with the Arabic derivations of Avicenna (Ibn Sina), Rhazes (al-Rhazi), and Averroes (Ibn Rushd) based on it, remained dominant throughout the Middle Ages. The empirical tradition kept itself alive either as folk medicine or practices outside the West. Although formal medicine has since broken out of a Galenic bubble as dramatically as astronomy burst out of a Ptolemaic universe, the Aristotelian puzzle of nature is still our reference point and theoretical threshold. Even after the isolation of DNA, in fact *because of* genetic reductionism, diseases have become more fixed, categorical, and incurable than ever—and that is despite groundbreaking gene splicing and modification for inherited diseases and disease dispositions. Microbiology and energy medicine are antithetical systems. I know a few people who practice both, but they change personae as well as hats to do so.

The most notable break in the fourteen-hundred-year rule of Galenism was instigated by Swiss physician Theophrastus Bombastus von Hohenheim (1493–1541), who took the name of Paracelsus not only to honor Celsus but to indicate that he had gone past him. His audacity was unshakable:

I found the medicine which I had learned was faulty, and that those who had written about it neither knew nor understood it.

They all tried to teach what they did not know. They are vainglorious babblers in all their wealth and pomp, and there is not more in them than in a worm-eaten coffin. So I had to look for a different approach.[13]

His quest led him through Spain, Portugal, England, Germany, Prussia, Poland, Hungary, Transylvania, Croatia, Italy, and France. As he walked from village to village and region to region, he interviewed midwives and herbalists, bathkeepers and magicians, doctors and philosophers, priests and knights. His ethnography restored lost medical traditions by recovering their scattered pieces. Paracelsus justified his long grail as an on-site education in the world's active medicinal methods: "What a doctor needs is not eloquence or knowledge of language and of books, illustrious though they be, but profound knowledge of nature and her works. . . . I do not compile from the excerpts of Hippocrates or Galen. In ceaseless toil I created them anew upon the foundation of experience."[14]

The Doctrine of Similars was axiomatic for Paracelsus: "Never a hot illness has been cured by something cold, or a cold one by something hot. But it has happened that like has cured like."[15] This led to prescriptions as literal as a sponge for bloating, crab's eyes for ocular diseases, and lapis lazuli for calcareous deposits (tartar) in the body.

Paracelsus dismissed prior disease etiologies and Contraries to reverse their effects. In his view, the body exists only as a whole, as the simultaneous activity of all its healthy members; hence, an illness occurs as a holistic entity too, not just a disturbance in a locale where it gets randomly noted or where it evinces the most trenchant pathology: "How then can the physician look for the maladies in the humors and assign their origins to them, since they are produced by the malady and not the malady by them? The snow doesn't make the winter, but the winter the snow."[16]

Likewise, the symptoms do not make the disease, but the disease the symptoms.

Alchemy

In the Paracelsan system, local conditions responsible for diseases provide their cures as long as a physician has the perspicacity to seek and recognize them *locally*. Because of his investigation of mines, Paracelsus was particularly sensitive to the mineral and alchemical basis of scourges; he proposed that the ailments of miners "are a spiritual entity caused by an emanation from the metal."[17] Their symptoms act like a mild form of metal poisoning and, according to Paracelsus, can be healed only by encouraging the metal's beneficial rather than pathological aspect as it is converted into a medicine—a precursor of mineral potentization. In his alchemical view, there is no difference between the metal's spirit and its chemistry and biochemical effects. He explained:

> Nothing else needs to be known to you in order to understand
> the matter, *corpus*, etc., of the disease than what the natural
> things of the earth and the elements indicate to you. If now
> you know the same, then you know the illness. Herein lies the
> anatomy, herefrom follows the medicine. For the medicine grows
> like the illness, and same and same yield each other's theory.[18]

From the way that the Similar of a metal drives out its toxic emanation in a miner's body, Paracelsus extrapolated a general taxonomy for deriving remedies from local plants, animals, and stones. Poisons were seminal to his pharmacy because they were *already* specified and biologically potentized; he wrote: "Consider, a spider is the supreme poison, on the other hand, also, the highest *arcanum* in chronic fevers."[19] Hahnemann would come to the same conclusion about not only poisonous spiders but also poisonous snakes and plants.

In his status as a proto-chemist, Paracelsus developed remedies not ordinarily associated with herbalism or alchemy. He established laboratory processes to turn animal, vegetable, and mineral substances into tinctures that he called Quintessences. Through a sequence of physical and spiritual stages enlisting flames, decanters, and ovens, he raised each potency into a new "body" that ostensibly rendered it vital and active.

All the pieces of homeopathy were there but combined in an alchemical rather than a pharmaceutical mode. They elicited many of the same aspects of substance that homeopathy arrived at centuries later. Though alchemical and homeopathic processes differ in ingredients, scale, and calibration, homeopathy is a transposition of alchemy into an algebraic field where astrological botany's duodecimal phases are synopsized in decimal succussions.

For centuries, alchemists as such sought the Quintessence of mercury and/or antimony in attempts to synthesize the Philosopher's Stone, a powder with which to make medicines and "philosophical" gold. Legendarily, when the powder was added to a piece of metal cut out of a pan or to a section of lead piping, a bubbling and hissing followed, and when the flames died down, a lump of gold larger than the original substrate glowed in the athanor. This foreshadowed Hahnemann's potentized microdoses of gold.

Alchemy was metallurgical and phenomenological by comparison to homeopathy's sanitized molecular laboratory, but it mapped the same subtle terrain of transmutation in nature. While alchemy used a repertoire of soils, minerals, waters, and reagents, homeopathy took place several octaves (or succussions) higher, where the energy of potions like snake's milk (*Lachesis*), *Sulphur,* and *Sepia* (cuttlefish ink) were bound in tiny bundles of sugar or alcohol. Potentized sulfur wasn't a form that Renaissance alchemists considered when they used the mineral as a reagent of mercury to turn salt into a subtler brine; they were chemists, not physicists. Yet before the microscope revealed universes within pond droplets and strings within dimensionality itself, scientists didn't consider scalar relationships or the esoteric nature of quantity. Homeopathic potentization can't be seen by eye or instrument. It is alchemy in an athanor smaller than a grain of sand!

The first tetrad of alchemical transmutation—the *nigredo* or decomposition and separation—took the alchemists' *prima materia* through calcination to putrefaction and coagulation, delivering a viscous or spongy black gruel. This was regarded as a purgation of substance, drying up its humors through its own natural heat (mineral coction), then catalyzing it by a separately prepared fluid. The residue was designated the Sign of the Crow for its dark satin hue.

The second tetrad potentized the porridge by a sequence of fixation, ceration, distillation, and sublimation. The dry matter was fused with philosophic, not metallic, mercury, which was derived from sulfur combined with what modern alchemist Fulcanelli called a "primeval celestial water." It left a pasty or syrupy mass, which was then poured into a bottle, left to dry, and dissolved in antimony vapor. During these phases, it progressed through a rainbow of colors, the alchemists' peacock's tail, until it was evaporated by drying and sublimation into a perfect whiteness, the *albedo*.

The third tetrad replicated the prior eight phases by fermentation, exaltation, multiplication, and projection. These separated and refined the powder. Fermentation meant sowing the substance with a metal (antimony, iron, silver, or gold), described vividly throughout alchemical literature as "feeding the thirsty lion and making him drink till his belly burst." Exaltation was sublimation of the burst lion's contents in an alembic. Multiplication sealed the outcome in a vessel with three or four parts of alchemical mercury from a prior phase to increase its quantity. Fermentation enhanced its virtue. The Philosopher's Stone was a dry red or golden powder or black pebble with glowing striations, an object that couldn't pass into the ledgers of chemistry because it could only be made paraphysically.

In projection, the stone was applied to other metals and turned them into silver or gold by a reddening phase, the *rubedo* or *iosis*, hence frying-pan and lead-pipe nuggets. The powder could also be used as a Quintessence for direct healing or making medicines.

Alchemy's hermetic chemistry is reflected in versions of preparation by contemporary *noms de alchimie* Fulcanelli, Lapidus, and Frater Albertus as well as in Rudolf Steiner's anthroposophical pharmacy. Albertus wrote that the traditional alchemical stone was "a crude yellow colored mineral that, when added to molten metal, was absorbed and brought about the transmutation." His own by comparison was "a glass-like crystal that radiates light," a mirror in which scenes of strange lands appear, "and any metal coming in the field of its rays will be transmuted into the next higher specimen, such as copper into silver and silver into gold."[20] This prism indirectly recapitulates the transformation of macro-alchemy into micro-homeopathy.

In sum, the relationship between alchemy and homeopathy is archetypal and has evolved through an era when neither is especially validated. The rubric under which they fall encompasses biological transmutation (elemental metamorphosis by living cells) and atomic physics and its mind-matter uncertainty states. The alchemical archetype explores tiers of causal energy that give rise to elements, periodicities, and isotopes, in principle anywhere in the universe. In homeopathic microdoses, the energy is both divisible and indivisible, and inseparable from its psychosomatic and telekinetic expressions in organisms.

The main correspondences between Paracelsan alchemy and Hahnemannian homeopathy center around the sublimation of curative aspects of common and simple mineral, vegetable, and animal properties and the attempt to activate the Quintessence, a potentization of substances that in their ordinary state have no transmutative or medicinal effect. Both traditionary sciences posit the transmutation of matter into energy. Additionally, one drop of either's "stone"— powder or pellet—is as good as a hundred drops. Half a drop or even a fraction of a drop may be *more powerful*. Just the smell—the aromatic essence—can be therapeutically effective in aromatherapy.

The science of biological transmutation and vital energy now stretches from atomic fission in stars and substrata of superstrings to transduction of potentized substances and portends a limitless release of energy from the infinitesimally minute. Nonlinear systems that stray far from equilibrium may not explain homeopathy, but they limn a universe in which it *could* have an explanation.

Signatures

Paracelsus selected his medicines according to not just Similars but also "signatures": intrinsic shapes in nature that resemble—not necessarily cause—the diseases they are selected to cure. He wrote: "Whereas things to come may thus be known before in the Elements, by that wherein the Evesters dwell; some Evesters will be in the water, some in looking glasses, some in crystalls, some in polished muskles; some will be known by the commotions of waters, some by songs and by the mind."[21]

Signatures can be anything from the color of minerals to the veins in which they occur to the ways in which plants grow. They can be signs emanating from one part or another of a plant; for example, the shape of hepatica's leaves might indicate its use for liver disease, while walnut as a kernel in a shell indicates its use for ailments of the brain, St. John's wort is prescribed for bruises and wounds because the holes in its leaves resemble pores, and aconite shows its use for eye diseases in its seed, which is small, dark, and round and contained in a white cuticle. Paracelsus laid down the "sympathetic" rationale: "As nature prefigures to us externally the mineral's nature in the rushes, in woods, and other plants, accordingly we shall also know that the salt in the body by its operation gives similar forms; from which it now follows that like heals its like, which is to say, equals form equal kinds of holes. And it has been shown with all types of holes that its like form has been its like medicine. Therefore it behooves the physician to know the anatomy of matching one thing with another."[22]

Sixteenth-century Paracelsian physician Oswald Croll provided supporting occult ontology: "Magically, Plants through their Signatures speak to the man of medicine who looks deep within, and they manifest their Insides, hidden in the secret silence of Nature, to him through their likeness: for there is . . . a means of demonstration through likeness, a means by which the Great Demiurge is used to manifesting things divine and occult so that they yield up the supreme likeness of ideas. . . . All plants, flowers, trees, and other things coming forth from the earth are Books and Magical Signs, communicated by the enormous mercy of God, wherein those Signs may be our Medicine."[23]

Croll and his contemporary Henry Cornelius Agrippa turned an esoteric treasure hunt into medicinal astrology.

Homeopathy mostly ignored hermetic signatures. It was not until the 1940s that Edward Whitmont, a Jungian therapist as well as a homeopath, organized them in a morphodynamic system (see pages 118–125).

Para-Paracelsus

Paracelsus's concordance—a unified field theory and a practical medicine in one package—was too vast for its time. In the hands of his followers, it fractured into alchemy, chemistry, herbalism, pharmacology, hermetic philosophy, physics, and magic. As post-Paracelsan alchemy merged with conventional pharmacy, it lost much of its connection to the Doctrine of Signatures and astrological botany. Yet its medicines became so popular that chemists following Paracelsus took over the drugstores of central Europe, an influence that later spread to the court of James I of England and the apothecaries of France despite a ban instituted in 1603 in favor of Galenic remedies.

It is no wonder that Paracelsus is viewed as the father of medical chemistry or pharmacy. Over time, many of his formulas were adopted by mainstream academic medicine, though purely on a chemico-mechanical basis. Coulter noted that "the salt, sulphur, and mercury, which for Paracelsus were spiritual principles, operational definitions of physiological processes, became identified with these chemical substances as produced in the laboratory and were ultimately converted into the acids and alkalis. . . . Therapeutic practice was generated by chemical theory. Mechanics and hydraulics fulfilled similar functions."[24] Of course, these later medicines were administered solely on the basis of "opposites" in keeping with Galenic principles.

A hundred years after Paracelsus, Flemish physician Jan Baptista van Helmont developed his own version of herbal alchemy. Like his predecessor, he prioritized folk remedies, "for truly the Arabians, Greeks, or Gentiles, barbarians, wild country people, and Indians have observed their own simples more diligently than all the Europeans."[25]

An incipient scientist more than a vestigial magician, van Helmont explained disease as an idea or form imprinted on the vital force, or Archeus (in his terminology), which then "frames erroneous images to himself which should be unto him as it were for a poison . . . which images or likenesses, indeed, as being the seeds of disease beings, should be thenceforth wholly marriageable unto him in the innermost bride-bed of life."[26]

Whether by direct reference to van Helmont or in the general spirit of Neo-Platonism, Hahnemann suggested a similar mechanism, though the Archeus may have a more exact match in the theories of osteopaths and chiropractors who propose disease and energy patterns transmitted from the spine, other bones, and the blood and cerebrospinal fluid to various viscera.

From van Helmont's point of view, empirical medicines did not work quantitatively against disease products because both were specifics, unique wholes. The remedies imprinted the "ideas" of their own Archeus on the "idea" of the disease, dissolving or otherwise overcoming its influence. Such ideas (signatures) are scattered throughout nature and generate not only the characterological bases of individuals and their disease entities but the morphologies of plants and animals and the seeds of medicines manufactured from Similars—botanical and zoological nature repeating in personalities and constitutions. This Renaissance variation on Hippocratic, Celsan, and Paracelsan themes foreshadowed Hahnemann. Disease "ideas" eventually led to homeopathic remedy pictures and have been re-derived in the "sensation" theory of contemporary Indian homeopath Rajan Sankaran (see pages 58–61).

For reasons of holism, van Helmont opposed compound remedies and other forms of polypharmacy. To him, disease was distinct in relation to the organism and also in what can cure it. "The sealing notes and impressions of diseases," he wrote, "do not cohere with species, but with individuals only."[27] This too is proto-Hahnemannism.

In general, van Helmont retained a paradigm of nature as a vital flux, embracing an unknowable set of causes and effects operating only as a vital whole. He favored cure through coction, but it is interesting that, this far along in the history of the concept, coction had become so conflated with not only digestion but the assimilative and fermentative processes of each organ (which by then had been explored through scientific dissection) that van Helmont himself made no distinction between the vital force as a holistic energy and individual mechanical functions. It was not until Hahnemann that the discrepancy was even recognized.

Iatrochemistry and Solidism

More notably in terms of the mainstream march of medicine, the seventeenth century brought a new mode of scientific reductionism and iatrochemistry, e.g., organisms as an extension of their chemical properties. It followed René Descartes's view that if enough experiments were carried out, all motions in the universe and causes and their effects could be understood. Despite unified fields and genome maps, we are still scanning and counting.

In Descartes's time, the discovery of the circulation of blood by the English physician William Harvey bolstered a mechanical theory of health and disease to which Harvey nonetheless contributed his own vitalistic interpretation: "The blood does not seem to differ in any respect from the soul or the life itself. . . . Nor is the blood to be styled the primigenial and principal portion of the body because the pulse has its commencement in it and through it; but also because animal heat originates in it, and the vital spirit is associated with it, and it constitutes the vital principle itself."[28]

Fractal geometries and differential algebras were gradually replacing vital energies and Platonic forms. Even Harvey's "spiritual" blood acquired a Solidist basis. Descartes wrote: "The food is digested in the stomach of this machine by the force of certain liquids which, gliding among the food particles, separate, shake, and heat them just as common water does the particles of quicklime, or *aqua fortis* those of metals."[29] The Cartesian Academy in France even attempted to apply this model to the Paracelsan theory of elements such that the characteristics of different salts were based on the shape of the corpuscles making them up (i.e., round for mobility and volatility, elongated and square for a fiery nature). It was not long before the actions of all drugs were explained by the size and shape of particles and the laws of motion, a precursor of valences of protons and electrons in atoms.

A Dutch physician of the time, Herman Boerhaave, wrote: "The solid parts of the human body are either membraneous pipes, or vessels including the fluids, or else instruments made up of these and more solid fibres, so formed and connected that each of them is capable of performing a particular action by the structure, whenever they shall be put in motion; we find some of them resemble pillars, props, cross-beams, fences, coverings, some like axes, wedges, levers, pullies; others like cords, presses, or bellows, and others again like sieves, strainers, pipes, conduits, and receivers; and the faculty of performing various motions by these instruments is called their functions; which are all performed by mechanical laws, and by them only are intelligible."[30] He rejected the notion of a vital force on the basis that "the material substrate cannot first accept the disease and then react against it unless permitted the attributes of autonomy and spontaneity."[31]

Physis and Anima

Empirical medicine was kept alive during the seventeenth century by an informal, widely dispersed guild of physicians, including Giorgio Baglivi (1668–1707), an Armenian-born doctor raised and educated in Italy. He noted that, despite adhering to Galenic theory, the mechanists were not always successful in their cures, often evacuating bile without affecting fever and trying to heal too many conditions by focusing on acids and alkalis when "many diseases have nothing to do with acids and alkalis. Man has a thousand ways of being sick."[32]

An earlier English doctor, Thomas Sydenham (1624–1689), complained that dissection merely showed a dead mechanism: "Though we cut into their inside, we see but the outside of things, and make but a new *superficies* [surface] for ourselves to stare at."[33] Inside the walnut's shell is not its essence but another shell.

Sydenham shared a belief in the physis and the Law of Similars— that is, that "fevers, evacuations, skin eruptions, etc., which occur in disease represent part of [the] healing effort." Fever is used by the physis "for the isolation of the tainted particles from the remainder of the blood."[34] Dysentery helps cleanse the intestines of morbific matter. Likewise, ulcers provide an escape route for harmful substances. The physician should assist vomiting and bleed women with suppressed menses.

One of the strongholds of vitalistic medicine was the school at Montpellier, in France, which branched off the teachings of German Georg Ernst Stahl (1659–1734). Stahl was a chemist as well as a physician, yet he rejected pure materialism and, in its place, proposed that an intelligent force called Anima regulated the body. The circulation of the blood could be viewed not just as a hydraulic function but as the impulse of Anima mediated through the nerves. It was by the movement of fluids that Anima rinsed out toxicities and kept the organism healthy.

In the eighteenth century, Théophile de Bordeu (1722–1776), a student at Montpellier, located himself somewhere between acceptance of Stahl's Anima and loyalty to the surgeons and physiologists of the medical establishment. Even as he upheld vital-force dynamics, he tried to characterize them physically. The Anima, he said, regulated the flow of fluids through the body as a *chair coulante* (circulating flesh), filling the pores and crevices, picking up extracts from the glands and carrying them to the organs. Bordeu wrote, "A knowledge of the composition of the blood is inseparable from a calculation of the effects it produces unceasingly upon the sensitive organs."[35] Secretion is not a brute mechanical force; the Anima guides it intelligently and selectively through each organism. Bordeu's research anointed him ex post facto one of the fathers of hormonal medicine, and he laid the groundwork for an understanding of the sympathetic nervous system and the involuntary responses of the body.

In line with the Hippocratic and Paracelsan traditions, Bordeu believed in treating by Similars rather than Contraries, and he revived an original form of coction. Quelling the symptoms at crisis, he said, ensured only a legacy of chronic disease. He proposed that mineral springs were medicinal because they could transform chronic diseases into acute ones by inciting coction. He even dignified the cure-all theriaca, which was made up of all the leftover medicines from an apothecary's shop at the end of a day. Like mineral waters, it was peppy and stimulative, capable of awaking the vital force from its languor. This was potentization without specification.

The Medicine of No-Medicine

Like theriaca, medicine itself was growing in creative chaos without a guiding principle. All the notions and theories we have described (plus others) had been floating around, interacting and overlapping in a sea of paradigms, tautologies, and paradoxes that had gone on for centuries unresolved, though sick people got well, whether because of or despite doctors. It was clear that Galenic, Cartesian, and iatrochemical medicine not only did not cure diseases on a consistent basis but were mostly unsuccessful in chronic cases. A new theory of cause and effect was needed. Empiricists had been able only to patch around an expanding mechanist philosophy, borrowing its metaphors in simplifications of healing processes. Meanwhile, mechanism was taking over not only medicine but all of science. This was the dilemma confronting Samuel Hahnemann.

Homeopathy was not its solution, nor was it the sole outcome of either empiricist or vitalist traditions. For one, it hardly speaks to much of Paracelsus's philosophy. It does not address alchemical or biological transmutation or elementalism and a theory of humors. It does, however, represent the third major watershed of a mystery tradition—the first being Greek and Platonic, the second being alchemical and Neo-Platonic. Like its predecessors, it was rogue and unexpected, but it generated a cohesive, holistic theory that has traveled throughout the world. Homeopathy became the most successful offspring of the merger of shamanic chemistry, diagnosis by coction, and the search for vital principles of substance. It resolved these by systematizing and repertorizing Similars and by turning the "Stone" of alchemy into molecular dilutions and potencies. In Hahnemann, empirical medicine found its Galen.

I now distinguish three homeopathies, all issuing from Hahnemann but representing different cosmologies.

The first is a medicine combining a materia medica, a repertory, and a dispensing of potentized pills.

The second is a metaphysical science based on the specified energy of microdoses, nanochemistry, and paraphysical information. Hahnemann formalized this system without recognizing the ontological implications of his pill preparation, let alone its requirement of a new property of matter.

The third homeopathy is conceptually and historically beyond Hahnemann; it is a general system of converting psyche into substance, mind into matter, and vice versa. Consciousness had to hit the ground in substance somewhere, and where it does, it releases a burst of steam. For dualists and rationalists, the steam—or whatever it is—exists but never bottoms out physically. It can't—quantum physics established that—but it also can't have hidden layers of atomic or subatomic medicinal potency. Scrub the homeopathic microdose as a candidate. Conversely, for vitalists and empiricists, a homeopathic microdose has no actual substance but performs as if it not only did but is more potent and curative for its *absence*. Bypassing all these dialectics, homeopathy became the first scientific medicine of no-medicine.

3

The Tenets and Rubrics of Homeopathic Medicine

Repertoires and Materia Medicas

Since symptoms are considered expressions of the vital force under assault, in homeopathy they are used as guides to finding matching remedies that accelerate a healing response. The diagnosis is not a medical diagnosis per se; it is a picture of a remedy that matches the symptoms of the sick person. Symptoms are the diagnostic messaging of the vital force indicating where it is at work and could use help. Treatment is then by a Similar, a remedy that will instigate nonpathological symptoms matching those of the disease—an "outrage" of the system.

Because homeopaths are searching for a match among a variety of substances potentially as large and diverse as nature itself, they must learn to read symptoms at the appropriate depth or vibration. Otherwise, everything looks superficially like everything else, for each potential remedy has a range of effects that matches some aspect of pretty much any disease. But it is language—semantics—that is vague, not biology, and there are also many human languages and styles of speech that have to mesh through symptomology and repertories.

Accurate repertorizing requires specification, capturing the disease and remedy essence, for repertorized "pictures" are the lone basis on which to select a remedy. Remember, in homeopathy disease taxonomy is irrelevant or secondary; the disease cannot be assigned to a prior category and cured by characteristics common to it—there is no remedy for *everyone's* chicken pox or cholera. Each ailment is specific to the occasion of its appearance in a patient, where, in interaction with the defense mechanism, it leaves spoor—signs, sensations—as to its nature and path, indications for a proposed cure. In Hahnemann's words:

> The disease, being but a peculiar condition, cannot speak, cannot tell its own story; the patient suffering from it can alone render an account of his disease by the various signs of his disordered health, the ailments he feels, the symptoms he can complain of, and by the alterations in him that are perceptible to the senses.[1]

While cultural bias predisposes us to interpret homeopathic language in allopathic terms, now as then, Hahnemann was refuting diagnosis by prior categories or current virulence. He bypassed the whole matter of the relative importance of symptoms with a master stroke. *All* symptoms are important because all symptoms are indications. The worst damage that an ailment causes may seem to require a doctor's attention—and well it should, for it may be life- or function-threatening—but it tells the prescriber no more about the remedy than a minor symptom or quirk, for both are expressions of a deeper-seated malady and a constitution. The disease itself lies beneath concrete manifestations, beneath divisions into mental and physical aspects, beneath the form of pathology. Everything in the organism's being reflects it in some fashion: a wart, a nightmare, a taste in food, a sensitivity to cold, diarrhea, weeping, anger, messiness, fastidiousness, fear of the dark, restlessness.

A homeopathic materia medica depicts the myriad remedies and their characteristics. Like the later Wikipedia, it is as comprehensive as its contributors make it. In homeopathy, that means cumulative contributions since Hahnemann. "Drug" pictures are expanding snowballs that reflect different styles of observation and emphasis gathered in decade-by-decade contributions.

Most homeopathic materia medicas have descriptors of symptoms that resemble deadpan lists in allopathic pharmacopoeias or psychiatric diagnostic manuals. These lists meld physical, mental, and emotional indications, making no operational distinction between a rash and a panic attack.

Repertories are materia medicas in reverse: encyclopedias or abridged encyclopedias of the collected history of two-plus centuries (so far) of responses to remedies (repertories and materia medicas are also sometimes combined in a single book). Even amateurs can find a remedy by keying characteristics and repertorizing them similar to the way in which a rockhound classifies an unknown specimen and puts it in a lineage by its color, crystallization, hardness, fracture plane, and means of formation. Is it sedimentary, igneous, or metamorphic? A "disease hound" will likewise key symptoms and characteristics one by one and arrive at a group of remedies that incorporate most or many of them. James Tyler Kent's 1897 magnum opus was the bible of repertories for a new century. A hundred years later, collective computer hard drives have created a database dwarfing Kent's.

Only an unskilled practitioner or beginner counts up items to pick a remedy by majority. An experienced homeopath looks for a distinctive configuration that reflects the essence of a disease and remedy—congruence, not volume. Sometimes a single sensation may best characterize a source.

Quite comically, I ran into the dilemma posed by centuries-long lists when I taught a course on alternative medicine at Goddard College in 1976. During our section on homeopathy, I told my students about James Tyler Kent's repertory.

"Good practitioners read character," I advised. "They don't just count indicia."

"What's indicia?" asked Jessie, a cut-up who had played the clown in a number of my classes.

"Citations that list all symptoms and other characteristics caused and alleviated by a given remedy. There are more than two thousand indicia for *Pulsatilla*. Don't jump on just the blatant ones. Listen up. Here's *Carbo vegetabilis*: 'Face pale, cold sweat; hair falls out by the handful; bluish, parched, sticky, loose teeth, and bleeding gums.'" Giggles.

"'Foul taste and odors from mouth. Cold knees at night. Ulcers burn. Discharge offensive.'" I struggled to keep from laughing.

"'Hemorrhages, indolent oozings; even the tongue piles up black exudate; oozing of black blood from veins.'" The room was a riot. Me too—it took almost a minute to regain sobriety and get the list going again. "'Extremely putrid flatus, incarcerated flatus, collects here and there as if in a lump; diarrhea horridly putrid, with putrid flatulence; blue color of the body with terrible cardiac anxiety and . . . .'"

"Jeez," exclaimed Jessie, "is the guy still alive?"[2]

Remember, a list of a remedy's attributes includes everything known to be caused by its raw substance, in principle in *every* healthy individual; thus, such a list is a composite of common and exotic effects. Indications for the most popular constitutional remedies, called polychrests, can go on for eight to ten pages in a tiny font. Of course, the sum of them never occurs together.

A few homeopathic authors have tried to circumvent fragmentation and decentralization by combining symptoms in characters resembling figures in literary works to elicit a living coherence rather than a diffuse list. The remedies perform like actors on a stage, landing somewhere between a casting call and a short story. M. L. Tyler's *Homeopathic Drug Pictures* has a bit of the literary flair and idiosyncrasy of her countryman Thomas Hardy. Catherine Coulter's portraits of homeopathic remedies could inhabit the novels of her fellow Russian Fyodor Dostoevsky.

Homeopathic Character Analysis

In order to paint an accurate remedy picture, a diagnostician tries to draw his or her patient out with a detective-like progression of queries: "What do you feel before a storm?" "Do you close windows to prevent drafts?" "Do you find your house chilly or stuffy?" "Do you have times of more or less energy in the day?" "In what position do you like to sleep?" "How do you feel when your collar is buttoned?" "What is your experience of wearing a tight belt around your waist or a tight collar around your neck?" "How well do you tolerate waiting for a train?" The homeopath asks about spates of jealousy or sadness, expressions of frustration or anger, fantasies, bucket lists, dreams. He may examine the patient's rashes, warts, or pimples. He inquires into the color and density of urine and stools. He observes whether the patient presents as neat or sloppy. If the patient is neat, is that just neat or fastidious? He may ask, "How do those around you think of you?"

Some of these are direct questions seeking direct answers; others are attempts to get the patient to reveal something of which even the patient is not aware. A good homeopath is also a good psychiatrist and prosecutor.

In practice, homeopathic diagnosis falls somewhere between a research project and an imaginal—not "imaginative"—character reading. Though conceptually and historically removed from homeopathy, psychologist Wilhelm Reich's classic text *Character Analysis* is an excellent introduction to how core character gets shaped around resistances. Reich depicted its expressions both through and beneath the artifices of presentation. In a sense, the character reveals itself by the ways in which it tries to disguise its nature and control social interaction, including dialogue with a physician.

Similarly in homeopathy, a verbal account of discomforts may be less useful than the manner in which a patient presents information or the patient's incidental office behavior. If we see the remedies as characters, we may note that though many are hypochondriac, talking about their ailments incessantly, they differ in subtle ways. *Nitricum acidum* is nihilistic and will produce new, more dreaded symptoms once previous ones are relieved. It exudes sterile anxiety with a conviction that no one can help under any condition. *Arsenicum album* is just as anxious about his health, but he is convinced that the doctor can save him if only he will hear him out and get to the bottom of it. *Phosphorus* babbles about ill health, but not especially to the doctor and not with any sense that either her health or the doctor make a great deal of difference. *Tabacum* has a melancholic dread. A single such recognition can suggest a remedy without further repertorization.

Homeopathy can give the appearance, to an outsider, of being obsessed with trivial and odd symptoms, but from the answers to their questions, practitioners are trying to elicit a picture of the state of the patient's body, mind, and emotions, both in a healthy state and when ill. The symptoms and details are used in the context of a repertory to key possible remedies (Similars).

Decoding Symptoms

When allopaths examine a diseased organ or a recently deceased corpse, they believe that they are looking as directly as possible at actual pathology. For homeopaths, there is no such thing. Physical symptoms are hit-and-run effects of an assailant that has burrowed back inside the energy field or departed with the cessation of the organism's vital force. Symptoms are the accessible evidence of "mistunement" of the vital force. If the "intruder" happens to track in a few grains of sand that show where he came from, forensics will emphasize these and ignore the lamps he has knocked over and bureau drawers he has pulled out. Of course, Hahnemann knew that a heart attack called for more urgent care than a wart or a craving for broccoli, but as expressions of a constitution they are equivalent. In fact, the craving for broccoli may suggest a medicine that angina or an emphasis on aortic symptoms does not. A treatment based on craving for broccoli will then improve the heart condition.

A patient who recently suffered a heart attack may be surprised to find a doctor more interested in the patient's hand gestures, ways of expressing frustration, or recent nightmare than the latest cardiology report. A homeopath is a homeopath is a homeopath, not a cardiologist. A healee has a singular constitution, and its weaknesses are expressed differentially at different times. "There are no diseases," declared Hahnemann in a variation of the Hippocratic doctrine, "only sick people."

Homeopathy could be seen as structural more than semantic. Tastes in food hint at what the person's coction is craving or avoiding. These give voice to mute organs that speak through the mind and larynx.*

Viewed another way, the visible effects of pathology that stand out boldly and categorize the common disease groups of allopathy define homeopathy's symptomatic phases. Treated antiseptically, they may vanish, deepen, and return. Yet standard medicine emphasizes these spinoffs and fills its repertories and pharmacopoeias with them. The categories they provide take on institutional lives: whooping cough, colitis, schizophrenia, acne, rheumatoid arthritis, and so on,

---

*See contemporary anatomist Bonnie Bainbridge Cohen's Body-Mind Centering approach to movement and consciousness for a summary of this psycholinguistic process.

losing the unique identities—constitutions—of the patients in which they have gestated.

Among quirky symptoms recorded in a standard repertory (with the medicines of which each is a charactertistic) are time passing too swiftly (*Cocculus*); crawling as of ants over the surface of the head (*Picricum acidum*); calls his boots logs of wood (*Stramonium*); moved to tears welling at the sound of bells (*Antimonium crudum*); symptoms worse at 2 a.m. (*Kali bichromicum*); wounded pride (*Palladium*); feeling of a mouse running in the lower limbs (*Sepia*); feeling of a living animal in the abdomen (*Thuja*); ridiculously solemn acts carried out in improper clothing (*Hyoscyamus niger*); and a woman dreaming of a large snake in her bed (*Lac caninum*).[3]

It takes a paradigm shift to view such sensations as not only relevant but diagnostically equal to a fever or stroke; it also shows how closely a homeopath must read the patient, avoiding pitfalls of rationalist disease categories. Hahnemann thought that ranking symptoms was a red herring that had predisposed physicians into fictive classes. For allopaths, the symptoms *are* the diseases, to be treated in a manner considered effective by evidentiary precedent. Accustomed to allopathic symptomology, patients similarly tend to demote minor symptoms and provide only those that were most vivid and painful.

Patients may become inured to their longstanding problems, so they discount them. No conventional doctor had been interested in them before. In some instances, patients even forget them or dismiss their role in future developments. Nineteenth-century homeopath Edward Tine observed: "Patients are so accustomed to their long sufferings, when the disease is chronic, that they pay little or no attention to the lesser symptoms which are often characteristic of the disease and decisive in regard to the choice of remedy. . . . Finally they leak out in some way and the patient says, 'I have always had it and did not suppose that it had anything to do with my disease.'"[4]

Odd as some of the above symptoms may sound, each has a reason. The body wastes no energy or semantics. It would not be able to produce sensations unless it *meant* them—that is, unless something inward "spoke" them. In an open-ended system of signs, unusual items usually carry more discrete diagnostic information than common ones. In his *Organon*, Hahnemann wrote: "In this search for a homeopathic specific remedy . . . the *more striking, singular, uncommon, and peculiar* characteristic signs and symptoms of the case of disease are chiefly and most solely to be kept in view."[5] In this, he preceded Sigmund Freud, the structuralists, and the whole of twentieth-century information and psycholinguistic science in recognizing what would be anthropologist Claude Lévi-Strauss's seminal syllogism, "Either everything has meaning, or nothing has meaning."[6]

A generation earlier, Freud had deciphered dreams, jokes, and compulsions as "the royal road" to the unconscious, meaning psychological behavior and mental diseases. Having begun his medical career as a neurologist, he recognized that human thought processes and their expressions are a small portion of our overall mental activity and that the nervous system binds a huge unconscious reservoir. He combined his insight about the unconscious mind with concepts from anatomy, animal behavior, neuroscience, social theory, and anthropology. Lévi-Strauss correspondingly deconstructed ceremonies, kinship structure, totems, and variants of myths as the keys to the unknowable essence of a culture.

Each of these disciplines (psychology and anthropology) is a formal decoding of unconscious infrastructures behind acts and customs. Coming a century before Freud and likewise a grand synthesis of prior systems, homeopathy foreshadowed psychiatry (inadvertently, of course)—not in its overall organization of meanings but in its attention to the dynamics of symptoms and emphasis on the "mentals" as a code for psychosomatic roots. Like Freud, Hahnemann took the sum of medical and psychological theory up to his time and reconceived it as pathways into the essences of diseases.

But Hahnemann and Freud were very different. Similar-based homeopathy and symbol-based psychiatry are systems that interpret unconscious messages within states of body-mind using their own discrete premises. Homeopathy differs from psychology in being hermeneutic rather than analytical; it is a system of signs rather than a pantheon of etiologies, so it remains discursive. Whether it is an authentic set of laws or a parochial fantasy is not the key issue; homeopathy's legacy of cures shows that, either way (nanotransmission or placebo), Hahnemann found an unintegrated aspect of our understanding of nature and of the psychosomatic basis of disease.

In practice, homeopathic diagnosis may function superficially like psychoanalysis, as symptom-taking even has a transference-like effect—for example, startling the patient's constitution into a vital response even before putting a microdose under the patient's tongue. But homeopaths are not Donald Winnicotts or Jacques Lacans, though both Winnicott and Lacan recognized the closed integrity of a psychosomatic system. Homeopathic rubrics would be familiar to most ontologically oriented psychologists, for (in different language) they entail object relations, transitional objects, mirror stages, algebraic symbology, predicate logic, Self and Other, and the working relationship between mind and body. Anthropologists have noted how, after a voodoo master names a disease to an innocent target, the person is killed by the name. That person can also be cured by a name.

Symptom Networks, Sensations, Templates, Songs, and Snakes

Homeopaths try to cure symptoms not currently being expressed by gathering them in a network. Similars have no virtue or rationale beyond their creation of such a network while mirroring its reflection in a remedy. The mirroring is what makes the symptoms distinctive and their reflection curative. In fact, the homeopath only has to know *one* item in the network. If it leads to accurate repetorization, the organism will do the rest.

Since many disease cores develop in infancy or are inherited, homeopathic diagnosticians may elicit symptoms that appeared only in childhood, even ones that have totally disappeared or were long ago allopathically cured. They are interested in discovering the chronology of a person's susceptibility through a lifetime. They may even venture as far back as the prenatal history of the patient and perinatal history of the mother.

While wending their way through possible remedies, diagnosticians seek the closest specific match on the basis of a comprehension of the wholeness of the disease and a matching repetorization and drug picture presented in the materia medica. Though (as noted) many remedies will partially mimic a range of conditions, they try to narrow their choice to a few and then pick the best, the so-called Simillimum.

Homeopathic symptomology has evolved since Hahnemann and further since Freud. In the twenty-first century, homeopaths have attempted to characterize the core constitution and its indications in new ways that encompass insights from evolutionary biology and contemporary philosophy, film, and literature. Homeopathic physician Rajan Sankaran, born in 1960 in Mumbai, India, excavates hierarchies and organizations in nature that appear in the symptoms (sensations) recorded in repertories. He distinguishes individual constitutions and their remedies as having plant, animal, or mineral characteristics, or melodies and songs; that is, their quintessential sensations occur in discrete patterns, propagating like tunes from deeper instruments. This reflects the way in which nature builds physical and psychological systems in layers of emergent phenomena. From a substratum of integral properties, more complex entities harmonize combinations of qualities speaking the same dialect and attracting each other's aspects. Likewise, suppressed dissonances and discordances lead to similar out-of-tune squeals and screeches, all echoing source notes from both mental and physical plexuses.

For Sankaran, each organism develops along an individualized typography of its root template that radiates into all aspects of its life and resonates with a characteristic energy pattern. It is this deep self—a karmically and genetically based whole—in which a disease occurs like a crack, an accumulation of dissociative factors in similar keys. The remedy then seeks to match that frequency or song and retune it.

Sankaran's plant-leaning constitutions are highlighted by their heightened sensitivity to shifts in the environment and their own chloroplast anatomies, which blend into each other much as light and soil are translated into distinctive leafing and blossoming shapes. The remedies reflect mostly botanical dispositions: algae, fungi, lichens, and mosses as well as flowers, shrubs, and trees.

Sankaran's animal songs encompass competition, survival, and sexual attraction. He further grades these into mammal, reptile, spider, insect, and bird natures. The formation energy of these so-called "isnesses" are vitalities generating form, direction, behavior, activity, and overall design in organisms, and then in zoological therapeutic properties and the diseases they treat.

Sankaran's mineral realm is a domain of structure: resilience, maintenance, degrees of resistance, and also *loss* of structure, all of which also characterize the formation of molecules up the elemental ladder from hydrogen and lithium to lead and uranium. Their subatomic alignments are the clay and loom on which all matter in nature is based. Sankaran wrote:

Thus the ordered structure of the whole periodic table represents and maps a journey from simple, light beginnings (first row) through progressive development, properties, and possibilities (middle rows) to increasing heaviness and complexity, which ultimately results in disintegration and decay (sixth and seventh rows).[7]

These elemental kingdoms repeat in the development of personalities, institutions, and entire societies. The more fully a person experiences the physical sensations of their own underlying kingdom and type, Sankaran believes, the healthier they are, and also the more they are likely to use transparent language while describing their symptoms, and the more likely it is that the homeopath will find a remedy that reflects the source sensations, leading to a more complete healing.

The homeopathic materia medica, in Sankaran's practice, is a postmodern index of personified morphologies transferred into living patterns like ripples in water—motifs by which a repertorizer matches a remedy to a constitution that embodies its formation energy. Sankaran notes, for instance, that when potentized *Sepia* (cuttlefish) was given to a healthy person, he dreamed that "he was escaping by running backward. . . . The animal expressed itself through the dream."[8] Similarly, limestone and echinacea find mineral and botanical expressions in human forms.

Sankaran recognizes similar harmonies, or songlines, and discordances in emotional development, life crossroads, survival responses, reaction types, and coping mechanisms. Each of these resonates through constitutions, behaviors, complexes, and susceptibilities. To identify them, he draws on observations ranging from dress styles, makeup fashions, and behavioral patterns to tattoos, dreams, and, his specialty, doodles on paper.

What Hahnemann and Kent understood as the animation of disease qualities is loosely what Edmund Husserl and Maurice Merleau-Ponty derived as aspects of phenomenology and proprioception and Sankaran summarized as sensations:

When each peculiar, individual aspect of the person is explored to the level of energy and sensation, we find that they all speak the same language and sing the same song. When the main complaint is examined in depth, when the person's dreams, emotions, childhood, fears, ambitions, and so on are probed deeper, each of them will lead us (amazingly) to the same sensation, though superficially they seem to be so different.[9]

As long as the tune can be recovered and replayed, health can be restored.

Another contemporary homeopath born in India, Vatsala Sperling, has extended this frame of reference into multiple interlocking patterns that fluctuate under the surface of not only homeopathy but allopathy, physics, biology, and symbolic psychology. One of her specialties is snake remedies. Snakes are highly patterned, active, determined life forms, so they provide a sound basis—living epitomes—for repertorization. Plants and minerals often steal the spotlight, giving false indication to the layperson that homeopathy is nothing but herbal intervention, but the materia medica includes a treasure trove of remedies from the animal kingdom. A potentized molecule is not finally animal, vegetable, or mineral but energy, space, and vibration. In fact, as homeopaths know, anything can be potentized because everything contains the energy of its manifestation. Sperling's message is: Do not forget snakes when potentizing the rest of the garden. On these, she is thorough and eclectic, honoring the maxim "All that slithers is not *Lachesis*." Not all snakes are venomous, so not all snake remedies are venoms.

Her own snakes are mostly nonaggressive and nonpoisonous, with a few venomous vipers and some alligators and some fossilized dinosaur remains thrown in (these can be potentized too). She captures the striking relationships between the behavioral and physiological traits of snakes in nature and natural history as well as human propensities, attributes, and demeanors, deriving vital-energy forms that reptile kingdoms contain. Then she applies these to client constitutions and ailments.

To repertorize snakes, Sperling discusses their anatomy, habitats, predation, flight, self-defense, and maternal capacity and habits. Among the human expressions she excavates in a materia medica of colubrid snakes are desire for safety, revenge, dependence soon after birth, patience, love for bright colors, female dominance, fear of falling from heights, self-promotion, intense but fake anger, substance abuse, fear of abandonment, paranoia, suspicion, parental abuse, feeling at a disadvantage, becoming still when encountering a predator one cannot avoid, appearing sexier than one is, and wanting to save one's skin and not get trampled.

Among the main features of nonvenomous colubrid snakes are their mimicries of venomous snakes with the sole purpose of survival: they appear as something they are not. Similarly, patients requiring remedies from colubrid snakes present a threatening picture, but they are in fact simply mimicking a threatening posture for the sake of survival.[10]

Provings and Polychrests

The most serviceable information about remedies is derived from their outcomes in healthy people. In a "test" subject with no significant illness, a homeopathically prepared substance manifests as a brief artificial disease called a "proving" because it "proves" what a remedy can cure in a sick person. Without a masking disease, a remedy plays true. This is in contrast to the initial effect of an allopathic drug, which is to dampen and reverse the symptoms without matching energy or provoking an immune response.

The name of a homeopathic remedy is the name of its proven

disease. It is also the name of the patient's type or melody. Patients are diagnosed as *Sulphur, Lycopodium, Arsencium, Sepia* (cuttlefish), *Calendula, Lachesis* (bushmaster rattlesnake), or some other animal, vegetable, or mineral that causes the same symptoms in healthy people. They are then treated by a microdose of its tincture. A patient treated with *Zincum metallicum* has a zinc disease even if allopaths call it chicken pox, laryngitis, eczema, or gastric diarrhea. Every pathological manifestation of the patient is *Zincum* at its roots. The patient's constitutional type and remedy are likewise *Zincum*.

Allopaths don't miss *Zincum*; they just don't see the larger configuration that defines a homeopathic picture. They might identify the nerve-related symptoms of the *Zincum* state as a neurological disease and find a separate psychiatric diagnostic label for *Zincum*'s fear of police and of being caught committing a crime, but all of these, as well as aborted exanthema (spreading skin rash), come under the greater *Zincum* state, which is nothing more or less than, to borrow Sankaran's language, the vital force mistuned to a *Zincum* song.

Zincum is sometimes recognized by complications in childhood diseases, eruptions that do not fully break out, with later neurological complications. It might also manifest as bedwetting (especially when it occurs near morning), asthma accompanied by farting (particularly in the evening), coughing in a reclining position, restlessness, and tics; in rare cases, sleepwalking; the fact that severe diarrhea does not bother the patient; a dislike of wine, fish, veal, and sweets; or a dream of a horse that turns into a dog.[11] While any of these rubrics may point to the remedy, a combination of them is determinative.

A fashion show of polychrests would feature *Eucalyptus, Antimonium, Allium* (onion), *Ferrum* (iron), *Mercurius, Sulphur, Silicea, Calcarea carbonica, Lachesis, Nux vomica* (poison nut from the strychnine tree), and *Cantharus* (blister beetle). See also the later discussion of Edward Whitmont's "coutures" of *Natrum muriaticum, Sepia, Phosphorus,* and *Lycopodium* (see pages 122–124).

Rhus toxicodendron, a polychrest prepared from the flowering sumac (a shrub, vine, or small tree), is distinguished by neuromuscular weakness approaching paralysis and by nutritional deficiency. It is also indicated when acute diseases progress in a typhoid direction (into scarlet fever, diphtheria, dysentery, and pneumonia) as well as in cases of poison oak. *Rhus tox.* patients are recognized by the fact that they are worse when resting, with the condition relieved by motion, and then that movement causes them such exhaustion that they are compelled to rest. As a result, they are constantly restless. Other keynotes include joint pain (especially between 2 and 3 p.m.), a sore or dry tongue (sometimes coated but not at the tip), swelling of the eyelids, and a short ticklish cough originating behind the upper part of the sternum. *Rhus tox.* is used for sprains and twists and also for herpes, chicken pox, and shingles.[12] Because it resembles so many other remedies that share at least one of its major symptoms, *Rhus tox.* is a poster remedy for selection not on the basis of single symptoms but by the relationships of elements in a symptom complex.

Another herbal polychrest, *Bryonia*, is prescribed for some of the same allopathically defined conditions as *Rhus tox.* but differs in that it is worse from motion (even to the degree of having vertigo), is irritable and anxious, and experiences extreme thirst; its symptoms wax in severity from the midevening into the early morning (with 9 p.m. being a particularly bad time).[13] Hahnemann noted that upon "slight mental emotion (on laughing) there suddenly occurs a shooting (itching) burning all over the body as [the *Bryonia* patient] had been whipped with nettles or had nettle rash, though nothing is seen on the skin; this burning came on afterwards by merely thinking of it, or when he got heated."[14]

Tarentula hispania, a spider poison, is recognized by its crazed and tormented behavior: socially unacceptable deeds often regretted later. These patients are excited by music and sometimes perspire from melody or color. They sing and dance, have fits of nervous laughter, and masturbate frequently. Pain and movement in the stomach are sometimes accompanied by a sensation of insects boring and crawling on the limbs. Yet a *Tarentula* microdose can be indicated without any of the above symptoms in cases of constipation causing a person to roll from side to side or tumors around the vertebral column.[15] Again, a person may have several indicative cues or a single characteristic one. Repertorization is too much like divination to be adaptable to health bureaucracies and centers for disease control, though in an ideal world, homeopathy and allopathy would find a way to work together.

Cocculus indicus, a woody vine and traditional fish poison, is administered in some instances of extreme melancholy, deep reveries, difficulty concentrating, or speaking hastily (even wittily) without concern or sense. It is used also for vomiting, waking with a start from a hideous nightmare, and a number of cerebrally based disorders. It may be given for flatulent colic that is worse around midnight, especially in the context of an itching scrotum or early menstruation.[16] *Cocculus* has some of the same paralytic and anxious symptoms as *Rhus Tox.* and sings and dances like *Tarentula*. French homeopath Didier Grandgeorge noted that *Cocculus* is often the remedy for people who attend to the dying and seek to know the secrets of life and death. Such individuals may be endemically nosy and are drawn to become doctors, nurses, and psychoanalysts.[17]

Another polychrest, *Nitricum acidum*, is often an inflexible person who insists on following rules no matter what. If chastised, *Nitric Acid* will invariably make its own punishment worse. It is unforgiving of others. It loves fats and salt, especially herring. Physically, *Nitric acid* includes chronic nasal discharges, otitis, white spots on nails, fetid perspiration of the feet, double vision, vertigo, and roaring in the ears. It is prescribed for brunettes more than for blondes. People requiring it are chilly and depressed; they may have small, painful pimples on the tongue; and they find swallowing difficult because a morsel always sticks in the pharynx.[18]

Of this corrosive compound, Edward Tine wrote: "A patient comes with a pallid face, a rather sickly countenance, tired and weary, subject to headache, disorders of the bladder and disturbances of digestion, and in spite of all your questioning you fail to get anything that is peculiar. You prescribe *Sulphur*, *Lycopodium*, and a good many other remedies in vain. But one day she says, 'Doctor, it seems queer that my urine smells so strong, it smells like that of a horse.' Now at once you know that it is *Nitric Acid*."[19]

Plumbum individuals are gloomy and depressed with, symbolically, a dense metallic ring (high on the periodic table); they balk at constraints. They tend toward loss of memory, paralysis, sleeplessness, limb pain, stickiness in the throat, and numbness. *Lead* is distinguished by pale gums (sometimes with a blue line at their margin), blue swellings on the torso, lightning-like pains in the lower limbs and belly button (shooting to other areas), anemia and emaciation, the sensation in the throat of a ball rising into the brain, a disquiet feeling that the abdomen and back are pressing together, an old-cheese smell to sweating feet, a hallucination that the feet are made of wood, urination drop by drop and scanty, and pain sometimes through to the bones.[20]

Pennsylvania-based homeopathic physician W. A. Boyson reported a classic *Plumbum* narrative from a patient: "'About six years ago I began to have crampy pains in my legs, sometimes twitching and burning and numbness. These pains were so bad that I could not sleep. For relief I'd get up out of bed, pound my legs, soak them in hot water, rub them with everything I heard of. I took a barrel of pills and gallons of liquids—no good. Finally I had a lumbar sympathectomy. That really was a mistake and I lost my sight for several weeks. The pain in my right toe became so severe that I had it amputated. Now my leg pains are worse than ever. How is that for a case?' 'Not bad,' quoth I, 'you have given me a beautiful picture.' A picture of what? Well, the five big remedies of central nervous system disorders are *Agaricus, Phosphorus, Plumbum, Picric Acid,* and *Zinc,* and this picture is that of *Plumbum.*"[21]

Pulsatilla has physical manifestations such as circulatory problems aggravated by stuffy rooms, late menstruation, and frequent urging to stool followed by bellyache. *Pulsatilla* is often given to children, no matter their physical condition, who cling to teddy bears, suck their thumbs, and in general have difficulty separating from their mothers. It is a remedy for diseases caused by suppression of an infantile or early-childhood unhappy experience.[22]

A purple and yellow meadow flower, *Pulsatilla* is also an emotional remedy prescribed for women whose lives are dominated by the people to whom they are devoted. A *Pulsatilla* may be quite intelligent, but her feelings trump her intellect. *Pulsatilla* is typically unsteady, moody, whimsical, and discontent; she is lachrymose, timid, and phlegmatic. *Pulsatillas* are said to favor old-fashioned blouses and the color blue. They are often blonde with blue or green eyes and round faces—note the vibrational resonance between dress style (an extension of the epidermal layer of the body and even the cell's extracellular matrix) and epigenetic expressions of DNA. Many *Pulsatillas* sweat on only one side of their bodies and/or are almost superhumanly thirstless. They hate fatty foods but love butter to the point of craving. Their pains wander, with rheumatism going from joint to joint. They may sneeze a lot, chatter in their sleep, and, though feeling chilly, find external heat intolerable. They tend toward hypochondria with great enough anxiety to want to throw off all their clothes.[23]

A psychological picture of the patient may be used in a search of physical symptoms that give a confirmation of the choice. For example, a clingy child who wants to stick to his mother, is upset in a stuffy room, and bites his nails could be a *Pulsatilla* child, and a yellow, bland discharge from the nose accompanied by digestive upset from pork fat and other starchy, buttery, sweet foods may confirm the choice.[24]

Finding the essence of *Pulsatilla* can still be dicey, for it closely resembles *Silica, Phosphorus, Lycopodium, Calcarea,* and a number of other remedies. Hahnemann's *Materia medica pura,* in volumes 1 and 2, lists about 2,700 symptoms for *Pulsatilla.*

If you find this basis of diagnosis excessive or resembling obsessive-compulsive disorder, you have not shifted to a homeopathic frame. If observed homeopathically, our human landscape is populated by *Zincums, Plumbums, Sepias,* and *Pulsatillas.*

In 2023, homeopaths in England took a shot at a constitutional remedy, obviously too late, for Bryan Kohberger, primary suspect in the murder of four University of Idaho students, based on his quirky behavior and physical look, eyebrows to body type: it was *Plumbum metallicum,* a man sung to by lead.

Homeopathic historian and prescriber Jerry Kantor has done similar analyses of Donald Trump, Vladimir Putin, and Hillary Clinton. While acknowledging that these are inexact without medical records or direct contact with the patients, he uses them to show how homeopathy encapsulates mind, body, and spirit.

In the case of Trump:

> Connecting the dots between a love of property and glamour, obsession with building walls, tendency to superficial relationships, compulsion to fire his servants, cupidity and ruthlessness, Fluoric Acidum is unmistakably Donald Trump's indicated remedy. . . . [These types] will push anything and anyone aside in the all-absorbing desire to shine and glitter. They love to be the big macho guy for everybody to look up to. They want to draw the attention with their big car and high position in the glamour world. They are very ambitious, want to climb up high and earn lots of money. . . . Fluorine is the lightest, the most active and reactive [element], forming and breaking relationships very quickly. This can be seen

in the symptomatology of Fluoric acid. The remedy state is flirtatious, has many acquaintances but no deep relationship.

Aversion to responsibility, sexual desire increased; attracted to strangers, and increased energy. A naive psychopath, prone to serious gambling. Delusion [of] servants he must get rid of. In other words, "You're fired!" Fluoric Acidum is the only remedy in this rubric. . . . Compulsion to break taboos . . . sexual exhaustion, weakly constitutions, sallow skin, and emaciation as well as a germophobia feature pertaining to the syphilitic miasm within which Fluoric Acidum belongs.[25]

When I asked him about Putin, Kantor wrote:

From recent reports whose reliability I cannot verify he has a GI tract cancer of some sort and Parkinson's disease as well. What has been reported is unsteady gait, falling down stairs, involuntary loss of stool. Anyone who has seen him can attest his face is pretty much a mask. Don't think I've ever seen him smile. If this were all I had to go on and knowing his geopolitics I would say for the moment *Conium*: lower body paralysis, facial hardness, resignation to death (and the "God of death"), a sense of entrapment (re Ukraine). Loss of life's "juice," enjoining a general hardness of viewpoint and body function. I also think he is a deeply insecure man drawn to control and tyranny as a compensation which would have indicated *Lycopodium* earlier in life. Also to consider would be *Plumbum, Mercury*, and *Syphilinum*. But I would go with *Conium*, knowing only what I know."[26]

In what he called "a stab at Hillary Clinton," Kantor concluded:

The constitutional remedy that Secretary Clinton needs is made from the venom of the American rattlesnake and is called *Crotalus*

Horridus. . . . On the positive side: An independent and adventurous spirit. Leadership qualities. Sympathy and a tendency to protect the weak (her work on behalf of children and minorities). Love of travel. Playfulness. A spiritual or moral bent. Good with language.

Qualities that can be either good or bad: . . . Emotionally intense but suffers from the need for self-control (true about all snake remedies). Handling of Bill's Monica Lewinsky affair tested and inflamed this quality. Cannot bear to be controlled. This is actually the core theme of the *Crotalus Horridus* remedy.

On the negative side: Dictatorial. Averse to contradiction. Vengeful. . . . Capable of a stony "don't cross me" stare. . . . [A sense of] victimization. . . .

Ms. Clinton's recognized food and drink preferences suggest the remedy *Crotalus Horridus.* These include creamy and spicy food, as well as red wine.[27]

Nosodes

A special class of remedies, prepared from potentized bacteria, pus, viruses, and other disease products, was added to the homeopathic materia medica in the early twentieth century. The nosodes, as these are called, include such unappealing substances as bacteria taken from bowels and gonorrheal and syphilitic discharges. *Tuberculinum* is made from tuberculous lymph nodes. Some early homeopaths considered it so loathsome they wouldn't prescribe it. Now it is a standard part of the repertory, especially for dealing with tubercular aspects of disease layers of different origins.[28]

Tuberculinum types are fundamentally restless but not in an aimless way; they long to be free of whatever they are doing or wherever they are, experiencing a constant desire for travel (to the point of globe-trotting), consciousness-expanding drugs, and sometimes competitive and physical sports. They are highly intellectual folks who crave new stimulation and, while being naturally curious, often lack depth of inquiry, mental patience, or the ability to sustain any one quest. Because of their hyperactivity, *Tuberculinums* keep changing the subject of their attention (attention deficit disorder in modern parlance). Another indication of this type is that no other remedy works for any length of time, and many seemingly correct remedies have only a temporary effect.[29]

Tubercular individuals are also susceptible to allergies, deathly afraid of animals (especially dogs), had acne as teenagers, and are improved from staying in the mountains (but not above 5,000 feet, which is too arousing for them). They love open air or riding in a brisk wind and tend to open windows everywhere, but afterward they are susceptible to persistent colds and catarrhs. *Tuberculinums* tend toward headaches and/or constipation followed by diarrhea, during which they suffer heavy sweating. *Tuberculinums* can also be emaciated, "thin as a rail," and hypersensitive to changes in the weather.[30]

People needing *Tuberculinum* as a remedy often have tuberculosis in their family history and a negative, allergy-like responsive to the BCG (tuberculosis) vaccine: the vaccination causes swollen glands; its scar gives off pus. However, *Tuberculinum* is not just a cure for tuberculosis or tubercular conditions; it is a distinct character type of its own, of which tuberculosis is but one of many possible manifestations.[31] In other periods of history, it may find a different miasmatic expression.

During the 2020s COVID-19 pandemic, homeopaths used potentized microdoses of viral phlegms from COVID-19-infected people, boosted monthly (instead of vaccines containing genetically transferred spikes bound in graphene oxides and boosted whenever health authorities decided). They were often reinforced by potentized T cells. Informal surveys by homeopathic suppliers indicated a prevention and recovery rate of more than 90 percent with this treatment.

The gold standard of any treatment's effectiveness is—or should be—its performance under game conditions, with inexplicable intercessions allowed, even encouraged. It is *not* performance against a so-called placebo in an experimental simulation in which factors of transference, projection, object relations, transitional objects, and empathic participation, let alone subatomic, nano, and quantum effects, have been ignored, cancelled, or manipulated—or inadvertently purged. Living systems are alchemically and psychically entangled. In some cases, the active component is too subtle and multivariate to pin down. Creative chaos and colloidal disequilibrium can't be replicated in a sterilized trial, so a catalyst may be excluded from its own test.

Systemic Responsiveness and Sequences of Disease Pictures

The organism's own defense mechanism is the first and best remedy and often quite sufficient. A homeopathic medicine serves only as an amplification and support of an innate immune response; it can't do anything on its own—by correlative logic, a vaccine doesn't defend against a virus, but it activates antibodies that do. When a patient is given a Similar, his or her immune system responds directly to the microdose. The Simillimum or near Simillimum matches the pathology. They meet and, in a sense, annul.

Disease and medicine can be matched without insight into the mechanism of the pathology or the biochemistry of its dissipation. That information is essential in understanding biology, anatomy, chemistry, and other systems bearing on the physical functioning of organisms and the workings of nature itself, but it is superfluous or incidental to healing by Similars, Hahnemann's first law of homeopathic pharmacy is "that it is only in virtue of their power to make the healthy human being ill that medicines can cure morbid states, and, indeed, only such morbid states as are composed of symptoms which the drug to be selected for them can itself produce in similarity on the healthy."[32]

Another way to look at homeopathic treatment is to posit that the disease itself is the best medicine. For reasons of constitutional inertia, environmental toxicity, social disruption, genetic weakness—whatever—this is no longer the case. While an organism is able to improve on its own within embryogenic limits, it cannot spontaneously throw off an entire illness that is sustained by its own susceptibility, so it will succumb in time. Illness or disease also does not so much match a susceptibility as it is acquired, maintained, and expressed because of an inherent weakness or out-of-tune-ness in the organism. In another sense, the organism is sick because it cannot "see" its own disease, which occurs in its blind spot. Plus, illnesses arise in layers, without a singular shape or frequency, so they insinuate themselves like Trojan horses.

By allying with the defense mechanism, a correct remedy jars the system out of its apathy toward a healing response. A series of additional remedies may be needed after the first before the full condition, layer by layer, ripple by ripple, is excavated and retuned.

Until then, the physician proceeds etiologically from each whole picture to the next. Every remedy, as it is introduced, changes the picture. It is briefly the Simillimum, the single remedy, but as soon as the picture changes, another Simillimum supplants it. Ultimately, a series of "single" remedies can unravel and dispel an entire syndrome. Yet they are always administered one at a time, for no grand cleansing is possible without respecting each layer and the systemic integrity with which it formed. Each new picture is interpreted solely in terms of its current priority and the response of the system to the prior remedy given.

Each prescription also assumes that the organism will make the best possible use of a microdose even if it is not on exactly the wavelength of the disease, and that its reorganization then will define and direct the next phase. Overdetermined and synergistic, remedies will continually reoptimize as the patient is organized around a less inward center of gravity. If the patient is reorganized around a deeper disease, the medicine has failed and made the condition worse. If the medicine is totally off the wavelength of the disease, most often nothing will happen. A far errant prescription does not alter the case—it is generic bathwater—whereas a near miss may cause a distortion that, if not antidoted, will make the picture muddier.

The resolution of one picture leads to the emergence of the next, for life is a series of organismic challenges that keep it vital and meaningful. Only death ends healing crises, at least on this plane. In reincarnational systems, death may be the most logical and normal resolution of a dilemma on the soul's path through successive bardos. The unresolved complex is reengaged in its next incarnation.

Much as past conditions can't be treated unless a resolution of present symptoms brings them back into view, chronic ailments in temporary remission cannot be diagnosed until they recur. Surrogates cast by Similars continually ripple and reform. A homeopath cannot predict what will appear next. Unwinding a disease is preferable to a recurrent or deteriorative condition that never gets resolved. A successful sequence may pass through eruptions, especially if the disease is deep-seated and has been suppressed by antibiotics or steroids. Superficially, things get worse as the layers of suppression are penetrated. The alleviation is a suppression. While "pain free" sells pharmaceuticals, cure is the truer goal. If flare-ups did not occur, the pathology could not be unraveled. An organism that is in static, symptom-free equilibrium may also be apathetic. Jonathan Shore, both a homeopath and an M.D., noted: "After taking a remedy it is important to watch closely for changes. Remedies may begin their action by an improvement in the emotional area, by an aggravation of symptoms, by a general improvement, or other more subtle responses. . . . Sometimes a good response is a small change in some insignificant-seeming symptoms that show us indications for the next remedy."[33]

The basic homeopathic rule is reapplied at each new level: Prescribe by Similars; take a total symptom picture; prescribe the remedy that would cause those symptoms; wait while the organism establishes a new equilibrium. Take a new picture; prescribe again if necessary. Each condition, as it comes into being, is definitive. It does no good to say "That was a clearer disease. Let's refer back." It is no longer *the* disease after a remedy had altered its picture. As long as the present picture is clear, a more attuned remedy can follow a less correct match. The only incorrect prescription, as noted, is a near Similar that confuses the sequencing of layers.

When a homeopathic aggravation occurs in a sick person, an artificial disease converges with an actual disease, and the dynamics of their fusion combine. Conversely, if a remedy is right, the patient usually senses that they are better. Even if overt manifestations are worse, intuitively things are improving and will continue to improve. Lay homeopath Theodore Enslin described how, when symptoms drop off, they go back in time:

> In the treatment of a condition, a conditioning which has gone on for many years, sometimes it is not possible to cure with one shot; it's not a miracle at all. That's one reason a good prescriber wants to know as much about the patient as possible: everything. So you begin a reverse process. You begin, very practically, with what is exactly there. When those symptoms are cleared, very often you will find that the patient has symptoms that are prior, of things that happened before that. And you keep on going. You go back to childhood. And there are many stories about the actual walking off of the last symptom. You get to the point where it will go right

off a finger, the last wart or pain. There are many case histories like that. Sometimes this process can take a number of years.[34]

Kent gave twelve careful "observations" to make after the medicine is given.

1. When there is prolonged aggravation of the symptoms, followed by the final decline of the patient, it means too strong a medicine: the action was too deep for the degree of deterioration that had already taken place, and the weakened vital force was unable to throw off the new attack. Since the medicine can work only through the vital force, the physician must assess how strong the vital force is before giving a remedy. The potency of the medicine must be harmonized, approximately, to the capability of the vital force.

2. When there is also a long aggravation, but one leading to slow and final improvement of the patient, the disease was deep but deterioration was not as great, and hence the medicine was appropriate. The aggravation was long because tissue change had already taken place.

3. If there is a quick strong aggravation, followed by rapid improvement, the remedy was correct, and no serious tissue change has taken place.

4. When there is recovery without aggravation, there may not have been any disease in the first place or the disease may have been relatively new and superficial.

5. Improvement and amelioration of the symptoms followed by aggravation indicate that the disease is deeper than the medicine and the medicine was acting only palliatively.

6. Short relief followed by return of the symptoms might mean the patient has antidoted the remedy by coming into contact with substances that neutralize the potentization.

7. If the symptoms are relieved, but the patient still feels sick, the medicine was wrong. There are latent organic conditions preventing a cure.

8. The patient proves every remedy. This may be an idiosyncrasy; it may also indicate an incurable condition. Kent suggests using a higher potency.

9. Proving: the method of bringing on symptoms in a healthy person by giving a medicine. Proving is a procedure for discovering new remedies and is considered beneficial in an immune-stimulating way to people who do it.

10. New symptoms might also indicate a proving, which would mean the wrong medicine had been used.

11. It is important to distinguish between a proving and the reappearance of old symptoms. When old symptoms reappear in the reverse order of their original occurrence (the eleventh observation), this confirms that the healing process is moving in the natural direction.

12. The symptoms move from without to within, driving the disease deeper. This indicates the doctor prescribed only for a peripheral condition, and in so doing hastened the disease process.[35]

Edward Whitmont emphasized the nondichotomizing, nondual component of single doses in *all* holistic medicines:

There is no malefic-beneficial dualism: toxic or potentially damaging agencies may also serve genuine healing when applied with due regard to organismic integrity. The needle in the hand of the acupuncturist, the knife in the hand of the surgeon, microdoses of arsenic administered according to the homeopathic simile principle all may heal when used as a means of harmonizing, balancing and reintegrating overall psychosomatic functioning. When aimed at isolated functions, however, they serve to forcibly change one part, hence evoking a compensatory imbalance of others. Then such remedies become irremediable.[36]

In 1990, I received a packet of *Magnesia phosphorica*, repertorized in part for a chronic flicker in my left eye. To the degree that I expected the macule to improve, I thought it would dissipate and then dissolve. Yet almost immediately after I put the microdose under my tongue, the flicker speeded up (which it never had till then) until it vanished by oscillating so rapidly I couldn't see it. After that, I reconceived homeopathic aggravations as energy blips that activate sensations. For all I know, the flicker is still going on, and was going on before I "saw" it, oscillating so fast I didn't notice it. Its slowing to visibility represented systemic apathy. By analogy, Earth is moving so fast relative to us—rotating, revolving, and otherwise traveling galactically and supergalactically—that we don't feel it.

About a year later, I began to experience optical migraines (without pain) for the first time, and I interpreted that as the next layer of the flicker. I now think that its earliest rung was a hypnogogic sleep disturbance in my childhood: objects changing size, density, and relation to space as my fingertips and parts of my face seem to grow fat and puffy. I fell from the sky into cities that grew out of dots as I approached them. Then the cities ended up in my imaginarily swollen fingers. Sometimes these events were followed by sleep paralysis.

Spasms, sparks, and space-time dysphoria encompassed both a greater disease and its remedy.

Miasmatic Philosophy and Esoteric Homeopathy

Homeopathy is not just a medical practice but a philosophical study of the relationship between health and disease. In esoteric homeopathy, diseases are layers, patterns imposed upon each other. The disease of any one person is built up of historically successive trauma—"plagues" or miasms. The same process of diagnosis that applies to miasms applies to the individual or collective health of a society or planet. The relationship of societies to germs, health, vital force, and the epigenetic field is also a "pathology measure" of each species in its terrain. It is exobiological in principle, applicable to any world in this universe.

A doctor must begin by prescribing for the current miasm, suspending treatment of deeper levels till they appear. If the treatment removes the outer level, the pattern will oscillate, find a new equilibrium—creative disorder—and then present a new picture to treat. The source miasm can only be approached layer by layer, like peeling an onion.

The deepest miasm is genetic, congenital, and evolutionary. An organism inherits the constitutional predispositions and weaknesses of its ancestors, species, and world. Onto the genetic level are inflicted the miasms of the womb, early childhood diseases, traumas, and conditions muffled by allopathic medicine or systemically suppressed. Onto this level is imposed a series of chronic and acute diseases and allergies (the latter of which may simply be heightening sensitivities of chronic conditions to external aggravation), and, finally, onto these are dispensed the environmental conditions to which the organism is exposed, including its social order and economic system, the psychospiritual phase of its society, toxins in soil and water, microplastics, forever chemicals, smoke particles, radiation, ionization, WiFi signals, stress, and whatever else is in play. Organismic integrity is reestablished regularly in relation to assault by biomes and habitats. Then each allopathic drug and vaccine brings a miasmatic universe of its own, as each iatrogenic event interpolates prior ones. These interlocking webs may be imbued in a variety of ways, but the patient is a dynamic expression of all of them. They have brought the patient into being and sustain the patient's world. Health and disease are expressions of vital responses to miasmatic phases.

Mainstream science also deals with environments, societies, organisms, microbiomes, and their combined ecology, but not as an integrated complex with pathologizing and self-healing equilibria. An ailment of the liver is an ailment of the liver, a job driving a bus is a job driving a bus, and a bus driver losing his job, causing his family to suffer, are each an independent event. If a bus driver develops a liver ailment and cannot go to work, the allopath attempts to heal his liver and return him to his livelihood. If the liver is "improved," the patient can drive the bus. He can reinhabit his job, support his family, and contribute to society and social welfare.

But jobs and social roles may be aspects of deeper diseases; thus, when healees start to get better, they may find themselves unable to fill the same positions in society. When they return to old pathways, their illnesses also return. A holistic treatment requires an adjustment of *all* circumstances, organic and environmental. The liver ailment and driving the bus are not independent circumstances but interdependent layers of the same condition imposed by environment and class as well as constitution. In esoteric homeopathy, full cure is impossible. Healing is measured by organismic resilience and miasmatic homeostasis. In a sense, allopathy is situational "homeopathy."

Social and economic crises are an aggregate result of untreated diseases driven inward. Crimes, wars, and sociopathy are manifestations of leprosy, smallpox, malaria, cancer, and the like—symptom complexes converted by generations of suppression. A morbific agent manifests when the overall civilizational process requires it.

In his acts of torture and erotic cannibalism, Jeffrey Dahmer was as sick as victims of AIDS or cancer because his system was unable to generate an immune response on the physical plane. His behavior was the apathetic reaction of his vital force to trauma, perhaps triggered by a childhood hernia surgery after which, his father claimed, he was never the same. He kept trying to reopen his body and get at his own organs.

Plagues are generalized healing aggravations. For instance, a palliative suppression of tuberculosis might lead to an increase in criminal activity—the work of miasms driven inward to the mental plane. In a prescient 1990 book, Harris Coulter proposed a direct causal relationship between some vaccines and social violence.[37] That concept goes beyond debate about DPT shots, thimerosal, and autism. Pornography, sexual transgressions, political polarization, kidnappings, child armies, civil disobedience, riots, insurrections, and wars likewise express miasmatic aggravations trying to resolve socioeconomic and ecological imbalances in the only way that organisms know how: by generating an immune response or, in Jungian terms, summoning the shadow archetype. An esoteric homeopathic way to interpret the insurrectionist events of January 6, 2021, in Washington, D.C., applies equally to the French Revolution and 2020's temporary autonomous zones in Portland, Oregon, and Seattle, Washington. History becomes a chronicle of vital responses to miasmatic states: revolutions, while destructive, remove layers of biological and social pathology and revive collective health. Despite their violations of personhood and the social order, we would be miasmatically sicker without them. The disturbances they express were long in gestation, some extending perhaps as far back as ancestral primates or mammals. That's the *big* big picture!

Guns mark a psychopathologization of the relationship between the individual and the collective. Aggrieved and otherwise dissociated individuals align their own tendency toward violence with the machine's lethal action. They have no other way to salvage their terminally depressed egos from rage paralysis, incel envy, or a sensation of having lost their own manhood (or gender identity). They go for flashes of apocalyptic disindividuation.

Guns allow miasmatic expressions. They were firesticks that blacksmiths forged from a combination of medieval explosives and flaming arrows, which had their own forerunners in Stone Age spears, slings, and bolos. Electrons have replaced sticks and stones, but homicidal projections are unchanged.

Miasms don't doom us to an infinite regression, but they point to how we became who we are. A chordate heritage shaped our early tissues, hormones, and agendas around an embryonic notochord, a larval lesion or primitive streak that led cell masses from a starfish's circular wheel to a worm's bilateral ladder. All agendas and symbols henceforth were hypostatized on that axis. Unresolved acts passed from fish to axolotls to bullfrogs to mice and wrens. We're descendants of the climbing-shrew line; birds, dinosaurs, and amphibians went another way. Each must procreate and provide offspring, so each spawns codes, turning them into acts, customs, and conditions. Social orders and geopolitics are emergent and self-generating, but they couldn't occur without miasmatic disturbances along the way. We are still animals, plants, and minerals singing animal, plant, and mineral songs. That is a measure of miasmatic depth.

Esoteric homeopathy encompasses germ theory, for Hahnemann developed his system before a conflict in medical ideology between terrain (natural immunity) and viruses, bacteria, and other adventitious intrusions. Far from being freelance invaders that increase and decrease in natural selection, bugs are miasmatic manifestations that respond to organisms (or societies) according to systemic weaknesses.

For instance, contagious ailments affect large numbers of contiguous people, but not all and not all in the same way. The health of both the herd and the individual determines the nature and expression of disease threshold in a biome. Except in Black Death–like scourges or biological warfare, morbific agents are secondary to individual responses of organisms; each immune system will use the occasion of a "bug" to express its particular disease layer and vitality. That's why each sick person requires individual treatment for the same infection during a pandemic. Homeopathy is characterological, not categorical.

In cases where a morbific agent is powerful enough to impose consistent symptomology on a large number of people, homeopaths may use a limited range of remedies or a single remedy for all people—the disease itself is too powerful and overwhelming an agent at a particular stage of history for individualized responses. Within a pandemic, homeopaths may decide to confront an assault on their patient with a pharmaceutical "toxin" like erythromycin (bacterially) or monoclonal antibodies (virally), recognizing that the sick person is not strong enough for a miasmatic cleansing. This is where mainstream allopathy and miasmatic homeopathy converge. From an esoteric standpoint, homeopathy is a creative use of artificial diseases to bring about human transformation and individual and collective health, while allopathy is a means of antidoting diseases to bring about a new layer of functional health. Both are part of Earth's miasmatic cycles. Likely entire species came up against hazards that killed off most of them, but the biological field itself found new pathways and resiliences; it hatched novel species.

Outlier psychologist Immanuel Velikovsky proposed that a locust-like cloud descending from the comet that became Venus inculcated many of humanity's miasms, and that's not the only cloud or descent of locusts in terrestrial mythography. A more recent "conspiracy theory" proffered that the COVID-19 virus was strewn from debris of a comet's tail over Earth's northern hemisphere. And, after all, comets contain the raw material of organic chemistry—water, cyanide, oxygen, amino acids—and have long been deemed nests of viral life.

An evolving biosphere doesn't need repertorized remedies; it repertorizes innately *in order to evolve*. Earth—Sol 3—provides substances, germs, toxins, pandemics, and the like to balance its own planetary constitution and restore system-wide homeostasis. It "understands" herds, tribes, biomes, and organisms in dynamic counterbalance with their own interdependent phases of vitality and apathy.

Since the advent of life on Earth, viruses and retroviruses have transferred RNA within microbiomes. They are natural chromosome-updating machines. Through their exchanges, our cells developed stem pluripotency, and their multicellular bundles have gotten recapitulated in diverse taxonomies. Birds' wings are human arms with different chromosomal gating that may have come from a viral or insect vector instilled during an infection.

Humans house bacteria, viruses, viromes, fungi, algae, trichocysts, vestigial protists, archaea, lysosomes, mitochondria, Golgi bodies, prions—rogue proteins that were once independent creatures—as well microbes and microbiota that are *still* independent (though captured and colonized), *and all these life forms' genes*. They participate with each other in microecologies while exchanging DNA indiscriminately. We also have a HERV (human endogenous retrovirus) library of nonhuman DNA, much of it made of diseases passed down through thousands of generations.

In a book on the microbiome, gastroenterologist Alessio Fasano and coauthor Susie Flaherty explained, "Our human genome has coevolved with trillions of constantly changing microorganisms found in and on the human body. . . . [W]e are the *product* of coevolution . . . with the metagenome (the gene array from our microbiome), which contains from 100 to 150 *times* more genes than we do"[38] (italics mine).

Vertebrates have borrowed from other chordates, jellyfish, fungi, oaks, and the like while differentiating into mammals and primates. Before that, alleles jumping species, phyla, and even kingdoms—DNA is a universal language—led to the differentiation of a primeval chordate blastula with RNA from insects, spiders, algae, club mosses, and snails. We are viral and pandemic in database.

Systems of remediation are required—and have come into being—

only as the human race has fallen out of balance with these innate processes of nature. Organisms in harmony with their environment's own nanodoses generate homeopathic cures without formal medicine.

The coronavirus pandemic that erupted in late 2019 was viewed miasmatically as a response to pollution, deforestation, and reduction of biodiversity. According to avant-garde physician Zack Bush, the modern world is triggering its own mutations. In his theory, COVID-19's RNA spike protein is a viral reading of pesticides in the agricultural industry (notably Monsanto's Roundup with its soil-killing glyphosate) as well as antibiotics pumped into factory farms (particularly our biological cousins, pigs), air pollution (disgorges of methane, carbon dioxide, and particulate matter), and a generally pharmaceuticalized habitat. The coronavirus didn't just come from bats. Bats were its vector, but the virus represents a holistic response of the biosphere and our genome.

Clumping with toxins, COVID-19 runs too much exogenous data through our protoplasm. This overload, not the virus, posits Bush, is what is making people sick. The hypoxia of COVID is cyanide poisoning in response to the choking of planetary oxygen—a hyperinflammatory autoimmune blowback or cytokine storm from cell overload. Yet, Bush reassures, most of those infected have their RNA updated without serious harm. They receive regular small COVID-19 variant loads and develop immunity as well as rudiments of new enzymes and organs. From his view, our species is responding to its altered planet by refreshing its microbiome, so the pandemic is a biological awakening, a transspecies metamorphosis, and a healing crisis. We are readapting to the planet and, in a sense, healing our own miasm. The pandemic is like a Zen master imposing lessons as well as a collective ayahuasca ceremony to escape stagnation. From this perspective, mRNA nanoparticles won't alleviate the pandemic; they will increase toxic overload and suppress an innate homeostatic response. They don't address the extracellular matrix, biospheric membrane, and atmospheric bubble around Earth.[39]

The miasmatic message is that we are going to have to live with our guests, invited or not, guests or golems. We are going to have to accept their gifts, gifts or not, and their price, incremental or absolute. We are loose in the same biosphere, we share a biome and microbiome, and there is no net vast enough or fine enough to get each of us out of the other's snares.

Microdoses and the Vital Force

When the precisely correct remedy (Simillimum) plucks the corresponding string of body-mind, the vital force uniquely recognizes and harmonizes with it. Homeopathic theory confers the power of dynamic readjustment not on remedies or organs themselves, but only on the vital force. Hahnemann wrote:

> This *dynamic* action of medicines, like the vitality itself by means of which it is reflected upon the organism, is almost purely *spiritual* in its nature. This dynamic property is so pervading that it is quite immaterial what sensitive part of the body is touched by the medicine in order to develop its whole action . . . immaterial whether the dissolved medicine enter the stomach or merely remain in the mouth, or be applied to a wound or other part deprived of skin.[40]

"Immateriality" is the eternal homeopathic elephant in the room. Microdoses are "spiritual" medicines. Despite their elaborate chemical preparation by a laboratory procedure, they are not drugs (though *legally* they are over-the-counter pharmaceuticals). The operative product, the pill, is such a high dilution of the original substance that nothing is left of that substance, or, in some cases, for instance in preparations of potencies below 12C, an infinitesimally tiny amount, not known to have any biomechanical effect, remains incidentally. Since the remedy does not operate in a material milieu, homeopathy is not a chemico-mechanical system. As noted, the potentized substance is more like the alchemical Philosopher's Stone.

I will go over the homeopathic method of preparation of microdoses multiple times from different perspectives so that readers will have a full understanding. A general understanding suffices for most purposes, but a broader, layered explanation allows one to think homeopathically and participate imaginally in the tincturing. Imaginality will also help if you decide to practice psychic homeopathy as described in chapter 7.

Note too that since neither homeopathic practitioners nor lab pharmacists fathom how the medicines work, a ritual adherence to Hahnemann's empirical phases of discovery and institutionalization supplants biochemistry or targeting by molecular mechanism. As long as the microdoses do work—as long as they seem to transfer medicinal information—they continue to be made in a traditional fashion. The same could be said, by the way, of many modern pharmaceuticals despite corporate claims of proven causation. Pill-less homeopathy wouldn't even be a possibility (per chapter 7) if we knew *how* the microdoses worked.

Any natural or man-made substance—plant tincture, animal product, mineral, disease discharge—that can be diluted or ground into a powder, and any form of energy as well, can be turned into a homeopathic remedy. However prepared, the solution is shaken vigorously (succussed) at each stage of dilution. To form each next decimal potency, one part of this dilution is then mixed with nine parts of a neutral medium (ninety-nine parts for the centesimal dilution) and shaken or triturated. The third decimal potency is made with one part of the second decimal and nine more parts of a neutral medium (ninety-nine parts for the centesimal). At this point in the decimal sequence the original substance has become only one-thousandth of the final pill. The third centesimal dilution produces a pill with one-millionth part of the original medicine.

In the *Organon*, Hahnemann laid out a precise methodology of trituration, dilution, and succussion and the exact ratio of original medicinal substance, neutral medium, and alcohol. Using this formula and following its unique steps—trituration, dilution, succussion—remedies can be potentized in 1:10 (decimal, abbreviated as *X*), 1:100 (centesimal or *C*), 1:1,000 (millesimal or *M*), and 1:50,0000 (quinquagintimillesimal or *Q* or *LM*) scales.

In each, the first three steps are repeated as many times as are necessary to get to increasingly diluted potencies—1X, 2X, 3X, and on, 1C, 2C, 3C, and on, and so forth.

Three different processes of dilution and succussion are used depending on whether the raw material is soluble in water or alcohol or not. Here are examples:

1. Dilution and succussion for water-soluble medicinal substances: One part of the water-soluble medicinal substance is dissolved in ninety-nine parts of water and succussed to get 1C. One part of the 1C solution is dissolved in ninety-nine parts of water and succussed to get 2C. The process is repeated again and again to get to 30C or 200C and beyond. Example, Sodium chloride, common salt.

2. Dilution and succussion for alcohol-soluble medicinal substances: One part of the alcohol-soluble medicinal substance is dissolved in ninety-nine parts of alcohol and succussed to get 1C. One part of the 1C solution is dissolved in ninety-nine parts of alcohol and succussed to get 2C. The process is repeated again and again to get to 30C or 200C and beyond. Example, essential oils from various spices.

3. Trituration, followed by dilution and succussion: Some sub-

stances are neither soluble in water nor in alcohol. For example, vegetable carbon (activated charcoal from carbonized wood). One part of the insoluble medicinal substance is mixed with ninety-nine parts of cane or milk sugar and ground, using a mortar and pestle, into a fine powder to get 1C. This process is repeated further to get 2C and beyond, and the successive grinding renders the insoluble substance soluble in water and alcohol.

If a frequency of energy—for instance electricity, X-ray, or sunlight—or a gas is used for making a remedy, alcohol is exposed to a form of it.

The purity of the raw material is presumed critical, as the entire molecular and submolecularizing process follows from there. For instance, the gold foil used to make *Aurum metallicum* must come from a reliable manufacturer; the same is true for sourcing plant materials for potentized botanicals. If the raw material is impure, its impurities will be potentized too, and a somewhat different remedy will be produced.

Insoluble materials are triturated—ground—manually in a mortar and pestle, or these days in a ball mill while being mixed, for instance in making the centesimal dilution, with ninety-nine times the amount of lactose as the raw material. Hard porcelain cylinders churn the material into a fine powder. Hahnemann Laboratories in San Rafael, California, triturates—continually grinds—dry materials for several hours to yield a 3C triturate used to prepare liquid potencies. The "Preparation" section of their website describes the process for preparing liquid potencies from triturates, soluble substances, and mother tinctures:

We prepare a one to one hundred dilution of the solution and then succuss this new dilution vigorously at each step. Succussion is the forceful pounding of the liquid dilution against a firm but resilient surface in order to fully develop its potential. Current scientific trials show the formation of nano-particle-clouds stabilized by silica from the glass container as a result of the dilution and succussion process. We require that trained lab staff witness the entire procedure to guarantee that each critical step was performed correctly.

At Hahnemann Labs we always prepare the first fifteen potencies in separate vials, which is the Hahnemannian method. We prepare the following potencies on our Potentizer designed by Michael Quinn, which ensures that each succussion is performed with the same number and with the same force of strokes to ensure that every medicine we make is of the highest quality.

The mystery of homeopathic preparation recalls not only quantum physics but divination, as Hahnemann Labs is not only a reliquary of Samuel Hahnemann but also of pharmacist Michael Quinn, whose expertise, craft, and sixth sense were preserved after his premature death in 2019:

> The engineers who built the equipment actually measured Michael Quinn's arm from elbow to closed hand in order to build a mechanical arm of the same length. They measured his movements while vigorously succussing the vial. The data was used to produce the drive system which pounds the mechanical arm against a firm rubber pad. Each potentizer is located in a separate room which is supplied by high purity HEPA filtered air to prevent cross-contamination, and driven by compressed air.[41]

Because exactly how information is put in the microdose is unknown, great care is exercised in replicating procedures and mechanisms that have yielded functioning pills—pills that lead to patient improvement.

This general process of preparation, totally unique to homeopathic pharmacopoeia, ensures that not even one molecule of the original medicinal substance is present in the dilutions—for example, the original medicinal substance is diluted ninety-nine to one over and over; only its healing signature is copied. As a result, even though homeopathic remedies list names like *Lachesis, Tarentula,* and *Belladonna,* they do not contain the harmful and toxic parts of the original potentized substance, only its therapeutic value. When, for example, *Belladonna* is prescribed as a homeopathically prepared remedy, it is able to mirror and then cancel the symptoms of crude *Belladonna,* a poison.

In the physical world, some substances are poisonous, some are nutritious, and some are inactive in the human body. Yet after homeopathic potentization, the majority of these physical properties depart, and new properties occur that are unexplained by biochemistry (even as molecules have emergent properties not evident in the atoms from which they coalesce). *Bufo,* a medicine made by dilution and succession from poison exuded by a toad, is an azoic fluid—molecules of lactose and alcohol containing the healing signature of the animal, not the toxin.

Although there is a rough resemblance between the behavior of a potentized substance and its physical base, the differences are great enough to establish a whole new system of biochemistry—hermetic medicinal chemistry—starting from substances' toxicology in material doses and translating, transducing, or even reversing some aspect of it as subtle vibrations in microdoses. For instance, coffee, consumed in material doses, causes exhilaration, excitement, and sleeplessness. When coffee is diluted, succussed, and potentized to remove the toxicity of the original medicinal substance, it is used to treat sleeplessness with excitement and racing thoughts.

During provings of homeopathic remedies, healthy people bring up symptoms caused by the remedies being proven. Yet trituration, dilution, and succussion ensure that there is *no* material medicinal substance present in the remedies, so the original substance is not itself the cause. Let us then consider: How do the provers bring up symptoms when the original substance is absent? It must be that the remedies carry nonmaterial memory along with the healing signature of the substance. Insofar as the original substance is diluted into non-existence and quickly passes from the picture, if anything remains it must be in the form of a message or specification that has passed to the neutral medium before dilution eliminates its source; information is transferred to the microdose. Perhaps the tincture transfers something like a template of itself or some of its properties to the surrounding solution, much in the way DNA and messenger RNA exchange information in the replication of living cells.

The nonmaterial memory contained in a remedy elicits symptoms just as if the provers were consuming the original medicinal substance. When symptoms similar to those elicited in a remedy's proving are encountered in a sick person, and then based on the Law of Similars a matching remedy is given, the nonmaterial memory of the original medicinal substance abrogates any disease symptoms, while the healing signature conveys a chord of wellness to the vital force.

Whatever their definition or explanation, homeopathic medicines finally cannot be considered drugs: they are parallels, vibrations, spiritual entities, intelligences, messages—blessings, to use Vatsala Sperling's term. Their existence is the best deal in a universe that is often clumsy or violent. If such a significant law of medicine and nature exists, for it to be dismissed or consigned to the dust bin of history is a waste of a principle of energy and congruence as well as a concession to brand monopoly.

The method of preparation of homeopathic remedies was Hahnemann's unique, prescient contribution to quantum physics or, more properly, paraphysics. The procedure may appear chemical, but it is so different from anything in standard science that most chemists do not even deign to investigate its mechanism. It is the best-known process—perhaps the only such process—for removing toxicity from natural substances and turning them into remedies.

If poison nut were the selected tincture for its tendency to produce symptoms in organisms like the symptoms of a disease, then the nut juice would constitute one-millionth of the actual medicine at the third centesimal dilution. By the twelfth centesimal dilution (or twenty-fourth decimal dilution), there is almost certainly no trace of the original substance in most of the medicine—no trace at all! There is no cuttlefish ink in the remedy *Sepia*, no mercury in *Mercury*, no gold in *Aurum*, no dog's milk in *Lac caninum*.

Homeopathy is certainly immaterial when the "pill" is projected psychically instead of physically, as it is by some homeopathic healers! Edward Whitmont tried writing remedies on a piece of paper or simply "thinking" them in lieu of giving an actual potentized microdose (see chapter 7). He explained the paraphysical basis of his prescriptions:

A homeopathic potency once produced lasts indefinitely and can always be perpetuated without any loss in intensity by simply adding new solvent. Nor can psychic induction be quantified or shown to be subject to entropy. Einstein's formula $E = m/c^2$ does not apply, there being no masses, energies or velocities.[42]

No mass, energy, or velocity means no ordinary domain of cause and effect. The process construed by Hahnemann, cutting the dilution at each stage, changes the original material in an unknown way. Whitmont continues:

In terms of our accustomed understanding of biology and physiology, it seems incredible that spasms are relieved by a dose of "no-thingness," an "absence" of something that in its material form would cause spasms. What of the corollary fact that when we further attenuate this "no-thingness" it becomes more intensely effective? How are we to understand that a "non-existent" dose of Spanish fly, a blistering and abortive agent in its material form, does away with the effects of second-degree burns and can even be life-saving and infection- and shock-protective in third-degree burns, and that it exerts this effect not from local application but after ingestion orally? How can we explain that a dematerialized potency of ordinary table salt, a substance we consume daily, regardless of this daily consumption, can alleviate sorrow and grief and their somatic effects as well? Or that *Arnica*, a plant growing on high mountain meadows, protects against the effects of mountaineering accidents and contusions, sprains, concussions, and physical but also emotional shock?[43]

Homeopathy provides a virtually paradigmatic instance of the phenomenon of inner-outer correspondence by nonmaterial conduction, a principle has been recognized and ignored throughout human history. We find similar rubrics in African drumming rituals, Navajo sand-painting ceremonies, Tibetan visualizations and thoughtforms, and various systems of healing by sound, color, prayer, and faith. Japanese Reiki as well as the polarity therapy developed by Randolph Stone in India, radionics, and even some apparently concrete treatments such as hydrotherapy, herbal baths, aromatherapy, and skeletal manipulation elicit the same inexplicable but consistent range of effects. We are looking at something that is real but impalpable. UFOs present humanity with the same dilemma, indicating less interstellar travel than the need for a new physics of dimensionality or a different relationship between mind and matter. Like homeopathic microdoses, UFOs offer a material glimpse of something that is fundamentally immaterial and/or interdimensional. Both manifestations begin in matter somewhere, but convert to energy before their coordinates can be captured and identified. The notion that the microdose paradox is merely extenuated placebo effects is as misguided as the belief that all UFOs are mirages or misidentifications of other objects. In this regard, there is no existential difference between water as a medium and air as a medium, or between the molecular sky and the stellar sky. Neither space's ambient phenomena can be reduced to hardware, nor do the "skies" have an intrinsically objective basis of being. Information transcends classification.

In their 1967 paper "Microdose Paradox: A New Biophysical Concept," G. P. Barnard of Surrey, England, and James H. Stephenson of New York City raised the salient issue:

In Great Britain, the dilution stages extend to 1000 on the centesimal basis, that is, a "dilution" of 10^{-2000}. In the U.S.A., the dilution stages are continued to "dilutions" of $10^{-20,000,000}$. Obviously, any therapeutic practice based on the use of dilutions of these orders of magnitude is manifestly absurd, unless the specific method of preparing these dilutions fortuitously exposes a natural phenomenon of profound biological significance.[44]

To assume that there is any original substance left after homeopathic preparation would be in violation of either Avogadro's law or some other immutable statute of physical chemistry. Avogadro's constant itself is a mainstay of physical science, based on research with gases originally carried out by turn-of-the-nineteenth-century Italian physicist Count Amadeo Avogadro. His statistically based ratio was made public in 1811, but its implications for chemistry and pharmacy were not recognized until a century later when it was named after its discoverer. Avogadro's law states that the number of molecules in a gram molecular weight of a substance is 6.0225×10^{23}. The 6.0225 is not the key; 10^{23} is. For, if a substance is diluted beyond 10^{-24}, with uniform mixing at each stage, there is in all probability nothing left of it in the sample used to prepare the medicine. Each dilution reduces the number of molecules of the substance, which begins at the unimaginably high figure of, roughly, six followed by twenty-three zeros, until by the twenty-fourth decimal dilution (one to nine each time) there should be not a single molecule remaining in any one pill. No doubt, if one or more hung on from irregular mixing, they would be in total jeopardy in the passage from the twenty-fourth to the twenty-fifth decimal. Even at dilutions significantly less than 10^{23}, substances should have difficulty levying any chemical activity. Furthermore, in ranges of 10^{-4}, chemists using advanced analytical techniques find traces of virtually every naturally occurring element in the periodic table (though these "contaminants" are not intentionally introduced or "derived by controlled dilution stages from a saturated solution"[45]). The background impurity level approaches the dilution level of the substance on which the solution is based. What is left of the substrate is less than a molecule of dust. Yet the homeopathic preparation has just begun!

As noted above, this process continues, usually to the thirtieth decimal, but often as far as the one-millionth centesimal, and there is no reason to assume it should stop there. This amount of dilution is beyond comprehension. There is already nothing left at the twelfth centesimal, and yet that substance continues to be diluted, one to a hundred, one to a hundred, one to a hundred, almost a million times more to produce the millionth centesimal. Furthermore, in millesimal scale, substances are serially diluted one part to fifty thousand of neutral medium up into the hundreds of thousands of times. It is less concentrated than dropping a sugar cube in the ocean. A bewildered Abraham Lincoln called it the "medicine of a shadow of a pigeon's wing." A century later, Whitmont put that shadow into the language of microdose physics:

Apparently, what we confront here is not a dilution in the ordinary sense, but another, as yet unknown, dispersion of the substance which while "dematerializing" on the molecular level preserves its specific dynamic characteristics and intensifies its energetic charge.[46]

Each dilution, according to homeopathic theory, *increases* the effective power of the original substance. An informed physician would not think of using the ten-thousandth decimal, let alone the one-millionth centesimal, except in the case of severe or deep-seated illness: healing beyond degree zero or using the spiritual realm to activate the physical realm *physically*. It is no wonder that homeopathy finds little acceptance in mainstream medicine. Even convinced homeopaths have expressed dismay at the bizarre principles of their own pharmacy. It is more like shamanism with masks and chants leading to abreaction. They go on practicing only because they get cures. Journalist James Gorman mused:

> In the end, you are left with a puzzle—experiments of disputed value, anecdotal evidence. The anecdotes are most suggestive. Why, after all, do so many patients and doctors have so many accounts of successful treatment with homeopathic medicines? Are they making the stories up? Are all of the accounts examples of the placebo effect? In fact, it is quite curious that the placebo effect is so maligned: regular physicians scoff at homeopathy, saying it's merely the placebo effect. Proponents of homeopathy insist that the positive results they see cannot be merely the placebo effect.[47]

As noted earlier, the mystery of how homeopathic remedies work is reflected in the conflicting injunctives given to patients with their pills. Some homeopathic doctors believe that certain strong substances can antidote—depotentize or devitalize—a remedy immediately or lessen its curative effects. These relapsing agents include allopathic drugs, recreational drugs (marijuana, cocaine, LSD), megadoses of vitamins, camphor, caffeine, food or drink within fifteen minutes of taking a remedy, electric blankets, and dental drilling. Thus, patients are urged to avoid chocolate, cola, Kahlua, all essential oils, pau d'arco tea, Bengay, Vicks VapoRub, Noxzema, Tiger Balm, or anything of camphory vintage.

Even doctors who believe that all or some of these substances interfere with therapeutic responses to homeopathic medicines set different ranges on the amount or degree necessary for devitalization. In one patient the remedy can be palliated by a single sip of coffee; another's remedy is antidoted by the mere smell of coffee; yet another must drink several cups a day for many months before there is a negative effect. But can tissue made healthier by an original potency be undermined retroactively over nine months later by coffee? Some homeopaths insist this is so—that the positive effects are literally reversed. More homeopaths deny that any common molecular substance can impede or invert a nonmolecular, spiritualized effect once it is triggered.

In response to my query about contradicting belief systems, Jonathan Shore told me, "The remedy is like a new seedling. At first, it is easily uprooted or washed away. Later it develops strong root systems and clings tenaciously to the body's tissues."[48] Another doctor confided that he regularly treated animals with the same success his remedies showed in humans mainly to reassure himself that his cures were not just suggestibility plus placebo. He did not, however, prove that he wasn't using telepathy!

Whitmont itemized some of microdoses' more startling transphysical nanocharacteristics:

It has been found that the medicinal properties of substances in their high potencies are immediately transferred to the walls of containers as well as to any inert substance upon contact. In many instances, particularly in life-threatening situations, the therapeutic effect of the potentized medicine has been observed to occur with a simultaneity that could not well be accounted for by physical absorption. I myself once observed a patient in deep coma subsequent to a stroke return to consciousness within minutes after placing a dose of the thousandth potency of *Opium* under her tongue (opium poisoning induces coma).

This phenomenon strikes me as less like digestive absorption than like an exchange of information or a conveying of a "memory" of specific dynamic characteristics in a field process, analogous to the "morphic resonance fields" that Rupert Sheldrake has described.[49]

It also could be likened to a form of radiation, psi "thoughtographic" projection, Kirlian fields, or wavelengths of light. Elsewhere, Whitmont wrote more speculatively about the relation between potentization of matter and psychosomatic transformation:

As substance is disrupted and made chaotic, vibratory rate and transcendental awareness are raised so as to reach into the realm of implicate archetypal order. We might see this as an analogy to the human processes of maturing and aging and the "potentizing" effects of dissipative, disturbing illness and catastrophic factors that "succuss," shake up, our personal lives. They disorder and break up existing inertial structure, upset and confuse our materially encoded sense of order and existence. If and when we can attentively live through this process, a refinement and differentiation of consciousness, tolerance and emotional wisdom and love can be achieved, one that reaches out toward the "telos," to the individuation goal of one's life.[50]

Insofar as the potentized form of matter, as described by homeopathy, is a unique and stable state, different from gas, liquid, solid, or plasma, it is theoretically possible to potentize any substance or radiation. In actuality, some substances are preferable, for they were in herbal and medicinal use for centuries before homeopathy was formulated. But experimental homeopathy continues to potentize new substances and learn their properties as hermetic medicines. This is done not only in the search for materials with unknown therapeutic qualities, but in response to the adjustment of pharmacy to a world in which both human and environmental chemistry is changing. The credos of esoteric homeopathy posit that, following the Law of Similars, the world will continue to produce—potentize—new forms of illness and simultaneously new medicines to treat them.

This would happen whether a homeopathic science existed or not.

Likewise as homeopathy is practiced in new regions, different local substances become available. For instance, after a disciple of Hahnemann brought homeopathy to India in the middle of the nineteenth century, local provings added panther, tiger, and leopard to the medicine chest. Other homeopathic experimenters have potentized cat hair, tobacco, opium, cocaine, media exposed to radiation or sunlight, HIV, their own sperm, sulfur dioxide, plastics (turning them from polluting microbeads into cleansing nanobeads), vaccines (when obligated to take them), and a wide range of spiders and other insects—in each case following the loose homeopathic rule that a substance that brings about an imbalance or pathology in material form is a potential remedy in potentized form.

Though not specified or prescribed homeopathically by the Law of Similars, microdosed entheogens like LSD and cannabis have become such a popular pharmacy that people use them in place of antidepressants, serotonin reuptake inhibitors, and sedatives for reducing stress and anxiety—at work, on dates, during sex, and approaching death.

Microdose theory goes beyond homeopathy or its algebraic formality. For instance, Edward Bach developed a series of thirty-eight flower remedies from dew collected off plants. Subsequent dew or potentized-water healers have extended his system to encompass a much greater spectrum and variety of remedies, also mixing them for complex effects. For prevention and treatment of COVID-19, Dave Dalton of Delta Gardens in Massachusetts made a flower essence blend of Black Pansy, Chestnut, Botswana Agate, Lungwort, and Tobacco.

Pegasus Products in Southern California offers starlight elixirs. These are formed by the modification of a telescope with silver-coated mirrors, which capture and imprint the energy pattern of each selected star, including perhaps the transmission of thoughts and healings from sentient beings dwelling in the far-off solar systems. These vibrations and patterns are collected in quartz bottles of distilled water placed directly in front of the eyepiece. The telescope's clock drive follows the chosen star as Earth rotates, keeping it centered within the telescope's viewing field. Inert gas devices are used to block any negative thoughtform contamination in the vicinity. This fine-energy mixture is then transferred to a lightproof container, with pure grain alcohol added as a preservative.

Again, conventional physics is overridden by potentization at humongous distances and scales. Freud said that there is no time in the unconscious; in the superconscious, there is no time *or space*.

Ruslana Remennikova, a former developer of pharmaceuticals at a drug company who became a sound healer and activator of double-stranded junk DNA, described an experiment for exchanging information with a pet fish by way of water:

I've had the pleasure of studying with [water and crystal researcher] Veda Austin one on one in a workshop and, on one occasion, was introduced to her team and learned more about their interpretation of the language of water. She tagged the hydroglyphs from her technique as "crystallography molecular photography." They are revolutionary and inspired my path in merging water consciousness with sound healing. A hydroglyph is frozen water symbology that could indicate a single or multiple meanings. Because my method involves the observation of sound on water, my technique incorporates musical presentation that pertains to the 12-stranded DNA as opposed to a placebo (freezing water without intention), imagery, or a visual aid. I also experimented with red dye in several cases but did not find it to influence the form of the crystallization. To build a relationship with water, I began with my goldfish, a watery intimate.

I had a goldfish for a couple of years; it lived in a five-gallon rectangle aquarium next to the window in the kitchen. My name for it was Little Fish. One day, I decided to take a sample of its water and freeze it in a glass petri dish to look at its shape and patterns. Using just enough aquarium water to cover the bottom of the dish, I experimented to find the sweet spot when the bottom layer of water freezes without the entire dish becoming stressed by ice. I was stunned to see the first crystallized form that the water revealed. There were many odd shapes, but one that stood out was a heart. I tried it again the next day and continued to talk to Little Fish. It appeared to be a lumped flower. The following day the imagery was more clear, and I saw two flowers beside each other. This time, I decided to consciously talk to water and asked how it would show a friendship. After repeating the same experiment, the crystallography showed two flowers next to each other.[51]

Somewhere between our projections onto nature and nature's projections back on us, links are generated, whether they represent physical cause and effect or paraphysical attunement. You don't have to believe in Little Fish's communications to accept the possibility of hydroglyphs and molecular intelligence. In the case of homeopathic preparation, the succussion (shaking) of the tincture after each dilution may "hammer" in a message and transfer a molecular signature, and then each successive dilution, with continued succussion, would charge the information, increasing its amplitude and frequency, potency by potency. We end up with tiny, white, chemically neutral sugar balls, but if anything like the above occurs, we also have the vitalized record of a potency. That imprint would contain not the chemical properties of animal, plant, or mineral, but something that precedes their expression and generates those properties, even as the invisible core disease precedes and provokes disease symptomology.

The so-called microdose phenomenon is embedded in known biological systems too. Morphogenetic changes during the development of organisms result from extremely small concentrations of substances. Protein manufacture by RNA transfer takes place from the positions of single amino acids in long, repetitive, palindromic chains. Enzymes in minute amounts also catalyze protein and tissue morphogenesis. Trace minerals such as selenium, germanium, barium, and cadmium have biocatalytic effects in ranges of just a few parts per 10^8. Fluorine to prevent tooth decay is added to public drinking water in amounts of 1 to 10^6. Even medicinal springs do not deliver significantly greater mineral content than this.

Gorman made his own survey of the microdose effect:

Thierry R. Montfort, president of Boiron [the largest homeopathic manufacturer in the world], says, "We still don't know how to explain the mechanism of action." Beverly Rubik, director of the Center for Frontier Sciences at Temple University, which publishes research on homeopathy, acknowledges, "Nobody knows how it works." There is only speculation on the mechanism of action. Dana Ullman . . . suggests that even in the lowest doses, "something remains: the essence of the substance, its resonance, its energy, its pattern." He also mentions a possible interaction with the life force "similar to what the Chinese call chi [qi]." According to Rubik, the homeopathic "signal" may be "informational and electromagnetic in nature."[52]

Ullman described a famous brouhaha around microdoses:

In 1988, an article by respected French immunologist Dr. Jacques Benveniste was published in *Nature* that created a whirlwind of controversy. A study which was replicated 70 times in a total of six laboratories at four different universities showed that microdoses of an antigen diluted 1:10 up to 120 times had a significant effect on white blood cells called basophils. Because basophils are known to increase in number when exposed to an antigen, the research-ers conjectured that homeopathic doses of an antigen would affect basophils.

In a story that is probably familiar to people who follow con-troversies in science, *Nature* editor John Maddox, magician James Randi, and NIH researcher Walter Stewart went to the lab which originated the research at the University of Paris South. Although this lab and others had worked on this research for five years, the *Nature* team felt that they had debunked this original research after their two days of study.

The press never reported on some crucial specifics of this debunking. The research which supposedly debunked Benveniste's work was conducted blind a total of four times. The first time the experiment worked just as the original researchers predicted. This successful experiment was never described or discussed in the press. The next three times, however, the experiment did not show any action of the microdose on the basophils. The press only reported on the three negative outcomes.

When a more stringently controlled trial was recently completed, the press ignored it, with the exception of the *New Scientist* which reported favorably on it. This new experiment was published in the *Journal of the French Academy of Science*. An important, new feature to this experiment was that the researchers first tested the blood samples to make certain that they were sensitive to crude doses of an antigen. Because this experiment was testing allergy hypersensitivity to a specific substance and because not all blood samples will show this sensitivity in regular crude doses, this additional feature to the experiment was essential. As it turned out, 39% of those blood samples which had the sensitivity to crude doses responded to homeopathic doses of an antigen, while 0% of the control group responded.[53]

Randi, a stage magician and professional skeptic, was included on the investigative team to determine whether some form of trickery was at play; he turned the investigation into a travesty with distracting stage-magic tricks and a display of disinterest and exhibitionism.

"We thought it quite probable that there was someone in Benveniste's lab who was playing a trick on him," Maddox said. Randi found no evidence of conscious fraud, however, and Maddox said a more likely source of Benveniste's results was "autosuggestions"—one or more of the researchers seeing what they expected to see or wished to see. Benveniste, replying to the report in the same issue of *Nature*, denounces the behavior and the conclusions of what he calls the "almighty anti-fraud and heterodoxy squad." He notes that neither Randi, Maddox, or Stewart has a background in immunology and claims that this ignorance caused various mistakes and misunderstandings in the investigation. More seriously, he charges that the investigation was more a witch hunt than a sober search for scientific truth. "This was nothing but a real scientific comedy, a parody of an investigation carried out by a magician and a scientific prosecutor working in the purest style of the witches of Salem or of McCarthyist or Soviet ideology," he told the French newspaper *Le Monde*.[54]

Benveniste put this farce in context in an interview on July 27, 1988: "We have always said there was a possibility of an error of methodology and that possibility is still open. I will certainly have these experiments done again. . . . Never, but never . . . let these people get in your lab. Scientists must not be treated like criminals."[55]

For the 1990s editions of this book, Ullman became my clearing-house for innovative paradigms to free homeopaths from their vitalism cul de sac. He wrote:

Quantum physics may help lay the theoretical foundations for how the homeopathic microdoses act. Bell's Theorem, an integral part of quantum physics, holds that things are fundamentally interconnected and inseparable. Various studies have concluded that interconnections exist and that some things can dramatically affect other things, even if only very small changes in one thing take place and even if these things are great distances from each other. Quantum physicists do not precisely know the nature of these interconnections, but some evidence suggests that homeopathy's Law of Similars and its use of infinitesimal doses is additional confirmation of this mysterious but real phenomenon.

The diluted homeopathic medicines may have distinct effects upon the diluent (water) even in extreme high dilutions. What this means and the implications of this on homeopathy is that the dilutions, even beyond Avogadro's number, may not erase the template or the memory of the original drug once it has been registered as present as a particle in a solution. The medicinal substance, in diluted form, may then have a "field effect" upon the solution in which it is being diluted and ultimately have a field effect upon the entire organism who imbibes it.

Macroscopic changes can occur in living organisms when specific key enzymes, hormones, or tissues are activated, even if only slightly activated. Modern chaos theory tends to support this observation. One of the basic assumptions of chaos theory is that minute changes can lead to huge differences.

It is presently recognized that living and non-living things have their own resonance. As science writer K. C. Cole wrote, "Planets and atoms and almost everything in between vibrate at one or more natural frequencies. When something else nudges them periodically at one of those frequencies, resonance results." Cole goes on to say that resonance means to resound, to sound again, or to echo, and the power of resonance is in the pushing or pulling in the same direction that the force is already going. A synchrony of small pushes can add up to create a significant change. A classic example of the force of resonance is witnessed in the phenomenon of soldiers walking in place over a bridge, causing it to collapse. . . .

An article in *Gastroenterology* has suggested that small doses may have a more significant effect than large doses because of a "therapeutic window." Such action is more likely when an organism is in a state of "metastable excitation," a hypersensitive state which is "cocked and ready to go" as soon as a specific stimulus triggers the avalanche effect. The homeopathic Law of Similars may be ultimately the link to finding a substance in nature, which when individually prescribed, can trigger this avalanche effect.

Using small doses of the wrong substance or the right substance at the wrong time creates little or no effect. This is why the incorrect homeopathic medicine doesn't do anything.

What is also interesting about resonance is that resonance is more powerful when there is a little friction—when the force is similar to though not exactly the same as the initial force. The resonance becomes broader, creating something similar to a chord rather than a single note. The relationship of these ideas to healing is that homeopaths find that the most effective homeopathic medicine is one that is the "most similar," not necessarily the "same" as the symptoms the person is experiencing.[56]

This would explain why homeopathy is not allergology or isopathy. It induces a range of harmonics rather than a linear relationship of antibodies and antigens. More than a century earlier, James Tyler Kent recognized the dynamic quality of the relationship between Similars and their potentized specifications:

Vital disorder cannot be turned into order except by something similar in quality to the vital force. It is not similitude in quantity that we want, in weights and measures, but it is similarity in quality, in power, in plane, that must be sought for.

Medicines, therefore, cannot affect the high and interior planes of the physical economy unless they are raised to the plane of similarity in quality. The individual who needs Sulphur in the very highest degrees may take Sulphur sufficient to move his bowels, may rub it upon the skin, may wear it in his stockings, can take Sulphur baths, all without effect upon his disease. In that form the drug is not in correspondence with his sickness, it does not affect him in the same plane in which he is sick, and so it cannot affect the cause and flow from thence to the circumference.[57]

When I asked Theodore Enslin about this phenomenon, he singled out the high potencies, the fully nonmaterial dilutions:

[These] are a division of energy in the sense that the low ones are not. Up to six or seven X, there is a recognizable amount of molecular structure left in the pill. In the high potencies, it's not substance at all; it depends entirely on a release of energy. Energy is divisible, but it's not divisible in the same sense that molecular substance is. These potencies are really quite dangerous. A good physician prescribing can give a high potency and in one dose clear up something that has resisted all kinds of prescribing for years, and it seems miraculous. Anyone handling that had better be pretty competent. I mean, there are things that no good physician would deny, that are not known so far as those things are concerned. Substances that have absolutely no effect in low potencies suddenly have a very high one in the high potencies. And they usually are far more marked mentally than any other way. The one that is the old warhorse of the thing is *Silicea,* which is nothing more than flint. In a low potency you can take flint, you can eat rocks until they make a hole in your stomach, and it will have no medicinal effect whatsoever. But suddenly you get *Silicea* at 30x or higher; you can take it to the CM [the one-hundred-thousandth centesimal], which is the ultimate, and it has a profound mental effect, something that is not present in the lower potencies.[58]

A 1974 publication of the American Institute of Homeopathy put the same microdose effect in quasi-pharmaceutical language:

The homoeo-discipline is concerned with the specific, the individual, the distinctive. In order to achieve that goal, the homoeomedical discipline endeavours to study the reaction of the organism to an incitant and not the action of the drug itself. In doing so it reverses the roles of organism and drug and places emphasis on the vital response. . . .

The point we wish to make is that the homoeo-discipline denies that the drug possesses any power or virtue, but postulates that contact between the drug and the living organism sets in motion an influence. The drug is not injected, digested, assimilated, or transported physically. In and of itself it can do nothing except under the highly specific circumstances: when the properties of sensitivity, irritability, idiosyncrasy are exquisitely developed, the vital reaction—which is a function of the host and not of the agent—takes place.[59]

Not of the agent! What does the U.S. Food and Drug Administration think? Gorman checked it out:

Homeopathic medicines are considered drugs by the F.D.A., but minimally regulated. By law, all new drugs must be tested for safety and efficacy. So far the F.D.A. has chosen not to enforce this provision for homeopathic drugs, because their harmlessness is generally accepted. In 1988 the F.D.A. did issue labeling and packaging guidelines, and defined what homeopathic drugs could be sold over the counter (essentially, those marketed for what are called self-limiting conditions, like the common cold). Although many critics challenge the efficacy of homeopathic remedies, to date the F.D.A has chosen not to give them priority. Daniel L. Michels, director of the Office of Compliance of the F.D.A.'s Center for Drug Evaluation and Research, emphasizes that this hands-off approach "is not to say these products are effective."

Perhaps the most vocal critic of homeopathy is William T. Jarvis, president of the National Council Against Health Fraud, an organization that is death on everything from health food to acupuncture. Jarvis says proponents of homeopathy are either "stupid" or "deliberately fraudulent." Claiming that "the F.D.A. has let the public down" by failing to make homeopathic medicines prove their safety and efficacy as do other drugs, he says, "If we had the money we would sue them." *Consumer Reports* has also called for testing of homeopathic medicines.[60]

Yet they *have* been tested—proven—for centuries, more than can be said for countless psychotropic drugs and other pharmaceuticals that are regularly prescribed without any set notion of where their ostensible medicinal effects come from. Homeopathic microdoses are the survivors of generational trial and error. Nonetheless, under the current reign of cynical skepticism, the zeitgeist can't tell the difference between corporate hocus-pocus and undiscovered principles of nature, presuming instead with scientism that anything not yet revealed must be delusional or fake. In truth, professional skeptics are not philosophically or pragmatically skeptical. They are the true believers, holding to their fundamentalist paradigms despite volumes of contravening evidence. What true skeptics are skeptical of is the notion that all agencies in nature and the universe have been already discovered or at least sighted.

The ostensible success of homeopathic medicine has suggested avenues of research to unconventionally minded biologists and physicists as new models for the activity of succussed microdoses have continued to be explored. In 1996 scientists at American Technologies Group in California found that a previously unknown type of stable crystal was formed when substances diluted in distilled water were shaken or stirred and then rediluted and reshaken. Shaped like lentil beans in flat-disk configurations and aggregating in clusters from 15 nanometers to several microns across, these entities were named I_E crystals (for "ice/electrical field") by physicist Shui-Yin Lo, though they are different from ice in geometrical shape, charge, and density.[61] "What's additionally interesting and initially confusing," said Dr. Lo, "is that the number of ice crystals actually increases as does their biological and chemical effect after each time we dilute and shake the water."[62]

In fact, diluting and shaking increased the amount of crystals in solution from approximately 1 to 2 percent to 10 percent.

The I_E crystals appear to carry some form of information and remain stable even at temperatures above one hundred degrees Celsius, continually breaking apart and reforming by dipole interaction, producing more numerous and larger crystals. To achieve this shearing, fragmenting, and crystallizing effect takes vigorous shaking, something like homeopathic succussion; simple chemical agitation will not accomplish it.

I_E crystals have thus far been used as additives to decrease smog and carbon buildup in engines and improve fuel efficiency. They have also reduced scaling and fouling in ethylene crackers (large plastic-manufacturing furnaces) and other heat-transfer equipment. Some scientists have found that they have a positive biological effect on fungal and bacterial strains—an increase in titers of microorganism-generated enzymes and a decrease in fermentation time.

Lo himself acknowledged the unresolved relationship of these crystals to homeopathic microdoses:

There seems to be something unique in water that undergoes extreme dilution, and we now have the laboratory evidence and even the photographic evidence to verify it. . . . Thus far, we have only systematically tested substances that have been diluted one-to-ten 13 times. Homeopathic doctors sometimes use medicines which are diluted one-to-ten 30, 200, 1,000, or more times, and we have not tested these extreme dilutions yet. However, I would not be surprised if I_E crystals are also observed in these doses. Based on our research to date, every dilution beyond the sixth has found I_E crystals in them.

The homeopaths were definitely onto something, but our discovery of I_E crystals may help their medicines become even more powerful, and these I_E crystals will probably have significant industrial applications, energy transfer benefits, cleansing uses, and ecological protection.[63]

It is as if there is more energy in the microcosm and its nanocosms than in the macrocosm with its cosmoses—string theory deluxe.

Experiments in entangling tiny life forms have shown the potential of converting matter into not only energy but information. In 2021 scientists at the Nanyang Technological University in Singapore quantum-entangled hibernating tardigrades with superconducting qubits. Each frozen tardigrade was placed between two capacitor plates of a superconductor circuit to form a quantum bit or "qubit"—a unit of information. When the sleeping tardigrade contacted Qubit B, it shifted the qubit's resonant frequency. The tardigrade-qubit coupling was then linked to nearby Qubit A. The qubits became entangled, and the frequency of the qubits and tardigrade changed in tandem, making a three-part entangled system.[64]

The laptops and smartphones of the future might be run on circuits of entangled qubits and stem cells. Microtubules, amino acids, proteins, and carbon chains could provide zetta- and yottabyte memory, storing data on singularity clouds in nucleic helices well beyond the capacity of inanimate silicon. If the entire database of the planet could be stored on the holographic hard drive of one stem cell from a tadpole embryo, then a disease epitome can be potentized in a meadow flower. As I wrote in my 2020 book *Bottoming Out the Universe*:

In string theory, entire universes are folded into one another based on their inherent topological structure; dimensions that come into being as degrees of freedom resolve their dynamical tensions, whatever that means under game conditions. Our own landscape arises from the behavior of quark-scale "objects" in spaces now lost to inquiry or passage. By the same rationale of disproportion, the

Big Bang pulled this whole cosmos out of a clown car tinier than a flea.[65]

Iris R. Bell, a psychiatrist and researcher in neuro- and biobehavioral sciences, has spent well over a decade investigating the nanoparticle basis of homeopathic medicines and the interaction of various alternative therapies and treatments with the organism as a complex adaptive system. Considering these two problems together from the standpoint of both high-dilution chemico-physical interactions and human psychosomatic and dynamic behavior systems, she has been working toward a unified model of homeopathic potency.

It may be that microdoses transfer information in a fashion not subject to laboratory analysis, rendering Bell's experiments futile in advance. Physical space may fold like tissue paper as it reaches from our plane to other dimensions until this whole universe of matter becomes a speck in a gigantic map itself reduced to a tinier speck, like the brilliance of clouds in a dell beyond time and space. Star elixirs and Little Fish messages may be the mere beginning of a breakthrough in the relation of mind and matter. In *Bottoming Out the Universe*, I proposed that DNA may have an Etheric state resembling its molecular double helix, and this may translate interdimensionally:

While the geometry of Crick-Watson-brand DNA operates as a self-contained carrier of heredity on the Physical plane, an Etheric twin-helical progenitor (uncannily like the serially twined *ida* and *pingala* nadis of the upper Etheric) propels its expression. In other words, mutually orbiting spirals represent an esoteric geometry through which Causal, Mental, Astral, and Etheric energies materialize into amino-acid-based codons. . . .

The thermodynamic landscape remains under full Darwinian

traction. There is no wiggle room between the two realms—one material, the other meta-material. Seemingly incommensurate systems meet at frequencies of the same energy: physical DNA germinates from Etheric DNA.[66]

Likewise Etheric or Astral energy gets transferred back into biochemical energy through a process discovered accidentally through the ages and systematized by Hahnemann.

It may also be that there is also an unexplored range of specified, physically transferrable nano-effects that transcend chemical and biological data otherwise flooding the environment. Bell explained her premise in the abstract of a paper with Mary Koithan:

The proposed active components of homeopathic remedies are nanoparticles of source substance in water-based colloidal solution, not bulk-form drugs. Nanoparticles have unique biological and physico-chemical properties, including increased catalytic reactivity, protein and DNA adsorption, bioavailability, dose-sparing, electromagnetic, and quantum effects different from bulk-form materials. Trituration and/or liquid succussions during classical remedy preparation create "top-down" nanostructures. Plants can biosynthesize remedy-templated silica nanostructures. Nanoparticles stimulate hormesis, a beneficial low-dose adaptive response. Homeopathic remedies prescribed in low doses spaced intermittently over time act as biological signals that stimulate the organism's allostatic biological stress response network, evoking nonlinear modulatory, self-organizing change. Potential mechanisms include time-dependent sensitization (TDS), a type of adaptive plasticity/metaplasticity involving progressive amplification of host responses, which reverse direction and oscillate at physiological limits. To mobilize hormesis and TDS, the remedy must be appraised as *a salient, but low level, novel threat, stressor, or homeostatic disruption for the whole organism.* Silica nanoparticles adsorb remedy source and amplify effects. Properly-timed remedy dosing elicits disease-primed compensatory reversal in direction of maladaptive dynamics of the allostatic network, thus promoting resilience and recovery from disease.[67]

Activated nanoparticle colloids could lead to a physico-chemical basis for microdose effects, though it is still a long way from there to the discrete premises of repertorizing. That requires complex adaptive systems. One critic accused Bell of "building a skyscraper on flimsy foundation."[68] In a partial defense of her procedure, Bell disputed:

The underlying assumptions are . . . that homeopathic medicines are ordinary, dissolved and diluted bulk-form chemical drugs in true solution that could only act pharmacologically with linear dose–response relationships. However, the trituration and suc-cussion procedures in classical homeopathic remedy prepara-tion may actually be crude manual methods that generate "top down" nanoparticles of source material. Nanoparticles range in size from 1 nanometer (nm) on a side up to 1000 nm or more, though much nanoscience research focuses on special acquired properties of small nanoparticles below 100 nm. Trituration with mortar and pestle is a manual method for mechanical grinding or milling, similar to ball milling used in modern nanotechnol-ogy. Like modern nanotechnology methods of microfluidization, sonication, and vortexing, manual succussions introduce intense turbulence, particle collisions, and shear forces into solution that break off smaller and smaller particles of remedy source material as well as silica from the walls of the glass containers or vials. The combined impact of these mechanical nanosizing procedures would be to modify the properties of the remedy, generating remedy source nanoparticles, as well as silica crystals and amorphous nanoparticles.[69]

Such an effect would also explain how cells in a blastula could transmit information during gastrulation from sources other than chromosomes, confirming speculations of epigenetic embryologists like Erich Blechschmidt and Stuart Pivar. Bell concluded:

> Homeopathic remedies are proposed as source nanoparticles that mobilize hormesis and time-dependent sensitization via non-pharmacological effects on specific biological adaptive and amplification mechanisms. The nanoparticle nature of remedies would distinguish them from conventional bulk drugs in structure, morphology, and functional properties. Outcomes would depend upon the ability of the organism to respond to the remedy as a novel stressor or heterotypic biological threat, initiating reversals of cumulative, cross-adapted biological maladaptations underlying disease in the allostatic stress response network. Systemic resilience would improve. This model provides a foundation for theory-driven research on the role of nanomaterials in living systems, mechanisms of homeopathic remedy actions and translational uses in nanomedicine.[70]

To me, the point is not whether Bell offers a viable explanation for microdose specificity but that a variety of potential experiments across an uncalculated range have been building on her pioneering efforts. She may have set her skyscraper on shaky ground, but she showed that there is *plenty* of such ground. As we have seen, a system like homeopathy cannot in fact work as substance. It gets its validity—its capacity to heal—from its reversal of unspecified mass. I would imagine that a medicine of "nothing"—which is what the American Medical Association (AMA) considers homeopathy—has unique potential in an age flooded with real, false, and artificial information, amped overproduction, vapid data and algorithms, and shelves of quicker-acting palliatives. Homeopathy tells us that a commodity bureaucracy is "nothing" also, and the life it endows is "nothing" as well. It and the other energy medicines replace the "nothing" of vapid informational noise with a dynamic "nothing": the power of uncompensated-for vital force. Homeopathy is allopathy's true enantiodromia—its unconscious opposite. It is also a clue to a nether universe of dark matter and dark energy—a realm shrouded in literal darkness and obscurity. Meanwhile, homeopathy's "dark knowledge" is cloaked in a conspiracy of silence.

Regardless of your beliefs about the natural world, we could certainly use an energy that continues to produce more from less. It might lead to new sustainable technologies beyond wind, solar, tidal, and other cyclical forces. If microdose principle works, then substances in nature contain an unknown, bottomless free energy different from but related to nuclear fusion.

Psychomorphology

Some homeopaths have attempted to establish psychosomatic links between substances and their microdose effects. The pioneer in such attempts, Edward Whitmont, was uniquely qualified by his combined practice of homeopathy and archetypal psychology. Beginning in the 1940s, he wrote a series of speculative articles on various remedies, arguing, in essence, that the underlying vitality that gives rise to the shape or character of the entity from which each remedy is extracted also gives rise to its healing virtue.

Whitmont proposed that pharmacy and psychology are linked on a morphological level encompassing not only Similars but signatures of shape, color, behavior, and animal, plant, or mineral character that cross levels of emergence and scale. When we concretize medicinal virtues in remedies or intuit curative relationships, we are discovering associations that objectively exist in the world of nature. A dynamic totality brings together these events and forms according to their own essential natures. According to Whitmont, "Even as the symbol is the image and expression, in terms of form and appearance, of specific psychic energies, so is the morphological manifestation or appearance of an objective function in nature the expression and image in the world of sense perception of its intrinsic functional dynamism."[71]

The Doctrine of Signatures describes relationships which the Doctrine of Similars miniaturizes and transposes to a submolecular realm. Dog's milk, poison oak, white cedar, and silver are medicines for reasons we may intuitively grasp through qualities expressed in both them and us at different levels of structure in nature. Our link is fractal and cybernetic and because neither their morphology nor our morphology is accidental. The discovery of homeopathic virtues, like the discovery of the DNA helix and the meiosis of cells, is not accidental either, for shapes in nature are organized by the same order and under the same terms as phonemes and syntaxes of languages, synapses of thoughts, and cognition of ideas. Traditional herbal and animal medicines come likewise from a level of psyche that is transpersonal and collective and includes the structure of botanical and animal forms in the same archetypal "meaning" set.

In this vein, Carl Jung wrote:

The assumption that the human psyche possesses layers that lie *below* consciousness is not likely to arouse serious opposition. But that there could just as well be layers lying *above* consciousness seems to be a surmise which borders on a *crimen laesae majestatis humanae.* In my experience the conscious mind can only claim a relatively central position and must put up with the fact that the unconscious psyche transcends and as it were surrounds it on all sides. Unconscious contents connect it backwards with physiological states on the one hand and archetypal data on the other. But it is extended *forward* by intuitions which are conditioned partly by archetypes and partly by subliminal perceptions depending on the relativity of time and space in the unconscious.[72]

To Jung, the objective psyche could transcend space and time and embody the *meaning* of any substance, not just its medicinal virtue. He never translated specific biological morphologies into absolutes, but at his personal suggestion, Whitmont arrived at a possible system of transconscious, transmaterial relationships combining psyche and substance. In Whitmont's cosmology, the potentized medicines embody archetypes that also shape the plants, animals, and minerals—in fact, all of nature. If one can tap the essence of anything, not just its procreative seed or crystal per se but its elemental source, then medicinal action can be liberated on the same plane. Stones, diseases, metals, bacteria, even human symbols are equivalent on this level. The impulse that gives rise to the precise form of an oak tree or an eel, under individualized environmental-embryological blueprints, gives rise under different circumstances to an ulcer, a virus, a style of pottery, a myth, a phobia, and a potency. Whitmont explained the underlying psychosomatic unity:

> It is as though all of our problems, disturbances and complexes also portrayed themselves in some form of explicate earth-substance-imperfection. Implicate order encodes or "explicates" itself in our psyches as complexes: as image, emotion and drive patterns that through their "incarnations" manifest as conditioned deviations from the archetypal "ideal" (father, mother, love, hate, transition, heroic fight, surrender, permeability, etc.). They incarnate likewise in the patterns of biological life energies and in the forms of animal, plant and mineral substances.
>
> These correspondences are not of a linear one-to-one nature,

however. A father crisis, for instance, does not correspond to a particular substance. The patterns are more comprehensive and their connections far from clear to us. A parental problem that activates a crisis in the realm of permeability—when it is a matter of defining one's boundaries, physically or psychologically—may, for instance, correspond to allergic states and to a calcium process. When the resistance of one's "fiber" is in need of restructuring, it may correspond to silicon or pulsatilla, the windflower. It may be "similar" to *hepar sulfuris* (calcium sulfide) when the issue is one of an interplay between imbalanced permeability (calcium) and "fiery" uncontrollable overreaction (sulfur) that expresses itself in inflammatory conditions. A tremendous amount of study and research is still necessary to clarify these areas. We have as yet too little understanding of the qualitative aspects of the substances that structure our world. Until now we have studied only *quantitative* compositions—the chemistry of minerals, plants and animal life— but short of the homeopathic provings, we have never yet systematically concerned ourselves with the qualitative "moods," "personalities" or "souls" (anthropomorphic terms for lack of more adequate ones that would refer to *their* life forces, Qi and "astral"-emotional fields) of the elements of our surroundings—let us say of antimony, silver, the rattlesnake, quartz or a gentian or poison ivy plant—or with the "soul" of our cosmos.[73]

His intuition was that each substance (signature) will naturally reflect some aspect of its healing archetype in its habitat, chemistry, affinities, and growth patterns. Homeopathic remedies are then sublimated from the tinctures of these plants, animals, minerals, and other material and reduced to the archetypal plane—that is, they are dematerialized so that they are in tune with the disease as archetype rather than its symptoms as pathology.

Whitmont called these quanta "psychosomatic wholes" or

"dynamic totalities"; they exist simultaneously in nature and psyche and complementarily in medicine and myth. Some characteristics of a plant, animal, or mineral must persist in the sensations of its constitution and the character of its disease and remedy. In discussing *Sepia*, for instance, Whitmont draws our attention to "the dynamic meaning of the shell-enclosed jelly."[74] This has a symbolic relationship to the alchemical vessel of *prima materia*, which is also the uterus, and the feminine receptacle of the self in both sexes. *Sepia* may then project a healing function for equivalent disorders—emotional, somatic, and psychosomatic. Whitmont continued:

> Even as a half of the cuttlefish's body must remain within the enclosing shell, in spite of all attempts to break loose, so also the temperamental, sexual and emotional tendencies which one would disown cannot simply be cast off; they can only be slowly and gradually transformed by developing a conscious understanding with which to complement the world of instinctive feeling which is woman's primary expression and experience. Wherever the gradual expansion gives way to a violent, protesting attitude, suppression takes the place of gradual transformation and pathology arises. Challenge to and suppression of the quiet, contemplative and receptive feminine qualities, symbolized by the "creative vessel," thus become the keynotes of the *Sepia* pathology.[75]

This is not itself the *Sepia* illness, but it is the underlying psychosomatic song that precedes the onset of pathology. Whitmont cited the irritable, fault-finding, spiteful quality of *Sepia*—the movement from antagonism to gentleness and affection, the oversensitivity, the premature aging. These come from a suppressed unconscious personality that has a concrete somatization simultaneously in a mollusk, a person, and *Sepia*. I described Sankaran's oneiric interpretation earlier in this chapter.

Following Whitmont's model, the *Natrum muriaticum* patient, the one whose disease is "salt," is inconsolable for a reason having to do with failure of basic assimilation of vital energies, and hence disintegration of life forming in the seed.[76] The *Phosphorus* patient is ecstatic but terrified of a coming darkness, speedy but easily exhausted, somehow stunted in growth and anemic.[77] But then *Phosphorus* also contains within it an extreme brightness, a luminescence that is not radioactive but oxidating.

Of the same mineral, anthroposophical chemist Rudolf Hauschka wrote:

> Phosphorus . . . shines and pours out light, but is also a condensing agent. . . . Nerves are built of protein high in phosphorus. Indeed, the nervous system as a whole is as clear a revelation of the phosphorus process as the circulatory system is of the aluminum process. Phosphorus flames give light, but are cold. Our nervous system endows us with the cool, clear light of consciousness; but it is also the transmitting agent for the formative impulses that shape the body's plastic organs. . . .
>
> The phosphorus process co-operates on the one hand with the silica in our skin, on the other with lime in our bony structure. The skin contains innumerable nerve-endings, which convey impressions of the world around us. Though silica creates skin surfaces, it is the phosphorus process that gives them surface sensitivity. It is to phosphorus that we owe awareness of our bodies and a bodily consciousness of selfhood. The skin, with its nerve inclusions, thus forms a boundary between world and individual.[78]

Diseases treated with homeopathic *Phosphorus* include ones of the nervous system, especially those with left-sided symptoms, which suggest the unconscious hemisphere of the bicameral brain; gastrointestinal irritations, including lightheadedness and desire for cold water that is then vomited; liver cirrhosis; diabetes; and general tubercular conditions.

The person suffering from *Phosphorus* is nauseated by the fragrance of flowers when too strong; this person is extremely jumpy, sensitive to touch, and disturbed by thunderstorms' phosphoric energy.

With *Lycopodium*, Whitmont focused on its habits as a creeping moss whose spores "do not moisten as they repel water. . . . They are extremely hard but burn with a very bright flash when ignited. . . . The spores germinate only after 6–7 years."[79] *Lycopodium* patients have high nervous tension; they are developed mentally but with a weak body. They crave open air and loosen tight clothing; they are dry, constipative, and noneliminative, with kidney and urinary symptoms. Their diseases progress slowly and inwardly, with a tendency toward cancerous growth. They are bloated and do not digest well; they have bad circulation and lack inner heat. This symptomology is locked in the club moss spore until its archetype is realized in a disease and its potentized substance is used as a remedy.

Whitmont emphasized, together, the physical manifestation of each substance, its makeup as a plant or animal or mineral, and its meaning in human symbolism and myth. For instance, with *Lachesis*, snake poison, he noted the serpent as the dark, underground function, the figure which, in Gnostic tradition, replaces Christ on the cross: "The serpent pathology is the unintegrated life impulse, the unintegrated libido, the unintegrated instinct split off and split in itself. . . . *Lachesis* is the penalty of unlived life."[80] Thus the *Lachesis* patient is egotistic, vicious, sexually repressive of others, and mean, all in frustration for the actual self not lived. *Lachesis* has intense pain everywhere, cramps, pressure, sensitivity, swollen gums and toothaches, and extreme excitability with irritation and disease in the sexual organs, especially the ovaries.

The *Sulphur* personality, in alchemy a crude earthy ferment that

can be transformed into spirit and gold, is characterized by skin eruptions, general congestion, and stagnation and contains raw uncom-
plicated psora, with a tendency to dirtiness, distraction, unfocused
genius, and mental brilliance with disregard for personal being.[81]

Psychosymbolic Transference

A homeopathic doctor and patient participate in a drama of amulets
(crystallized essences), grails, and narrative mythologies resembling a
Navaho sand-painting rite or Aboriginal Aranda cave initiation. One
physician concluded a diagnosis with the following assessment:

> Gold is an interesting thing in the history of man. It has been
> hoarded as wealth. People have worn it as jewelry and struggled
> for possession of it. It is associated with the sun. It is found often
> in quartz, and near the surface of the ground. Pans in rivers trap
> gold particles. It is purple in the colloidal state and used for stain-
> ing glass in cathedrals. Gold anchors the value of money systems.
> Without the anchor, value disintegrates. *You* have a disease called
> *Aurum,* gold. I will give you its medicine.[82]

These archetypal references link human, mineral, and nature in
an act of shamanic transference—a convergence of doctor, remedy,
substance, symbol, and vital force.

Modes of shamanic transference resemble potentization in terms
of both abreaction from masks, chants, altars, and empowered images
and "interaction among psychological, biological, spiritual, and external factors in spontaneous healing."[83] Explanations of informational
specification and transduction are as varied and nonlinear as those
offered for Hahnemannian nanodoses. For instance, masks used by
shamans for healing in societies as widely separate as the Iroquois in
the Northeastern Woodlands, who call them (in English translation)

False Face masks, and the Balinese of Indonesia, who call them Rangda (Demon Queen) masks and assign their production from pule trees to consecrated carvers. These carvers are said to induce spirits from living trees: masks are cut directly in the live tree and removed, decorated, and personified only after the tree's spirit has entered, or successed, into them.[84]

The Mouse Woman of Gabriola, a petroglyph cut at an unknown time into a natural stone stele in Nanaimo on Vancouver Island, British Columbia, has "large ears, whiskers, breasts, and possibly a tail." It has one hand raised and stands at the entrance of a grove. People pressing ailing parts of their bodies against the simple, crude image have felt heat and then experienced dramatic improvements of serious bone, muscle, and skin ailments.[85] Whether this is psychosymbolic telepathy or telekinesis (or both), it represents instantaneous field states that move from universal unity—innate interdependence—to individual points of transformation. Chaos fields similar to those that organize cyclonic spots on Jupiter and Saturn may bring informational sets into correspondence with one another.

4

Homeopathy and Modern Medicine

Disease Definitions and Cures

This chapter attempts to square multiple paradoxes and contradictions from earlier versions of this book as well as progressive levels of my own understanding of homeopathy. Some of my prior work presented undeclared thought experiments and hyperboles regarding the relationship between homeopathy and allopathy. I have adapted these, modifying and contextualizing them. I haven't cut them because their genesis underlies this book, and modernity is itself a living paradox in which we each participate, rectifying its contradictions sometimes hourly. It should be no surprise that homeopathy introduces a "wicked paradox" at more than one level. Health and medicine are an existential as well as a practical search for well-being and meaning with no absolute endpoint, only an evolution of truth mysteries.

Homeopathy differs from mainstream medicine at the most rudimentary level of operational definition, retaining the Hippocratic tenet that the disease itself is unknowable. That doesn't mean that we can't see pathologies; it means that signs of disease processes—their effects on organs and functions—are not the actual diseases.

Doctors can alleviate and, in many cases, remit these effects, but the core malady remains and will seek another expression.

So much for the armada of memes that modern medicine took more or less intact from the rationalists without reexamination. Modern anatomy is more sophisticated, but it has been put into the same prefabricated boxes.

According to homeopathic definition, the diagnoses and diseases of standard medicine are classes of pathology representing weaknesses in defense mechanisms of organisms. Core diseases arise *only* individually and can neither be put into general classes nor cured according to modes assigned to classes. If the life essence—what sustains a living entity and keeps it healthy and self-healing—is transcendental and holistic, then the conditions that degrade it are likewise too subtle and "spiritual" for physicians to perceive. Dissections, even vivisections, show only cellular and molecular expressions in tissues.

To put the matter in ontological perspective, if medical biologists could track disease chains to sources, they would also be able to create life in a test tube. You can no more see a disease than you can see a life force. You can find DNA's twin helix by triturating amino acids, immunoblotting proteins, and applying crystallography and win a Nobel Prize, but that is not the same as seeing life or a vital force.

The pathological force operates in the same range. Its expressions leading to maladies and syndromes are, in essence, vibrations of the healing energy that have been mistuned. We are viewing not sicknesses but symptomatic discordances: health trying to reassert itself by healing crises.

Everything I say henceforth in this chapter should be taken in this context. Hahnemann was seeking a song that plays throughout the universe. That is homeopathy's strength and also its limitation: its laboratories are more like orchestras than mills. Homeopathy can change people's vibrations, but it cannot make drywall, WiFi, or prostheses. Keep that in mind as you read, for civilization is not a given;

it is how we are presently convening on Earth. Humans have smelted televisions and jets out of minerals, but they have not changed the baseline vibration of life and matter.

By homeopathic theory, pathologies oscillate simultaneously on three planes: physical, emotional, and spiritual. From there, they take distinct forms according unique predispositions—constitutions, ancestral lineages, lifestyles, metabolisms—of individuals. Those predispositions give rise to a diversity of ailments, some resembling each other in different individuals, but none of them are *the disease*. You can conceptualize health and illness in different ways to understand how homeopathy might work, but they will always be metaphors for a three-billion-year-old nonlinear process on Sol 3, a process that is interpolating levels of organization as it integrates and deepens in its expressions.

In the transfer of a disease from a material to a psychosomatic plane, the new inflammation tends to occur at roughly the same level or a slightly worse—more mental and deeper—one, but it can never improve. The defense mechanism and vital force of each individual determine whether the disease will spread on the same plane or be passed to a more interior one. Either way, that's the "QR code" that a successful homeopathic constitutional remedy must mirror and activate.

A digestive ailment may appear to vanish without a trace, but the patient is suddenly restless. A conventional doctor would consider the two unrelated; the homeopath looks for a constitutional link—for instance, that the disease came closer to the organismic core; it jumped to the emotional level and expressed itself as anxiety. The patient felt worse because he experienced the disorder globally even though the digestive malaise cleared up.

Years ago, a homeopath told me about treating a patient who had been chronically ill before joining a satanic religious sect. Soon after taking a remedy, she lost interest in religion and developed multiple sclerosis. It was as if the ailment moved to a new corresponding point on the physical plane, protecting the mental domain. Whether this constitutes an authentic causation or is a syllogistic placeholder for a dynamic process too deep to interpolate is almost irrelevant in terms of diagnostic and medical procedure.

Homeopathic treatments can't fit into statistical models or double-blind experiments. Fifty cases of fever cannot be given *Ferrum phosphoricum* or *Aconite* to see if the microdoses have a biomedical effect. Each case of fever has to be particularized individually and the remedy chosen based on the Law of Similars. One case of fever might get *Belladonna*, another *Aconite*, and another a remedy not usually prescribed for fever. So, what is the double-blind target and what is the arrow?

In his *Lectures on Homoeopathic Philosophy*, published in 1900, American homeopath James Tyler Kent put the matter axiomatically:

> Causes exist in such subtle form that they cannot be seen by the eye. There is no disease that exists of which the cause is known to man by the eye or by the microscope. Causes are infinitely too fine to be observed by any instrument of precision. They are so imma-terial that they correspond to and operate upon the interior nature of man, and they are ultimated in the body in the form of tissue changes that are recognized by the eye.[1]

"Ultimated" is no longer a commonly used verb, but it is an ideal descriptor for latent disease complexes. Tissue changes are the visible result of vital healing (or diseases) on an inner plane. The change may not show up in labwork or a CT scan or MRI. If it does, it won't be identified with the energetic effect of a microdose (or with an osteopathic palpation or acupuncture needle). Yet disappearing goiters, abscesses, and sores, mended broken bones, and healed guts have been documented soon after homeopathic treatment, though homeopaths rarely get credit for the improvements. This is a dilemma at the core of modern medical theory and reifies the gap between materialistic and energy medicines. There is no simple way to bridge the gap either; the systems must, at best, operate in concert, producing or failing to produce cures in individual circumstances with only cover stories for epistemologies.

Homeopathic Homeostasis

In homeopathic biodynamics, the organism is presumed to generate the best possible (i.e., least destructive) response to a disturbance in its vital field—that aspect of life forms that osteopath John Upledger nicknamed "your inner physician," meaning "your internal embryogenic gyroscope." The organism's response to a disease may at times be symptomatic, but it will always be the best defense it can muster under the circumstances. Tissue dysfunction or deterioration, even pain, is a system-wide recognition of the presence of a pathology and an optimal attempt to reestablish homeostasis with the least damage to vital organs. Fevers, coughs, inflammations, and even ulcers are seen as positive responses, preventing more serious ailments from arising and lodging. They are beneficial except when they begin to cause their own irreversible tissue damage.

If the best possible response is frustrated by systemic weakness or palliative treatments, then the organism will find the next best possible response—that is, an optimal integration in the new situation. Although a curtailment of symptoms would be considered "cure" in allopathic terms, homeopathically it is often viewed as a suppression of the vital force and its homeostatic response. Breaking the inner physician's homeostasis (or "gyroscope") is what leads to chronic illness. The difference between the best possible response and the second best (or between any two sequential responses) may be the difference between an eventual cure and lifelong relapses. A pathology is the patient's ally, not the enemy.

As a disease expression spreads, it tends (by homeopathic interpretation) to change in the following manner: exterior organs improve, internal organs are affected in their place; symptoms move from the periphery of the body, for instance the fingertips and toes or skin, toward the center of the body, notably the heart and nerves; symptoms also move upward toward the head; life-sustaining systems (liver, heart, brain) are attacked last in the process; the acute becomes chronic, with more severe and new acute phases; temporary alteration of function becomes permanent alteration of structure; and pathology moves from the physical plane to the emotional plane to the mental plane, its ultimate expression being insanity and loss of reason.

In instances of the correct remedy, a healing aggravation will be followed by swift and deep cure that works its way back out, symptom by symptom, from the invisible to the visible, as described by Edward Whitmont:

No matter what the nature of the disturbance and the point of its appearance, it "wanders" through the whole organism from periphery to center, from less vital to more vital organs. A cure also operates in total-body fashion, but conversely, dissolving pathology in the opposite direction—from within outward, from the center to the periphery, from the more to the less vital parts. Demonstrating the non-local character of illness as well as the locus of healing, the cure moves also in the time dimension, reevoking and subsequently abolishing symptoms and disorders in the reverse order in which the purportedly "separate" and "unconnected" disturbances originally occurred. The cure moves backward along the time scale, even over a whole life span. Former, less serious conditions that are thereby shown to have been earlier manifestations of the same, seemingly different disorder may temporarily return, only to be abolished automatically as the cure proceeds.[2]

This is the homeostasis by which a disease is actually a healing crisis and the first stage of self-cure.

A homeopathic sequence indicating improvement might be a heart attack followed by mild pneumonia (as the disease releases its hold on the heart and diffuses into the lungs), then rheumatic arthritis as it is dispersed to the joints. Its ultimate stage might be a return of childhood eczema. If the original condition was severe, the inflammation may remain in mild chronic form for the patient's lifetime, a weakness grafted permanently onto the system. Still, dermatitis is less debilitating than the same expression in the lungs or heart.

Conversely, homeopaths have compiled retrograde sequences from personal and collective historical observation: for instance, first herpes on the lips, then canker sores in the mouth, then canker sores deeper in the digestive tract, then duodenal ulcers, then colitis; or first a urinary infection, then a kidney infection, then cystitis, then nephritis, finally kidney failure. A gallbladder surgically removed drives its pathological expression inward into depression. A skin disease is converted into a kidney disease, then a phobia, though the dermatologist is exonerated. The skin disease *was* depression.

Ullman stated the principles of the homeopathic approach in contemporary language:

Hans Selye, the father of modern stress theory, asserted, "Disease is not mere surrender to attack, but also the fight for health; unless there is a fight, there is no disease. Disease is not just suffering, but a fight to maintain the homeostatic balance of our tissues." . . .

Different stresses upon a system cause it to adapt to that stress. An organism responds in at least two ways to a stress: it has general adaptive capabilities, and it also has the creative tendency to transcend previous defenses and develop new and potentially more effective means of reducing the pathogenicity of a stress. The system seeks to create a new level of order through fluctuation. "Order through fluctuation" is a common description in physics of how systems adapt to change, and yet, few scientists or physicians have considered that the body creates symptoms as a way that the organism seeks to create a new level of dynamic homeostasis.

From this perspective, therefore, a symptom does not necessarily represent the organism's collapse due to a stress or infection. Rather, a symptom is an adaptive reaction of the organism that represents the best possible response the organism can make based upon its present resources. It is, for instance, widely recognized that a cough is the body's efforts to clear the bronchials, that inflammation is the body's effort to wall off and burn out invading foreign bodies, that fever is the body's way to create an internal heated environment which is less conducive to bacterial or viral growth, and that the symptoms of a common cold are a response to viral infection, with the nasal discharge as the body's efforts to flush out dead viruses and dead white blood cells. Such are the body's impressive self-organizing, self-regulating, self-healing efforts.

With this understanding, the homeopathic Law of Similars is completely logical. Instead of suppressing symptoms, which then inhibits the organism's inherent defensive reaction, a homeopathic medicine is prescribed for its ability to mimic the symptoms of the sick person.

Just as the best way to control the skid of a car is to steer into the skid, perhaps the best way to heal ourselves of disease is to steer our body's own defenses into, rather than away from or against, symptoms. By aiding the body's efforts to adapt to stress or infection, the organism is best able to heal itself. Stewart Brand's description of homeopathy as "medical aikido" is thus perfectly apt.[3]

The Homeopathic Distinction between Diseases and Symptoms

What the allopathic physician might consider a relapse, the homeopath welcomes as the reversal of iatrogenic suppression according to the therapeutic law that older pathologies recur in reverse order when present ailments are cured. If, after allopathic treatment, a person with kidney disease has less albumin in his urine, the assumption is that the kidneys are working better. If the patient feels worse, the doctor attributes that to a side effect of the disease or a matter for a different specialist.

Suppressed renal disease may be followed by greater discomfort, and a real cure will require, on some level, a brief, superficial return of prior kidney symptoms. This hierarchy was set down by Hahnemann in 1810 in the *Organon,* his textbook of homeopathy:

> All diseases are, in fact, diseases of the whole organism: No external malady . . . can arise, persist, or even grow worse without . . . the cooperation of the whole organism, which must consequently be in a diseased state. It could not make its appearance at all without the consent of the whole of the rest of the health, and without the participation of the rest of the living whole (of the vital force that pervades all other sensitive and irritable parts of the organism); indeed, it is impossible to conceive its production without the instrumentality of the whole (deranged) life, so intimately are all parts of the organism connected together to form an invisible whole in sensations and functions.[4]

At the time that Hahnemann wrote this, holism (an understanding of the universe and nature as consisting of interacting wholes rather than a sum of parts) could still be assumed and used as a basis for diagnosis and treatment. Nowadays holism has to be renegotiated and, in a sense, re-staged every time it is cited. Hahnemann's statement sounds radical only because medical and scientific thought has gone in an algorithmic rather than a holistic direction.

Theodore Enslin told me about a man who went to a homeopath in Philadelphia and, as he was leaving, turned and asked, "'Uh doctor, I notice you only gave me one medicine. Now is this for my feet, for my teeth, for my eyes—' and oh, about a dozen other things—and the doctor looked at him and said, 'Your name is Miller, isn't it? That medicine is for Mr. Miller.'"[5]

Symptomatic intervention rather than activation frustrates the organism's innate holistic healing response. That is why palliative care for chronic and psychological diseases tends to make their chronic states worse as well as more systemically trenchant. If the visible pathology is not the real disease and its alleviation is countertherapeutic, then mainstream medicine is involved in a series of superficial palliations leading to more serious ailments. Doctors merely displace symptoms to subtler planes and less optimum channels of expression, each of which they (and, of course, their administrators and insurance companies) consider a separate event—or claim—because of its location in a new organ of the body. Each time a disease is cut off from its preferred mode of expression, it is driven deeper into the constitution. Rationalist medicine with its disease categories and cures is a wild goose chase for imperceptible geese. To extend the metaphor, I might note that the geese are flying in formation with their own extrasensory or telepathic gyroscope.

Allopaths don't think that way. They don't believe in constitutional cores or a supranormal vital force with vibrational expressions. Each symptom complex is seen as a new ailment—separate entropic effects of genetics, toxic exposure, or chance (Murphy's law). If homeopaths want to claim they can cure something more profound, mainstream medicine leaves them with the burden of proof that something more profound exists.

Standard medicine, in addressing perceptible pathology, must, by homeopathic logic, *always* force disease deeper because it continually deprives the organism of its best defense. A worse pathology invariably replaces a suppressed one. The older one may have been "cured" allopathically, but only because the organism's defense response has retreated to a stasis imposed by palliative drugs. While suppressed symptoms lead to new pathologies, the core disease never gets resolved; removing its better outlets drives it deeper into the organism. Since allopathy doesn't recognize disease transposition, the doctor declares a cure when a symptom is eased or dispelled.

Allopathic alleviation is temporary and peripheral. Suppressing symptoms may hinder the disease's advance but also stifles the dynamic function of organs without provoking an immune response. The most significant and lasting effect of an allopathic pharmaceutical may turn out to be its *side* effect, which is not only chronically suppressive and aggravating but expensive (in part because of the need for regular refills). Allopathic patients are encouraged to become pharmacy-dependent. Symptomatic medicine is so widely accepted that people no longer know what true health is. They don't blame the medicines, they blame themselves, conceding inherited or acquired defects requiring continual fixes. Economic interests have locked in their own unexamined medical paradigms.

Take for instance the following hypothetical sequence: A sick person goes to an allopathic doctor. His disease is treated, and he is considered cured.

The next time he is sick, he goes, perhaps unaware of the difference, to a homeopath, who views the new illness as primarily the suppression of the earlier disease. Homeopathic therapeutics require a return of that disease, which was ostensibly cured, its treatment paid for or covered by insurance.

Homeopathy condemns allopathic treatments and drugs as palliatives while claiming that they almost always make their patients sicker even if they provide a temporary relief. If they prolong life, they do so at a weaker vibration, leading to vitiated societies populated by people who never feel quite healthy, in balance, or fulfilled. By homeopathic standards, the patient is a victim of poor medical treatment. By allopathic standards, the patient was cured and came down with an adventitious new ailment. If he should return to the allopath, he would be told there is no such thing as a constitutional disease and that the two physical ailments he has contracted are different diseases. If an intervening homeopathic treatment caused a "relapse," the AMA-approved doctor will try to alleviate it—suppress it—again. If the patient should return to the homeopath after that, the homeopathic doctor, believing that shifting symptoms of an underlying vibration are part of the healing process, will prescribe another aggravation. On this carousel of double binds, a choice must be made. The allopathic establishment made that choice more than a century ago collectively for the public. I am not saying that it was the "wrong" choice; it wasn't. I am saying that it was the nonhomeopathic, nonhomeostatic choice. Complementary medicine provides a way to straddle the horses and ride both as far as they will cooperate with each other.

Conversely, a loyal patient of a homeopath might consider her rash to be a minor annoyance, even restorative, after having experienced the same disease in her heart. If her angina were suppressed allopathically, it might lead to suicidal ideation.

Seventy years ago, James Tyler Kent warned that if we continue to treat skin disease palliatively, the human race would cease to exist. This is a colossal exaggeration by usual standards. But homeopathy considers the skin—the ectodermal membrane contiguous with the brain and nervous system—a drainer of poisons and the first line of defense against diseases taking deeper root. If the outer layer erupts in sores, rashes, or malignancies, it protects the organism. Hence, skin diseases are never trivial and should not be excised dermatologically.

I considered pathological suppression in the case of my mother's older brother in 2001. After a pacemaker was installed in his chest and he was prescribed a daily regimen of pharmaceuticals—a reasonable allopathic course of treatment—my uncle jumped off his balcony to his death shortly after returning from the hospital. There were contributing factors—my mother's similar suicide sixteen years earlier, the attacks of 9/11 a few days before—but in a holistic world all causes combine in an interrelated field, which is perturbed by medical treatments as well as by world events. The greater external environment may not be controllable—it usually isn't—but the heart's response to it is subject to either suppression and enervation or tonic and rejuvenation. That courage and love are associated with vibrations of heart tissue is a homeopathic as well as a neurological and ayurvedic intuition.

In my uncle's case, heart disease may have turned suicidal, or, more properly, angina and suicide may have been aspects of a single wave aberration. In his own era, Hahnemann offered the example of suppressed syphilis. First the external chancre is removed palliatively, and the physician is satisfied, but the disease is deprived of its outlet. It may fester at the same level for several years, but eventually it will lodge more deeply, damaging the nervous system or the brain. In the first appendix of this book I have provided a case study of my daughter's childhood eye disease because it played a central role in my homeopathic education and brought into play implicit strain patterns in the conflict between homeopathy and allopathy.

Sane Asylums

Biochemists and psychiatrists these days conflate pharmacologies with moods and behaviors in ever shorter loops. Every antianxiety pill or antidepressant drug is a variation on a GABA-serotonin theme in an attempt to enhance or suppress neurotransmitter activity, bypassing homeostasis and cellular intelligence. Pharmaceutical companies throw broad-spectrum drugs at pigeon holes in a manner unchanged since the 1940s and 1950s, when my mother's doctor, William Hitzig, prescribed her a palette of opiates and other sleeping pills, all of which augmented, leaving her with acute insomnia.

During the Middle Ages, the depressed and insane were considered in disfavor of God, who was punishing them for their sins. In the words of literary author and lifelong sufferer Andrew Solomon, "The melancholic's despair suggested that he was not suffused with joy at the certain knowledge of God's divine love and mercy. Melancholia was, in this view, a turning away from all that was holy. Furthermore, deep depression was often evidence of possession; a miserable fool contained within himself a devil."[6]

A devil in the brain was desecrating the beauty and joy of God's creation.

The current spectrum of drug cocktails and digital illusions is even more medieval and melancholic. People were once taught how to make sacred boundaries and protect themselves from both physical and transpersonal energies. Churches may have persecuted witches and magicians from backward views of spirits and satanic energies, but they did confer a sense of transdimensional energy. No psychic roses, holy water, or golden suns are carried on the streets of Materialism. Pedestrians stroll into psychiatric and psychic buzzsaws and come away with invisible wounds and traumas. Demonic vibrations and crises of possession are ignored.

Author Solomon wondered if it was even accurate to view madness as a consistent "externally ordered sequence."[7] The truth, he concluded, is that "the individuality of every person's struggle is unbreachable. . . . [It] retains an unquenchable aura of mystery. It is new every time."[8]

New every time is the homeopathic motto. Yet the depressed, schizophrenic, bipolar, phobic, and uncategorizably insane are housed together, crowded into a single institutional category and hell realm that would appall even the Pope. There they act in ensemble, affirming and triggering one another's terror. They are effectively in prison, for they cannot leave. They scream, flee paranoid visitations, and weep and fart without restraint. They try to mutilate their own bodies with any sharp or hot thing because physical pain is a welcome distraction from mental pain. They try to kill themselves, so they end up in padded cells or suspended in nets. There is no exit from spaces more suggestive of Philip K. Dick's dystopias than the rococo realms of Dante's *Inferno* or demonology of Hieronymus Bosch.

In his 1961 book *Madness and Civilization*, philosopher Michel Foucault described a pendulum in the Western world: it oscillates between trying to establish a dialogue with madness and trying to punish or disgorge it. Freud and Maslow had had their shot; now the gendarmes were back, and they intended to burn, poison, and exorcise with a vengeance.[9]

But if that was the game, a real exorcist would have been better trained and more proficient. Homeopathic potencies weren't even considered. Jerry Kantor has written extensively on the success of Hahnemannian "sane asylums" during the late nineteenth and early twentieth centuries in lieu of the much faster-growing "insane" brand. For using microdoses of Similars to treat mental diseases, he singled out New York's Middletown State Homeopathic Hospital and Philadelphia's Hahnemann Medical College. He also described a nineteenth-century network of homeopathic drugstores and standard pharmacies with homeopathic options, including Chicago's Corneau-Diller Drug Store patronized regularly by Abraham Lincoln and his wife Mary Todd Lincoln (for her migraines and insomnia)—hence the president's one-liner about a "shadow of a pigeon's wing," decades ahead of general recognition of homeopathy's phantom pharmacy.[10]

The Crisis of Modernity

You don't have to believe in homeopathy to see a profound medical crisis. As one of my own allopathic doctors remarked, "We are in a new dark age of medicine." Another told me, "They couldn't have more effectively destroyed the medical system if they had tried." These were scientistic loyalists, yet people at all levels of medicine are alienated and frightened by a machinery that dwarfs or trivializes their humanity, while taking the power of health and well-being out of their hands, either as physicians or as patients.

My Amherst College class, full of doctors and medical research-ers, debated this matter in an alumni class forum running during a period from mid-2022 into 2023. Ophthalmologist Richard Klein, an informed advocate of mainstream medicine, nonetheless gave this explanation of the current "doctor's dilemma" within the new medi-cal megastructure in response to a classmate's query about insurance company ethics:

It's getting more complex than your description of provid-ers vs. patients vs. employees. First, "providers" (in terms of who's in charge) are no longer the traditional providers of our youth—physicians and nurses and PTs, etc.—but rather Hospital Conglomerates, Private Equity firms, and Insurance Companies that own most of what used to be traditional providers' business. The traditional providers are now replaceable widgets in a huge system. The entire health care system has devolved into one whose sole purpose according to the owner/providers is market share and profit. Patients are the pawns in the system, and traditional provid-ers are rapidly becoming the same. Here's one sad example of how patient welfare took a backseat to profit/marketability in a large hospital system I know well: The hospital's bioethics committee spent hundreds of hours developing a bioethics manual which set

standards for the hospital system. Before publication, the bioethics manual had to be approved by the hospital system's marketing
department (!). They blocked its publication, and instead published
a slick manual about how the hospital was a "center of excellence."
So, physicians and bioethicists were trumped by a gung-ho MBA.
It was basically a "fuck you" to the traditional providers and to the
patients.[11]

This is not just a feature of the medical world; it is a result of
continuous stratification, consolidation, restratification, and recon-
solidation at higher levels of organization into structural hierarchies
similar to the process that anthropologists describe as elevating homi-
nids from bands to tribes to chiefdoms to states. Here, though, it is
transnational corporate consolidation under a capitalization so deca-
dent that it would have shocked even Karl Marx.

Our classmate Sid Schwab, a successful surgeon, voiced similar
dismay over the decline of his branch of the profession since his grad-
uation from medical school:

When I first went into practice, my future partner asked me how
many operations I'd want to do per week to feel fulfilled. Having
just been chief resident on the trauma service of one of the U.S.'s
premier trauma centers, where I'd done at least fifteen per week, I
said, I don't know—ten? You'll kill yourself doing that many, he
replied. Six a week is perfect: decent income, enough time to enjoy
life.

That was when docs could bill whatever they wanted, payers
paid, say, 80 percent, and docs could "balance bill" patients for
the difference. I won't argue fees were reasonable back then, but it
wasn't long before one could bill whatever they wanted but payers
paid what *they* wanted and you couldn't bill for the difference. And
"what they wanted" was around one-third of the so-called fees.

By the end of my career, before I burned out, I was doing fifteen to twenty operations per week and barely maintaining income in the face of nearly yearly cuts. For the most part, the same applies to hospital bills, which is why so many have folded.

I don't know how much a surgeon ought to make compared, say, to a baseball player or, for that matter, an internist or an NYU professor. But I do know that for decades the only attempts at cost control have been to cut reimbursement to "providers" (love that term, just as I love "clients" replacing "patients") and there's only so much blood in that turnip. I burned out from a combination of overwork and what was probably an overly acute sense of commitment to my patients and to keep providing the kind of high-quality, cost-sensitive care I always did, despite it being entirely unrecognized and unappreciated by payers, whose criteria for having docs on their "panel of providers" was accepting their latest cut to reimbursement.

Rewarding quality care is an ideal which is, I think, too complicated to be meaningful.[12]

The same basic point was made in a different way by a friend undergoing regular chemo treatment for an aggressive cancer. When told that they would skip weekends, he asked, "Do the cancer cells know when it's the weekend?"

There is a reason why traditional First Nations medicine people didn't accept payment for their services; the power to cure was considered a gift from spirit. They paid it forward. Otherwise, their healing frequency might drop into density and evaporate entirely. The principle remains the same: medicine loses power when it becomes a commodity.

Trouble is, most scientists and doctors don't recognize spirit, density, and hexes, nor do they acknowledge the vital force, the memory of water, telekinesis, potentization, synchronicity, vibration, prayer, thoughtforms, holism, the power of Similars, nonlinear effects, or the fluctuating line between medical healing and medical hexing. They assume that a product developed by Moderna, AstraZeneca, Johnson & Johnson, or Pfizer will automatically be more effective than a nosode potentized homeopathically from a microdose of viral sputum, though they can't say why. They try, but they can't succeed because they are operating at a symptomatic level after actual causes have been (to re-quote Kent) "ultimated in the body in the form of tissue changes."

For instance, a vaccine has to whack every mole and cover every gap like Aesop's wind trying to blow a man's coat off. A potentized nosode has only to smile like the sun: its radiance goes everywhere. I'm not saying that is proof of homeopathic effectiveness; I'm just "saying" because, otherwise, how did life get here, in the middle of nowhere, and what is consciousness? Are we robots or earth angels?

Placebo doesn't mean "the joke's on you." Mind may be the most powerful force in the universe.

A myth of life extension and consciousness singularity drives the ambitions of ordinary health care. A progress-oriented neoliberal establishment seeks to regulate conception, pregnancy, birth, life, death, and the afterlife. Consumers no longer even prefer to be human; they strive to be more (or better) than human—prosthetic-enabled cyborgs to be serviced, fed, wired, hooked up, bathed, and bred by transhuman networks. When their body fails, they can be downloaded with their memories into a cloud, stored on a hard drive until a technology for reconstituting them is available, or they can live in an AI-regenerated hologram with holograms of their pets and crawlers of their favorite tweets and posts, as long as their posthumous bank account funds an AI probability wave based on their life.

In a reigning zeitgeist in which health can be improved only by material methods, the scope and cost of repair must increase exponentially with new advancing technology, which takes it on deeper and deeper probes for an invisible entity: life, disease, health, consciousness. Any quest for an equivocal object (like the big bang's background noise of the universe) must grow exponentially more expensive at each level of investigation and analysis. As long as there is no limit to the complexity and design of equipment deployed, there is no limit to its potential cost. Diseases have become so deeply imaged and dissected that a supporting cast of laboratory, pharmaceutical, and surgical workers is required for those in hospitals, in waiting rooms and on waiting lists for an expanding range of medical specialties, each with their own anatomy range and billings.

Even if homeopathy didn't exist, the modern medical complex has created a state of futility and resignation for both patients and doctors.

It is not just, as presumed by politicians and concerned citizens, that the treatment of disease has become more expensive because of the improvement of technology and the expansion of health care and longevity; it is that the medical profession has launched a Mars-voyage-style expedition with the public as not only funders but guinea pigs. The price of a tautological system of diagnosis and health care must continue to skyrocket because there is no end to which materialists will go to forestall their material demise.

Though advanced research into pathology has become unsustainably expensive, actual health care has not improved except in postponing death. Unfortunately, prolongation incubates more exotic and previously unknown diseases, including mental and neurological conditions that rob life of pleasure. The longer individuals live in a devitalized condition, the more they are fodder for an onslaught of painkillers, palliatives, and other consumerist tchotchkes—just walk the aisles of any Walgreens. A visit to a Rite Aid or WalMart shows the enormity of our commitment to an attack on pain. It is existential now and has replaced a quest for health and well-being.

The ultimate anti-holistic, materialist fantasy has been personalized by those who have accumulated far too much money to spend in a human lifetime, so they fund attempts at artificial life extension or cryogenic preservation of their bodies or brains in hopes of a future time when medicine will have advanced to the point of making longevity a consumer item.

If the actual disease is invisible, all the high-tech research is for naught. If symptom-oriented treatments turn minor conditions into syndromes for which patients must be treated again and again, then the medical profession is an extortionist scheme. The "sting" would outdo any con game in history. Patients are volunteers in a clinical trial for the next quadrillion-dollar payoff (that's the decimal after trillion) in Big Pharma's bid to increase its market share in an ultimate narco-state. It is a matter of who controls the planet, biosphere, and future. Post-academic sociologist Daniel Pinchbeck laid our predicament on the line when discussing COVID-19 and his path, as he put it, "from vacillation to vaccination":

A good deal of my resistance to mass vaccination—in particular, with the mRNA vaccines—was based on a vague, ominous sense that we are being pulled into a technocratic, transhumanist control system . . . from which we can never escape. . . .

When I imagine an endless series of variants accompanied by an endless series of boosters, I toggle back to the conspiratorial view. I find it infuriating that this meshes ideally with the profit model of the pharmaceutical companies. It would reward the bizarre, inappropriate smugness that Bill Gates expresses in interviews. I feel deeply suspicious of Moderna, for instance.

Stéphane Bancel, Moderna's CEO, has a reputation for cutthroat corporate practices. . . . On Clubhouse, I heard Bancel speak arrogantly about how they consider mRNA to be the "software of life" and see the vaccines as "platforms" for future drug developments. Moderna's website states that they "set out to create an mRNA technology platform that functions very much like an operating system on a computer." The boosters, then, will be like system upgrades.

If these vaccines turn out to compromise our natural immunity, people may feel forced to get these new shots every three to six months in order to remain healthy or even just survive. I find this horrific. It seems the height of hubris to treat our intricate biology as an input/output machine, like a computer. I suspect this will backfire on us eventually, as so many of our other technologies have, from plastics to GMOs to fossil fuels. . . .

Capitalism/post-industrial society tends to take everything that was once intrinsic to our free existence as human beings, exploit and outsource it, then sell it back to us for profit.[13]

Next time you wonder why QAnon acolytes, trucker convoys, and populists tramp through the heartland tweeting and honking for "health freedom," consider the obeisance to technocracy, Big Pharma, and Big Insurance, which has turned once-thriving subcultures into opioid wastelands while making Sacklers and their fellow Aristos* into billionaires. You can hide a sophisticated con in commodity science these days. Blowback from this and the health freedom movement have flipped opposing liberal and conservative views, turning former Democrats into Republicans and vice versa, while generally scrambling twentieth-century ideologies.

When sacred activists, eco-futurists, cranial osteopaths, organic arborists, transcendent musicians, morphic resonators, anarchist astrologers, and selfless it-takes-a-village and welcome-the-stranger friends in food banks, homeless shelters, and centers enfranchising

---

*I use the term Aristo, from "aristocrat," to describe members of the oligarchy: politicians, corporate executives, technocrats, and some pop and sports stars.

the poor and powerless support GMO vaccines as the sole responsible and effective response to a mutating coronavirus, citing high-level, socially conscious technocrats and biotechnicians as their witnesses and corroborators, while right-wing agitators, militia members, bikers, and conspiracy theorists set up biodynamic and herbal clinics and schools of crystal healing in the hinterland in the name of health freedom, then we are truly in a Tower of Babel. When anthroposophists, noni-fruit vintners, and energy healers flee Berkeley and Kauai, once ground zero for alternative medicine and the free-speech movement, and head for Sandpoint, Tulsa, Houston, and San Miguel de Allende, the cult of progressive scientism has ended. Where we go from here depends on political, economic, demographic, and social factors that can't be predicted, but that is also where we came from.

Impossible Knowledge and Iatrogenic Illness

It should be clear by now why a full rapprochement between standard medicine and homeopathy is near impossible. On principles alone, without even addressing microdose pharmacy, homeopathic theory dooms most (nonemergency) medical treatments to superficial symptom suppressions that in no way reflects the true dynamics of disease. In treating mirages, allopathic physicians condemn themselves to obsolete categories. Hahnemann wrote the epitaph for rationalism in the *Organon,* but it went pretty much unheeded: "Two thousand years were wasted by physicians in endeavoring to discover the invisible internal changes that take place in the organism in diseases, and in searching for their proximate causes and *a priori* nature, because they imagined that they could not cure before they had attained to this *impossible* knowledge."[14]

Yet that "impossible knowledge" is the basis of the world's medical systems—their institutionalization, funding, and research, their electron microscopes, magnetic resonance and ultrasound machines, and microsurgery, and, more recently, their CRISPR-based biotech—use of clustered regularly interspaced short palindromic repeats of amino-acids in a system deciphered from a bacterial gene editing system to edit human chromosomes and get at diseases' nucleic origins. This technological progression makes the National Institutes of Health, March of Dimes, Centers for Disease Control, and Harvard Medical School legitimate, respectable organizations—a presumption that the more "knowledge" we gain about biochemistry and genetics, the more effective medical science will be, no matter the costs or health and social consequences.

Allopathic pharmacy is not only the dominant medicine bundle in today's health care networks but represents 10 percent (and climbing) of the world's gross national product, second only to energy and food and with a far lower cost of goods sold, and hence a gargantuan profit. It is invaluable in a society that commoditizes goods, labor, and well-being. George Vithoulkas, a contemporary Greek homeopath, elucidated a range of symptomatic dynamics overlooked in the mainstream:

Since allopathic drugs are never selected according to the Law of Similars, they inevitably superimpose upon the organism a new drug disease which then must be counteracted by the organism.

Furthermore, if the drug has been successful in removing symptoms on a peripheral level, the defense mechanism is then forced to re-establish a new state of equilibrium at a deeper level. In this way, the vibration rate of the organism is disturbed and weakened by two mechanisms: 1) by the influence of the drug itself, and 2) by interference with the best possible response of the defense mechanism. Consequently, if the drug is powerful enough, or if drug therapy is continued long enough, the organism may jump to a deeper level in its susceptibility to disease. The real tragedy is that the defense mechanism of the individual cannot then re-establish the original equilibrium on its own; even with homeopathic treatment, it may take many years to return to the original level, much less to make any progress on the ailment.

It is a strange but true paradox that people who have been weakened by allopathic drugging become relatively "protected" from certain infections and epidemics. This, of course, occurs because the center of gravity of susceptibility has moved so deeply into the more vital regions of the organism that there is not enough susceptibility on superficial levels to produce a symptomatic reaction. In such an instance, this is not a sign of improvement in health, but rather a sign of degeneration.[15]

From a homeopathic view, allopathic medical care has driven disease inward to such a degree that we now see an epidemic of pathological expressions—cancer, heart disease, mental illness, various scleroses, and autoimmune diseases like lupus, rheumatoid arthritis, and mast cell, along with a prolongation of life. Anti-inflammatory drugs and steroids, psychotropics, tranquilizers, antibiotics, chemotherapy, radiation, biotech experimentation, and widespread industrial and electromagnetic pollution have led to novel malignancies, immune, autoimmune, and iatrogenic disorders, and exotic states of chronic illness, depression, anxiety, violence, dysphoria, and sociopathy. Harris Coulter believed that this process, over generations, spawned AIDS from suppressed syphilis.[16]

Older, sicker people, their diseases driven inward by earlier treatments, require ever more expensive medical care and drugs, ultimately paid for by society in the form of higher taxes and insurance rates. Each individual is also a participant in an ongoing lottery, encouraged to gamble on the results with insurance companies. They bet with their money that they will get sick and with their body and life that they will stay well. Either way, the individual wins, and either way, the individual loses.

It is difficult enough for the average patient to accept that a doctor has limited insight into the cause of their illness, but to allow that such knowledge if attained is of little help in the *actual* treatment of diseases makes energy medicine look like witchcraft, recalling Carl Sagan's warning about a return to "a demon-haunted world."

Our own world is haunted by *mechanical* demons. Though medical science has evolved, the advance has been almost solely technological and ideological. The deep understanding of health, vitality, and self-healing has, if anything, trended backward. By a homeopathic view, the range of chronic and mental diseases plaguing modern civilization comes from a failure to address actual diseases and their causes, which has led to waves of negative feedback, not only in individuals but in families, cities, biomes, and ecosystems. A homeless encampment is a mass disease formation.

It is not that allopathic physicians are fools; any competent doctor recognizes natural immunity. Psychiatrists understand that an organism develops a neurotic or sometimes a psychotic state to allow it to function at all, and that without those symptoms its psyche might fissure. Where allopathic doctors go astray, by homeopathic standards, is in choosing a seemingly arbitrary point at which to break off an appeal to the defense mechanism and begin intervention. The doctors take on the role of coction, homeostasis, and the inner physician, and of embryogenic restoration itself, especially when they replace one of nature's genetic splices with their own. Allopathic patients have come to expect doctors to solve or reset somatic timing for every condition that their biological systems can't. That's the job description, a syndrome of a society that beguiles its citizens by nonstop entertainment. Though not apparent at first glance, medicine has become an offshoot of the entertainment industry.

I am posing a medical caricature, a fuzzy-logic parable, to get across a polarity: the proximal causes of pathologies do not always indicate their best treatments. Maybe they should; in practice they don't. Health is more slippery and more elusive, and life is unpredictable and entangled—hence both miracle cures and remissions.

There is a reason why the health care system functions as well as it does: homeostases are imbedded at multiple levels and, because of natural resilience, the vital force and (if you believe in such things) the Etheric plane can instill healing from *all* treatments. The mere introduction of new information lets the embryogenic field realign and reinvigorate. The state of science in Hahnemann's and Kent's eras did not allow them to consider these broad implications, so they recognized only the homeopathic aspects of their own cures.

Homeopathic Allopathy

If homeopathy and other energy medicines were the baseline system rather than allopathy, allopathy would still have a role. Complementary medicines currently work in concert with allopathy. Furthermore, a homeopathic cure sometimes comes only at the expense of the patient's immediate well-being, plus a remedy is counterproductive if the patient cannot integrate it. A mental disease driven back onto the physical plane in a debilitating way is not a cure. Even homeopathic physicians may decide *not* to treat a certain depth of ailment if they feel that a patient has no space into which to expand—to make space for the remedy—and can live a healthy life otherwise. They practice allopathy as homeopaths—they practice *medicine.*

Drugs, surgery, and scientific triage not only reduce suffering and limit organ damage but can translate into therapeutic-field effects by unloading a physical or psychosomatic stress pattern. They can be used effectively to halt infections, free arteries, and reduce obsessive-compulsive thoughts. They slow pathologies that were once incurable or fatal. Modern medicine intervenes successfully in situations as wide-ranging as Tommy John surgery for baseball pitchers and quarterbacks to prostheses for war victims to prolonging life after severe injuries and poisonings. Allopaths train ambulance crews, run emergency rooms, and answer 911 calls.

Once a healee is stabilized, a more holistic treatment, if still desired, is available. To the limits of a person's overall physical and mental capacity, a transition from suppressive drugs to energy medicine is as much at their disposal as twelve-step programs are for alcoholics forswearing alcohol and heroin addicts junk.

Despite the current "zombie apocalypse," we can no more replace allopathic drugs overnight with homeopathic Similars than we can replace oil with wind and solar power without instituting a new belief system and infrastructure. But we are far removed from a consciously breathing, agriculturally sustainable civilization ready to live ceremonially and tap subtle bodies and vibrational fields, and we are also are not headed that way. People who consume canned capers and chemical-suffused corn (or nachos and McNuggets), all of them laced with sweeteners and additives grown in depleted and contaminated soils, or raised on factory ranches or in toxic fish farms, are also addicted to pharmaceutical as well as recreational drugs. Likewise, lifestyles with competitive, materialistic goals lead to a health care system that provides a fix-it, tranquilizer-addicted, mood-altering, workaholic mentality.

In the 2019 movie *The Sound of Metal*, a drummer in an ear-splittingly loud metal band goes deaf and heads immediately to an audiologist to get his ears fixed. Ruben intends to keep on playing and wants to know how much getting his hearing fixed will cost. A cochlear implant at $80,000 results in a contraption attached to the back of his head that bypasses his ears and translates sounds directly into his brain without depth of field or filtering. He finds himself in a realm of clatter, clank, and screech. After initially preferring that route over residency in a deaf commune and learning sign language and practicing stillness, by the end of the film he disconnects the device and blisses out in silence. It's a metaphor for the entire health care system.

Allopathy is where society is, so it is where disease and treatment are; they match energetically. The homeopathic critique posits an idealized Erewhon as an antidote to medical utilitarianism. That is not a possibility, nor does homeopathy present any plausible pathway there. Insofar as homeopathic philosophy addresses nature and society as a whole, allopathic medicine is itself a necessary phase of miasmic treatment, homeopathic in its balance with the society in which it has arisen. In an ironic sense, allopathy is capitalism's Similar, extending the life spans of its consumers.

The problem was never allopathy; it is fundamentalist materialism, technocracy, and worship of algorithms. Nihilistic beliefs lead to nihilistic medicines—not poor medicines but medicines based on intersections of Darwin's law (random selection) with Murphy's law (anything that can go wrong will go wrong).

Should there be any truth to the homeopathic critique of our age of progress, when people are relieved not to have been born in a time of incurable diseases and dread plagues, then we need to rethink both the map and the territory. We have come a long way in terms of treatment and technology, but we have also fostered a grand illusion: that linear progress is possible without simultaneous retrogression and deficit along other lines. As twentieth-century philosopher Alfred North Whitehead pointed out, civilizations don't experience their backgrounds; instead, they explicate them uncritically. Unexamined paradoxes—wicked problems and hyperobjects—define entire epochs.

Surgery, radiation, and pharmaceuticals are less vectors of healing than crisis management, disaster prevention, symptom alleviation, and life extension. Real healing means transduction of disease into freedom. In that regard, the homeopathic microdose is also a metaphor for activating laws of cure. A deep jolt induces an organism to change by breaking into not only its morphogenetic codes but its semiologies, like Rudolf Steiner's alphabet of eurythmy that dances out a cure by spelling it.

The most powerful medicines are autonomous, latent, and part of the biology of being. The lighter and more internal the treatment, the deeper and truer its healing effect. The original elixir is our nightly dreams, for other mammals too. Natural laws of cure go from the inside out, from the body to the psyche, and from a subwave to its long wave.

What is left for us now, as in other mysteries, is to return to the birthplace, the proverbial scene of the crime.

5

Samuel Hahnemann and the Fundamentalist Basis of Homeopathy

Hahnemann's Early Life and Pre-homeopathy Career

Samuel Hahnemann was born at midnight, April 10–11, 1755, in the German town of Meissen, near the Polish and Czechoslovakian borders. The Hahnemann family had migrated there from the west a generation earlier so that Samuel's father could work at the local porcelain factory. So-called Dresden china had been innovated by Johann Bottger, an alchemist, in 1710, as a "day job" during his search for gold, and the Saxon porcelain industry was located at Meissen on the Elbe River, close to rich clay beds. A factory was established at Albrecht Castle, and in 1743 an art school was added. Writing in his journal at the age of thirty-six, Hahnemann described his origins:

> I was born on April 10th, 1755, in the Electorate of Saxony, one of the most beautiful parts of Germany. . . .
>
> My father, Christian Gottfried Hahnemann, together with my mother Johanna Christiana, *née* Spiess, taught me how to read and

write whilst playing. My father . . . was a painter for the porcelain factory of [Meissen], and the author of a brief treatise on watercolour painting.[1]

Hahnemann was born as well into the centuries of German strife. During the Seven Years' War ending in his eighth year, the army of Prussian king Frederick II decimated the porcelain factory and supply chain, impoverishing Saxony. Hahnemann's later homeopathic work shared a milieu with Napoleon's march across Europe.

Spiritually and scientifically, Hahnemann was educated in the German occult tradition, not by initial study plan so much as by his time and place in the world and then by his life quest. To the south, in Switzerland and Austria, Paracelsus had practiced and preached 250 years earlier, and Carl Jung and Rudolf Steiner, 150 years later, went on similar quests for spirit in matter. With each of their interrogations, a new riddle formed from prior enigmas. It is a process based on prior processes, not a soluble puzzle. Like the twentieth-century Austrian physician Wilhelm Reich and other less fabled mage-scientists, Hahnemann started with matter and mostly materialist intent and came to spirit, to vital energy, by default.

Though his boyhood studies were interrupted by war and by his father's demands that he acquire a bread-and-butter trade rather than amass mere book learning, Hahnemann emerged from his adolescence eclectically educated, for he continued to study with fanatical diligence on his own. At age sixteen, he was taken into the local state secondary school in Meissen by its rector, tutoring pupils in Greek and Latin in exchange for his own tuition. He graduated at twenty with a dissertation (in Latin) on the construction of the human hand. From there, he attended Leipzig University. By the time he was ready for some sort of career, he was already trained by eighteenth-century standards as a physician, biochemist, and anatomist—separate specialties then (and still, unfortunately, today). Few students truly master all three, but those that do gain a whole picture, whereas those who specialize must rely on secondhand knowledge from the others.

Recognizing the fractured and feckless state of the medical world, Hahnemann chose not to practice out of fear of doing more harm than good. He supported himself by translating. From age thirty to thirty-four, he translated and published more than two thousand pages, most of it from non-Germanic languages, with a few articles of his own on sores, ulcers, and drugs. Almost a third of that opus was a rendering of the twelfth-century letters of Abelard and Heloise—a medieval French theologian and his student—from English into German, a nonscientific undertaking that shows the breadth of Hahnemann's knowledge and skill. He noted dryly, "By teaching German and French to a wealthy young Greek from Jassy in Moldavia, as well as by translations from English, I procured for myself for a time the means of subsistence."[2]

Hahnemann's pre-homeopathic medical translations included physiology texts, descriptions of experiments with copper, a work on hydrophobia, two volumes on mineral waters and warm baths, and various writings on practical medicine. His analyses and deconstructions emerged from his scholarship. For instance, at twenty-seven, as a relative amateur, he translated a French treatise on industrial chemistry, correcting chemical errors in the original and adding additional techniques in footnotes. He had assimilated a biochemical overview. There is a reason why homeopathy spoke in refined chemistry, characterology, and differential diagnosis from the beginning. Its fluency came, in part, from a maze of ancient languages and foreign labs and included ignored work of obscure botanists and physicians of different eras, nationalities, and tongues.

Translation is also a disciplined meditation on the structure of language, the roots and etymologies of meaning, and transfers between codes and their dialects. Hidden meanings in one dialect emerge like glossolalia in their conversion into others. Homeopathy sometimes seems more like subtexts of multiple codes than a single scientific system.

Much of Hahnemann's translation research was not even medicinal or related to healing, so homeopathy reflects a synthesis different from any of its parts or lineal precursors. It was never wholly "medicine"; it was a theory of nature, life, and civilization, as universal and groundbreaking in its way as Darwinian biology, though not part of same crescendo of materialism.

Hahnemann did not plan to spring "homoeopathy" (as it was originally spelled) on the world as a novelty, but the old masters continued to lecture and overlap in his mind and he knew from his studies and hands-on experience that contemporary medicine was a muddle; it was better to return to the drawing board and recombine wisdom traditions. Greek alchemy, European herbalism, Arabic chemistry, and various local pharmacies—though each of their contributions to homeopathy is cloaked in the amalgam—were intrinsic to it and fused into new forms by Hahnemann's synthesizing.

It is not as though the founder merely reapplied old texts to "modern" medicine either. He made a fresh system by virtue of a mastery of the ancient medicines he studied. And he did more than bring back alchemical, herbal, and chemical tropes; he reinvented them in a simultaneously scientific and archetypal context. In the brief and mute hiatus between the end of academic hermeticism and the birth of hardcore professional science, he coaxed a single last child from their union.

The Origin of Homeopathy

From age thirty-five to thirty-eight, Hahnemann translated several medical, agricultural, and chemical books, notably materia medicas from English, French, and Italian. His last such volume, fourteen years later, in 1806, was Swiss physician Albrecht von Haller's *Materia*

Medica of German Plants, Together with Their Economic and Technical Use, from a French version of the original Latin. Hahnemann's expertise, by then, included plant identities and their medical uses, ethnomedicinal compounds, and Indo-European variants. When, in 1810, in his fifty-sixth year, he was required to give a public lecture as a prerequisite of teaching at the medical institute in Leipzig, the audience presumed a passionate defense of homeopathy, his trademark by them. He surprised them with a discussion of the ancient medical uses of hellebore, quoting from German, French, English, Italian, Latin, Greek, Hebrew, and Arabic sources that included doctors, herbalists, and natural philosophers. It was a tour de force of not only medical theory but botany, etymology, and comparative mythology.

It was, however, in Hahnemann's earlier 1790 translation of the Scottish physician William Cullen's *Treatise of the Materia Medica* that a new science emerged.

Cullen had a solidist mechanical view of the body. He believed that diseases were caused by variation in the "flux" of nervous energy. As primary organs, like the heart and brain, became blocked and irritated, they communicated their distortions to other parts of the body, leading to general debility. Since the organism was essentially an irritable jelly, the point of medicines was to stir and arouse the gel, stimulate it, and set it into corrective spasms. If an ailment developed from the direct pressure of agitated blood, for instance, it should be relieved by bloodletting. Inflammation was treated by either acid or alkaline blends, each to counteract a surplus of the other.

Cullen's prescriptions were always Contraries based on redirecting motions of a relatively simple solid. Diagnostically, his tendency was to pare the number of diseases to classes of inflammations and blockages and to put any deviations into subcategories. That way, the range of possible medicines was fixed by the degrees of spasming needed to clear the metabolism.

Cullen was a follower of Georg Ernst Stahl and the early

Montpellier school of vitalists. To arrive at solidism, it was necessary only for him to replace Stahl's Anima, a natural, harmonious, self-corrective healer and regulator, with a material rendition of irritability. Cullen and Hahnemann clashed by fate in Hahnemann's notes appended to his translation.

Cullen rejected the notion that Peruvian bark (quinine) can have a specific (i.e., intrinsic or vital) effect in the treatment of intermittent fever; instead, he held that it is a composite tonic, bringing together bitter and astringent qualities that combine to produce its effect. The translator balked here, and in a footnote to page 108 of volume II of Cullen's book, he offered a different solution:

By combining the strongest bitters and the strongest astringents we can obtain a compound which, in small doses, possesses much more of both these properties than the bark, and yet in all Eternity no fever specific can be made from such a compound. The author should have accounted for this. This undiscovered principle of the effect of the bark is probably not very easy to find. Let us consider the following: Substances which produce some kind of fever (very strong coffee, pepper, arnica, ignatia-bean, arsenic) counteract these types of intermittent fever. I took, for several days, as an experiment, four drams of good china [cinchona, a quinine source] twice daily. My feet and finger tips, etc., at first became cold; I became languid and drowsy; then my heart began to palpitate; my pulse became hard and quick; an intolerable anxiety and trembling (but without a rigor); prostration in all the limbs; then pulsation in the head, redness of the cheeks, thirst; briefly, all the symptoms usually associated with intermittent fever appeared in succession, yet without the actual rigor. . . . This paroxysm lasted from two to three hours every time, and recurred when I repeated the dose and not otherwise. I discontinued the medicine and I was once again in good health.[3]

In other words, the remedy had a discrete, systemic effect, unaccounted for by any of its component properties. Hahnemann was calling out something that seemed obvious to him. The debut of homeopathy in a footnote indicates that he intended scholarship more than innovation. Healing by Similars was a time-honored way of treating disease. As a medical translator, Hahnemann had come across it countless times in his reading. To that, he added a forceful antirationalist experiment—his first publicized proving. The implication was obvious: forget prior categories and test each substance anew empirically. To his peers this sounded arrogant and self-aggrandizing. They asked, "Are we to try all medicines on ourselves at mortal risk?" The footnote needn't have led to homeopathy, but through a series of serendipities and synchronicities it did. It took a master medicine man and scholar, though, to recognize and, in turn, apply them.

Hahnemann served in a number of medical positions in his early career, but he gave each up and always returned to translating and research. In 1781, at twenty-six, he married the seventeen-year-old daughter of the local apothecary in Gommern, and after he spent time working as a medical officer of health in Dresden, the couple moved to Leipzig to be near the university. It was here that Hahnemann translated Cullen, but the controversy he stirred was not homeopathic at all.

In 1792 Emperor Leopold II of Austria died under emergency treatment. Because of the political delicacy of the situation, the three doctors involved wrote and published a description of the emperor's illness, its treatment, and the ensuing demise of the patient. Hahnemann responded in a Gotha paper:

> The bulletins state: "On the morning of February 28th, [the emperor's] doctor, Lagusius, found a severe fever and a distended abdomen"—he tried to fight the condition by venesection

[bloodletting], and as this failed to give relief, he repeated the process three times more, without any better result. We ask, from a scientific point of view, according to what principles has anyone the right to order a second venesection when the first has failed to bring relief? As for a third, Heaven help us!; but to draw blood a fourth time when the three previous attempts failed to alleviate! To abstract the fluid of life four times in twenty-four hours from a man, who has lost flesh from mental overwork combined with a long continued diarrhoea, without procuring any relief for him! Science pales before this![4]

It goes without saying that his words alienated many of his medical peers.

Hahnemannism Is Not Homeopathy

A pragmatist as well as a holist, Hahnemann combined Christian and medical asceticism and was scrupulous about lifestyle and diet. In an era of poor ventilation in houses and little understanding about contamination, he insisted upon exercise, nutritious meals, running water, and open windows. Vitalistic beliefs did not dissuade him from classifying microbes, toxins, and agents of infection.

The rules of hygiene that Hahnemann laid down, though apparent to us now, were mostly unknown or ignored in the medical world of his time. For instance, he insisted on scraping clean a wound and on bandaging with alcohol-soaked cloths; he prescribed fresh air, exercises, cheerful company, warm and cold baths; he encouraged doctors to prepare their own medicines and be directly responsible for their effects. But he was panning for knowledge they didn't have.

A similar request today—when physicians prescribe pharmaceuticals and vaccines based mainly on the second- or thirdhand testimony of industry salespersons, advertisements in professional publications, financial inducements, and peer consensus—would be even more ludicrous. Modern doctors learn relatively little in medical school about activity at a subcellular level (that's in a different building), and their day-one-to-graduation education takes place within a rigorously allopathic model of cure under a sworn pledge to its AMA guild. They prescribe not molecular biochemistry but a set of abstract pharmaceutical memes. If doctors are no more than liaisons between the pharmaceutical industry and patients, then medicine has been subsumed in biochemical materialism, and the vital force has been downgraded to cyborgian status. The progression of this hierarchy can be traced back to Hahnemann's time.

Yet it is an irony of medical history that the man whose system has weighed most strongly against basic germ theory was an early advocate for boiling utensils used by patients with contagious diseases and isolation of those patients from others (either in a hospital or in a private house). Hahnemann identified ailments caused by the poor hygiene as well as the iatrogenic diseases from the unproven medicines of his time. Mercury dosing, bleeding, and venesection along with freely flowing sewage—a "common shore" (as it was satirically called) in lieu of wastewater treatment—led to eighteenth-century skin outbreaks, intestinal disorders, and likely also mental diseases, epilepsy, and co-seizures. Hahnemann criticized hydrotherapy (cold-water treatment) and mineral baths as ineffective and deemed the era's indiscriminate pharmacy and bloodletting unwarranted medically, excessive as well, and of little value.* He denounced standard modes of treatment of mental patients: cranial surgery or incarceration. Doctors then took the provocative language of mental patients literally and responded to insults with insults of their own and to asocial acts as if they were crimes needing punishments. Hahnemann maintained that aberrant behavior was an expression of disease, no

---

*Hydrotherapy and bloodletting have been reexamined since and been found, in some naturopathic quarters, to have circumscribed virtues, though less than claimed for their broader application in Hahnemann's time.

different from physical expressions, and that the words of mental patients were invaluable clues to their cures.

Hahnemann advocated public health as a civic and personal responsibility and wrote books and pamphlets supporting it, in one of which he declared:

> In order to save fuel and high rents, several miserable families will often herd together, frequently in one room, and they are careful not to let in any fresh air through window or door, because that might also let in the cold. The animal exhalations from perspirations and the breath become concentrated, stagnant and foul in these places; one person's lungs do their best to take away from the others all the small amount of life-giving air remaining, exhaling in exchange impurities from the blood. The melancholy twilight of their small, darkened windows is combined with the enervating dampness and musty smell of old rags and rotting straw; fear, envy, quarrelsomeness and other passions do their best to destroy completely what little health there is; all this can only be known by one whose calling has compelled him to enter these hovels of misery. Here contagious epidemics not only go on spreading easily and almost unceasingly if the slightest germ has chanced to fall there, but it is here that they actually originate, break out and become fatal even to more fortunate citizens.[5]

This same description would apply today to swaths of Africa, Asia, South America, and the Australian outback as well as slums and tent cities in the heart of modernity.

The Mystery of Health and Disease

Throughout his career, Hahnemann remained a mixture of the esoteric and empirical: a mage and EMT. During the years preceding the writing of the *Organon*, he was unsettled, continually trying to come to terms with professional medical practice. After his time travels through the West's medical epistemology, he found himself facing a hodgepodge of doctors knowing little of their predecessors or their own traditions. Following a stint battling with the authorities at a mental hospital in Gotha, he spent ten years alternating between city and country, attempting to earn a living as a doctor. His career was marked by both miracle cures and controversies. His insistence on manufacturing his own medicines and practicing his own brand of cure alienated both apothecaries and fellow physicians. In one much-publicized case, a certain Prince Schwarzenberg died after leaving Hahnemann's care for the bloodletting of his own physicians. Hahnemann walked in his funeral procession, not to show respect as much as to dramatize his innocence in the death.

These were painful times in which he witnessed illnesses and deaths among his eleven children. Having scoured all the systems of cure he knew for remedies, he concluded, in despair, "After 1,000 to 2,000 years, then, we are no further!"[6]

What was missing was a logic addressing the variety of pathologies and providing a consistent strategy for treating them. The Hippocratics had developed functional medicines, but their backup science was a gnarl of contradictions, ex post facto rationalizations more than applicable etiologies that guided development of new pharmacies. Medicine since then had chased Aristotelian questions in self-contradicting circles. No one knew why one disease expressed itself in fever, another in chills, and what the heat of a bath or the spirit of a tonic actually *did* in reducing a pathology.

Hahnemann did not accept Paracelsus's occultism, yet he was drawn to his Law of Similars. He took seriously the possibilities of Quintessential pharmacy (per his Cullen footnote), while he rejected alchemy and astrological botany per se as unscientific mixes of mythology, misread signatures, and speculation.

More than any of his contemporaries, Hahnemann realized how profound and intricate a matter disease was and how unequipped a linear science was to deal with its nonlinear aspects, though that terminology was not yet in use. Pathologies were catacombs. Compared to such adversaries, Napoleon was a schoolboy. While Hahnemann was writing the *Organon,* he reflected on his path in a letter to a friend, a professor of pathology:

For eighteen years I have been deviating from the ordinary practice of the medical art. . .

My sense of duty would not easily allow me to treat the unknown pathological state of my suffering brethren with these unknown medicines. If they are not exactly suitable (and how could the physician know that, since their specific effects had not yet been demonstrated?), they might with their strong potency easily change life into death or induce new disorders and chronic maladies, often more difficult to eradicate than the original disease. The thought of becoming in this way a murderer or a malefactor towards the life of my fellow human beings was most terrible to me, so terrible and disturbing that I wholly gave up practice in the first years of my married life. I scarcely treated anybody for fear of injuring him, and occupied myself solely with chemistry and writing.

But then children were born to me, several children, and after a time serious illnesses occurred, which, in tormenting and endangering my children, my own flesh and blood, made it even more painful to my sense of duty, that I could not with any degree of assurance procure help for them. . . . Whence then was certain help to be obtained?—was the yearning cry of the comfortless father in the midst of the groaning of his children, dear to him above all else. Night and desolation around me—no sight of enlightenment for my troubled paternal heart.[7]

The contemporary response to this lament is to note that Hahnemann was born a couple of centuries too soon.

Similars and Plant Spirit Medicines

Homeopathy as a discrete modality and term arrived modestly, well under the radar. In his "Essay on a New Principle for Ascertaining the Curative Powers of Drugs, and Some Examinations of the Previous Principles," published in 1796, Hahnemann rejected cure by Contraries as attacking only symptoms, not diseases. He dismissed virtually all exciting, inciting, cleansing, heating, and cooling actions of medicines, declaring them extraneous to the means of their alleviation. He distinguished the healing power of all substances solely as their capacity to *effect* (not *affect*) specific illnesses. He asserted that the organism had sequential responses to properly prescribed Similars: aggravation from the similarity, followed by stimulation of the vital force. Cures were simply intensifications of symptoms in order to help a body complete its healing process.

Hahnemann underwrote his claims, as noted, by testing substances on himself and recording the "artificial" diseases they induced. He emphasized poisons because of their tendency to provoke a quick, discernible response. His publicized provings of small doses of aconite, strychnine, and belladona were as inconsonant with the medical profession of his time as they would be today.

In the same essay, Hahnemann proposed a theory of disease interaction and layering: A severe chronic condition could prevent an acute disease of less severity from gaining hold over a system, but this was unhealthy even if it reduced symptomology. The more severe disease might form on top, and the older symptoms would eventually return. This type of thinking is almost totally absent in today's world of medical specialization.

Hahnemann noted the partial correlation of vaccination and

homeopathy; for instance, inoculation of smallpox not only protected against smallpox but often cured unrelated diseases, including deafness, dysentery, and swollen testicles. This was not, Hahnemann thought, a justification for vaccination of large populations, taking no account of individual constitutions and their defense mechanisms. He also felt that an individual who could successfully be inoculated against a disease would likely be immune anyway and more completely cured by a Similar, whereas a person responsive to the inoculation would develop chronic disease from the presence of a foreign pathogen in his system.

This contention flared up anew in 2020s debates about COVID-19, herd immunity, and genetically modified vaccines. During this recent pandemic, mass vaccination took place without medical record-keeping or physician oversight—one-size-fits-all jabs—and no cross-referenced checks for adverse outcomes. I acknowledge that this statement is subject to debate and, though I don't want to distract from my overall argument, vaccines play a key role in the larger homeopathic discussion, and I want to tie that in to current events.

A modern argument against modern mass vaccinations foreshadowed by Hahnemann is that isopathy can lead to antibody-dependent enhancement. Though enhanced initially, people's immune systems are dulled by an augmentation of data, leading to a reduction in overall immunity, while wrongfooting the body's T cells to vigilance without regard to a range of viral intruders, including variants from the inevitable mutations. When a widely scanning immunity network is redirected to specific adaptive immunity, antibodies binding to the pathogen can function as a "Trojan horse," *allowing* it into the cells and causing a virus to spread more widely. Meanwhile, "leaky"—incompletely targeted—vaccines propagate more infectious strains in the same way that overuse of antibiotics breeds superbugs—by putting selective pressure on an invasive organism while allowing it to escape herd immunity. Some viral loads leak through, allowing mutations.

Similars proved effective during the viral pandemics of both 1918 and 2020. Potentized microdoses have no ordinary structure so they can't augment and likely don't encourage mutations either. They work solely in terms of vital activation. If they don't activate the vital force, they effectively don't exist. Unspecified, they are truly nanodoses of nothing. If their successes could be confirmed by scientifically accepted data, it would alter the current debate about obligatory vaccination.

More than a century before vaccination was formalized as a medical procedure and philosophy, Hahnemann spoke out for homeopathic specification against generalized shots. Two of his statements taken together address the matter axiomatically: "Similar symptoms in the remedy remove similar symptoms in the disease"[8] and "This eternal, universal law of Nature, that every disease is destroyed and cured through the similar artificial disease which the appropriate remedy has the tendency to excite, rests on the following proposition: that only one disease can exist in the body at one time, and therefore one disease must yield to the other."[9]

Again, this sort of hierarchical logic is pretty much absent in today's medicine. The notion of the singular disease (or cure) and its holistic interaction with the organism has been lost in a mélange of specialists diagnosing additively, with polypharmacy following. People's bedside tables and medicine cabinets are cluttered with essentially incompatible and polarized pills, as if these could combine their effects beneficially according to each one's pharmaceutical directives. Few think any longer in terms of health as a discrete singularity like electricity or gravity (or consciousness), hence needing singular catalysts like Simillimums. The consequence has been chemical "wars," self-annulling augmentations, and iatrogenic diseases from pile-on biochemistry.

Interestingly, entheogenic practitioners cite related polypharmaceutical conflicts. As psychoactive plants meet each other in the bodies and psyches of recipients, they take on personalities and vie for seniority. One practitioner told me that iboga usually takes charge over ayahuasca, kambo, or peyote as if it were the more dominant molecule (like the alpha wolf or alpha baboon in a pack). But, shamanically viewed, entheogens are living botanical essences with innate intelligences, hierarchies, and "moral" codes. Pharmaceuticals have no intrinsic ways of establishing "right" territories. By contrast with plant spirits and their psychic allies, they are manufactured like widgets and have no biochemical compass or way to clear fields of competitors for their own function. My divergence here is to put Hahnemann's discoveries in a context with futuristic as well as historical ramifications. We may still not have arrived at a comprehensive energy-medicine landscape or identified homeopathy's place in it, neither as a Hahnemannian system with a materia medica and repertory nor as specified energy in all forms of nanodose and entheogenic healing.

Similars are not spirit molecules; in fact, they are not molecules at all, but they operate in a correlative vitalistic context.

Microdoses

Hahnemann did not just adopt homeopathy in 1796 and never look back. He was tentative in his reliance on Similars; for instance, he mentions, in a case of treating tapeworm, attempting more than sixteen allopathic medicines before, in desperation, administering white hellebore for its potential to cause a colic like the patient's. The result was such a violent colic that the patient almost died, but afterward improved rapidly and remained well. This confirmed the power of Similars over Contraries in vital-force-activating effectiveness and bringing about deep, sustained health.

In order to evoke a milder response, especially from poisons that had unique therapeutic power, Hahnemann tried diluting their tinctures, hoping to locate the level at which they still had an effect and their aggravation was least. As expected, he found that greater dilutions caused the least aggravation, but they also had decreasing medicinal value. Then he tried shaking the vials at each dilution. It is uncertain what led him to improvise in this way, and there is no analysis and explanation in Hahnemann's writing, although different traditionary sciences, including alchemy and Chinese medicine, use tympanic interaction with substances for potentization. Ethnographic literature records primitive peoples preparing medicines by pounding, grinding, blowing on, aiming at the sun or stars, scraping with coral or ivory, punching once with the fist (in the case of leaves), and (in the case of pollen) suffocating a bird in the medicine before its use—all to wake the spirits in the substance or bring transdimensional entities to attach themselves to it. Most Indigenous doctors believe that medicines contain no power in themselves but obtain it from contact with spirits or ancestral realms.

In the early 1990s, I went to a traditional Chinese apothecary in Oakland with a prescription from an acupuncturist in hànzì characters and had the "pharmacist" scoop and hand me a bunch of shells. When I looked dubious, he took them back, then crushed and pounded them into a powder by mortar and pestle. I was watching a forerunner of succussion.

The well-read Hahnemann had likely encountered versions of this method. He did not have to believe in shamanism or magic to take cues from them; he knew how to be "found" rather than "lost" in translation.

His results with the new dilutions were startling, and they are still startling. The smaller the dose, not only the less the initial aggravation, but the more their medicinal effects increased and the more profound the secondary healing. A delighted Hahnemann pursued this counterintuitive phenomenon to its limit. His original homeopathic doses were at times as high as seventy grams of substance per thousand, but commonly five grams. From 1799 to 1801 he began using notably smaller doses—1/5,000,000 of a grain of opium and 1/432,000 of a grain of dried belladona berry. During his lifetime, Hahnemann only went as far as the thirtieth centesimal ("It cannot go on to infinity," he fretted,[10] but he was already at infinity, and he had opened a Pandora's box). Rima Handley, in her biography of Hahnemann, guessed that he knew exactly what he was unleashing on the world:

> Hahnemann seemed to have realised that he had achieved something remarkable when he wrote in alchemical terms of the process of dilution and succussion as having liberated the "medicinal power ... from its material bonds" and said that the "attenuations" were "an actual exaltation of the medicinal power, a real spiritualisation of the dynamic property, a true, astonishing unveiling and vivifying of the medicinal spirit."[11]

Hahnemann already understood that diseases had a dynamic quality to them. That is what shifted him in the direction of dynamization (potentiation) of crude medicinal substances using the process of dilution and succussion. If matter was being made more dynamic by these preparations, then his belief that diseases were not material states but dynamic disturbances was being experimentally confirmed. Serial dilution and potentization of medicines were vibrational realignments with imperceptible discordance patterns. Hahnemann concluded that he had found and released the vital presence in substances—who wouldn't? He wrote:

> Now with respect to the development of physical forces from material substances by trituration, this is a very wonderful subject. It is only the ignorant vulgar that still look upon matter as dead mass, for from its interior can be elicited incredible and hitherto unsus-

pected powers. . . . Medicinal substances are not . . . masses in the ordinary sense of the term, on the contrary, their true essential nature is only dynamically spiritual . . . is pure force. . . . Who can say that in the millionth and billionth development the small particles of the medicinal substances have arrived at the state of atoms not susceptible to further division, of whose nature we can form not the slightest conception?[12]

Who indeed can say? Albert Einstein, Max Planck, Wolfgang Pauli, and Werner Heisenberg would ask the same basic question. Homeopathy is not mere algebraic vitalism. Hahnemann was unknowingly reinventing Paracelsus's quintessential physics while foreshadowing micro- and nanosciences.

In addition, the paradox of increase in potency with an increase in dilution does not occur on a linear basis or by monotonic progression. Instead, there are plateaus and jumps resembling rhythmic variations, 10^{-400} being generally more powerful than 10^{-2000}, but $10^{-20,000}$ being significantly more reactive than either. Furthermore, overly enthusiastic repetition of homeopathic doses seems to halt activity.[13]

Currently the thinking in this area is that when doses are repeated too often, the vital force determines to stop receiving further copies of the same healing message, like a ribosome saying to transfer RNA, "No more messaging, sir. You are repeating yourself."

The unique microdose aspects of substances do not behave like their more material herbal properties. Homeopathy is not just cure by Similars; when crude medicinal substances are dynamized and potentized, they are turned into dynamic remedies. When chosen on the basis of Law of Similars and given in minute doses, the remedies bring about vital healing without inverse offshoots or aggravations.

Augmentation of Similars could explain why many homeopaths insist on only one dose. Ideal dilutions respond harmonically to different planes of substance and illness—it is a matter of vibration rather than dosage, like the segregation and specification of a blastula through its stages of differentiation.

Microdoses would one day scuttle homeopathy from within by taking remedies out of the hands of conventional pharmacists and splitting Hahnemann's followers on the nature and limits of dilution. Mainstream criticisms of microdose principle were utter and scathing from the get-go. German doctor Hermann Schnaubert wrote satirically:

> Death has no further power over man, the homeopaths have taken away his sting! For, if shaking and rubbing a dead medicinal substance, reduced to an unimaginable size, can give an effective power passing all comprehension, surely nobody can be surprised if he sees dead men brought to life by shaking and rubbing, sustained appropriately.[14]

This critique was inevitable once homeopaths realized that they didn't have to place limits on degrees of succussion. If each dilution were successively more powerful, the ultimate promise and potential payoff must be immortality. However, since remedies work only through the defense mechanism and vital force, they can't raise the dead. Homeopathy's spiral logic eluded the medical and pharmaceutical majority made up of circular thinkers.

When the new fad of microdoses first arrived in America with immigrant European physicians, and doctors began to realize what was at stake in their own profession, the response was as American as Barnum & Bailey. Harris Coulter summarized some of medical blowback:

> One doctor estimated that a volume of water 61 times the size of the earth was needed for the 15th dilution. Others talked in terms of the Caspian or the Mediterranean, of Lake Huron or Superior.

One man calculated that 140,000 hogsheads of arsenic were dumped every year into the Ohio and Mississippi Rivers from the poisoning of rats in Pittsburgh and St. Louis, that this raised the Mississippi water to the 4th dynamization, but that it apparently had no effect on those living downstream.[15]

These appraisals overlook discrete alignments of microdoses with diseases in quantum-like packets of information. The potentized pill, emptied of substance, transfers something like a zip file of information into a cellular network structured to receive it. Homeopathic dosing transcends Mississippi River dosing in the same way that the first unicellular organism, the autogene, must have coalesced in the tidal waters. If life is the vital force agglutinating by its own elemental chemistry, the autogene was its first homeopathic proving and underwrites all later ones! Yet science does not deal with teleodynamics, morphic resonance, or psi phenomena, and homeopathy, though scientifically reasoned, is trapped on its own vitalist-empiricist fence. Coulter quoted from two other scornful accounts:

According to this view it is the spiritual influence of the sabre that pierces the body, not its material form. It is the spiritual influence of the club that breaks the skull. It is the spiritual influence of fried onions that causes an attack of cholera morbus.

And:

This spiritualizing of matter by trituration is an insult to modern philosophy, and in reference to this spiritualization and tendency to mysticism, it is the mere adventitious result of habitual modes of thinking in Germany [where] science is as much pestered with spirits as poetry is.[16]

James Gorman offered a contemporary version of the same bewildered skepticism:

> Joel Gurin, science editor of *Consumer Reports,* a critic of homeopathy, doesn't think most people understand "the enormity" of what homeopathic theory asks one to believe. He says: "One must believe that water in some way undefined by modern science, has a memory which can be changed in a meaningful way by progressive dilution and shaking, that this 'trace resonance' in the water has a biological effect, and that all these remarkable and challenging facts were observed by a lone German physician a couple of hundred years ago. To me that's a big leap of faith."[17]

Unless one presumes that systematic succussion potentizes microdoses, the results of homeopathic treatment have no ordinary explanation. But, as I have noted many times, homeopathy was practiced because it worked, not because it is explicable. Hahnemann the doctor spawned thousands of disciples who tried his remedies with the same beneficial results. The "great riddle" is not just homeopathy; it's medicine, life, consciousness, and the elusive placebo effect. A common refrain, today as then, is "No one knows how any pill works." Much of allopathic pharmacy is placebo plus side effects too.

Hahnemann as Bête Noire and Myth

From 1805 until 1812, Hahnemann lived in Torgau, Saxony, near his own birthplace on the Elbe, where he treated patients and, early on, wrote his *Organon,* the cornerstone of homeopathy. It was published in 1810. Given its radical proposition, the work was reviewed generously at the time, the common opinion being that the author had much of importance to say about the Law of Similars, a time-honored principle, but tended to extend it too. Doctors were complacent enough not to recognize the attack on their own methods, so Hahnemann was viewed only as an eccentric with a homeopathic specialty or fad.

His frustration at being, in essence, ignored led him to return to Leipzig and a public stage. With the lecture on hellebore delivered in 1810, he won the right to instruct medical students, as described above. In the winter term of 1812, the sage of homeopathy, fifty-seven years old and nearly bald, socially awkward (these days he would likely be dismissed as "on the spectrum") but dressed elegantly, presented the full science of his "new age" medicine, class after class. Word spread, and the audience for his lectures gradually grew. Some of it was admirers, but Hahnemann was also considered an entertainment, a buffoon, and a demagogue whose theatrical raging and blaspheming of other doctors delighted people because his outrage affirmed their own frustrations. Behind his back, he was belittled and quietly mocked by medical colleagues whose approval he no longer cherished. At the university he acquired a group of loyal disciples from among the medical students. He taught them to prepare their own medicines by collecting plants, minerals, insects, and the like, and making their dilutions and successions by hand. Together with them, he organized the first controlled provings and began a materia medica.

Wrote one student:

We lived very happily together, caring very little for the hostile glances and remarks of our colleagues. We stuck to our studies faithfully and honestly and gathered together occasionally in our teacher Hahnemann's household some time after eight in the evening. . . .

This was then the little circle formed round Hahnemann which even under the best of circumstances had to tolerate much mockery and irony and in malicious cases, hatred and persecution, not only during the student years but far beyond them. I can always remember very clearly how Hornburg was worried in his Final Examination by the old pates and only just managed to escape being plucked, whilst miserable thickheads, not fit to wipe Hornburg's boots, passed cum laude and are now flourishing aloft here—narrow-minded but successful physicians.[18]

The homeopathic brand was being born. Handley notes:

Hahnemann's stature as a practitioner now also increased as he became more practised in his new art. With the new medicine he was able successfully to treat typhoid fever, the great scourge of the time. The efficacy of homeopathy became particularly apparent in 1813, after the bloody Battle of Leipzig between Prussian forces and Napoleon's army, retreating from the fiasco of Moscow. After three days of fighting just outside the city, there were 80,000 dead and 80,000 wounded. The streets were choked with refugees, it rained incessantly, food supplies were short and the drinking water polluted. Of the one hundred and eighty victims whom Hahnemann was able to treat, only two died. This convincing demonstration of the power of homeopathy was fully documented in Hahnemann's 1814 paper, "Treatment of Typhus Fever at Present Prevailing."[19]

Hahnemann's flourishing practice in Leipzig aroused medical jealousy and opposition. Not the least galling aspect was the financial benefits accruing to him and his disciples.[20] Despite Hahnemann's fame as a healer, homeopaths never won more than temporary and conditional rights to dispense medicines in Leipzig. Local apothecaries fought to maintain their control over all pharmacy in the city, homeopathic too, though they in no way understood the preparation of microdoses. Hahnemann continued to insist on making his own remedies, for they couldn't be fashioned correctly by ordinary druggists.

Handley reports that "on February 9th, 1820, Hahnemann was brought before the court and accused of encroaching upon the apothecaries' privileges by dispensing medicines. Despite his defence on March 15th, 1820, the judgment of the court was that Hahnemann was 'to cease the distributing and dispensing of any and every medicine to anybody . . . and to give no cause for severer regulations.' Without being able to prescribe and dispense, Hahnemann could not practise."[21]

In the United States, the FDA holds the same potential power today over not only homeopathics but all herbal remedies, vitamins, supplements, and off-label uses. It keeps homeopathy in a suspended state of irresolution with only tacit permission, for it has no real capacity to assay spiritual doses, only to ban what it cannot explain by the rules of foods and drugs.

In 1821 Hahnemann retreated to Köthen, in Anhalt, north of Saxony, where he lived under the protection of Duke Ferdinand, whom he had treated successfully. Gossip preceding him warned the populace of an evil magician, so stones of greeting were cast through his windows. It is no wonder that Hahnemann became increasingly apocalyptic.

Miasms

In Köthen Hahnemann wrote his last major work, *The Chronic Diseases, Their Peculiar Nature, and Their Homoeopathic Cure*, which appeared in 1828. Like Freud's *Civilization and Its Discontents*, also a late book by the founder of a system, and Wilhelm Reich's eleventh-hour screeds (*The Murder of Christ: The Emotional Plague of Mankind* and *The Mass Psychology of Fascism*), it is a pessimistic evaluation of humankind. All three believed that pathology was ingrained, though only Freud called life itself a condition. Since civilization, with its ego and superego had suppressed the id's animal nature, Freud said, psychoanalysis could offer no more than temporary and superficial relief. Reich compared diseased individuals to trees that had grown up crooked and could not be straightened without replanting the roots.

Hahnemann made his case before the twentieth century's mass genocides and world wars. Years of practice had shown him that intrinsic disease was not as curable as he had hoped, even with the Law of Similars and microdoses. He explained this persistent pathology as a collective disease, a cumulative miasm. The widespread reaction against homeopathy was a symptom of an emotional plague. Most early homeopaths were able to overlook this gloomy prognosis in the prosperity of successful practices, but later generations drew darker conclusions.

If Hahnemann's *Organon* is a sourcebook of practical homeopathy, his *Chronic Diseases* is a scripture of doom. In this oracle of medical philosophy, he seeks the original meaning of disease—any disease. He defines psora, or itch, as the primal malady, and leprosy as its florescence when suppressed. External symptoms of itch—rashes, pimples, sores, boils—were readily cleared up, but their internalized aggravations persisted. Deprived of its outlet on the skin, itch penetrated and weakened inner organs. Psora were also inheritable at any level to which they had been suppressed. Thus a child is born "healthy" only insofar as it has no external manifestation, but it carries within it the psoric potential accumulated in generations of its lineage.

Hahnemann rewrote history as mankind's progressive internalization of psora eventually penetrating mental and spiritual planes, from where they were exteriorized as cultural products—not only (in modern times) plagues, genocides, insurrections, and *interahamwe* but rap, hip-hop, graffiti, TikTok, avant-garde art and dance, even energy medicines. Hahnemann went on to ascribe seven-eighths of all chronic diseases to suppressed psora—psora so deeply suppressed that a succession of remedies is needed to unravel the archaeology of the disease in any individual. AIDS, Ebola, and Lyme disease, viewed homeopathically, are expressions of an internal plague manifesting on an external plane; so are oceanic garbage patches, nuclear weapons, and species extinctions. In *Chronic Diseases*, Hahnemann wrote:

Mankind . . . is worse off from the change in the external form of the *psora*—from leprosy down to the eruption of itch—not only because this is less visible and more secret and therefore more frequently infectious, but also because the *psora,* now mitigated externally into a mere itch, and on that account more generally spread, nevertheless still retains unchanged its original dreadful nature. Now, after being more easily repressed, the disease grows all the more unperceived within, and so, in the last three centuries, after the destruction of its chief symptom (the external skin-eruption) it plays the sad role of causing innumerable secondary symptoms; i.e., it originates a legion of chronic diseases, the source of which physicians neither surmise nor unravel, and which, therefore, they can no more cure than they could cure the original disease when accompanied by its cutaneous eruption; but these chronic diseases, as daily experience shows, were necessarily aggravated by the multitude of their faulty remedies.[22]

Most homeopaths view *The Chronic Diseases* as a statement of the unrecognized importance of skin ailments and the danger of repressing them dermatologically. They take its miasmatic aspects more metaphorically. Yet Hahnemann was not a dermatologist:

So great a flood of numberless nervous troubles, painful ailments, spasms, ulcers (cancers), adventitious formations, dyscrasias, paralyses, consumptions and cripplings of soul, mind and body were never seen in ancient times when the *psora* mostly confined itself to its dreadful cutaneous symptom, leprosy. Only during the last few centuries has mankind been flooded with these infirmities.[23]

Autoimmune diseases, connective tissue disorders, and chronic fatigues head the same list today.

The other two chronic miasms, syphilis and sycosis, according to Hahnemann, are relatively modern; they emerge from complications of psora and are usually treatable with homeopathic *Mercury* and *Nitricum acidum* (syphilis) and *Thuja* (sycosis).

On one level syphilis and sycosis (from the Greek *sykosis,* from *sykon,* "fig," not *psyche,* hence figwort disease, i.e., gonorrhea,* not psychosis) are venereal diseases. Their relationship to psora is tied to their inheritability and genital expression. They overlie psora and are the field in which it is camouflaged and expressed. In a sense, they are nothing more than venereal-genetic transductions or complication of basic psora.

In another sense, though, their entanglement suppresses the natural pattern of the psora and bumps it into more inharmonious vibrations. While psora abound and are infectious on an unimagined level ("the hermit on Montserrat escapes it as rarely in his rocky cell, as the little prince in his swaddling clothes of cambric"[24]), the overlaid miasms require either genital contact (fluid exchange) or transfer through offspring. They penetrate deeply on emotional and spiritual planes, and their venereal symptoms can interact with prior psoric disturbances to amplify pathology and insanity. The psora are incurable until a successful remedy is prescribed for their overriding complications. Hahnemann explained:

> Only when the whole organism feels itself transformed by this peculiar chronic-miasmatic disease, the diseased vital force endeavours to alleviate and to soothe the internal malady through the

---

*Sycosis generally describes barber's itch and scrofula, neither of which are venereal or gonorrheal.

establishment of a suitable local symptom on the skin, the itch-vesicle. So long as this eruption continues in its normal form, the internal psora with its secondary ailments cannot break forth, but must remain covered, slumbering, latent and bound. While the external symptom is left in place on the skin the general health of the organism is not immediately threatened, but the illness, nevertheless, continues to grow. If the surface symptom is removed, "cured," the disease may become latent for a while, but will eventually be forced to return or seek another outlet, perhaps in a more important organ.[25]

A homeopathic homily states that it was the syphilitic predisposition in Beethoven that allowed him to create beautiful music—and the syphilitic miasm in us that hears it as beautiful.

As a text, *The Chronic Diseases* is a voluminous compilation of psoric symptoms followed by sixteen hundred pages of antipsoric remedies and their indications. The later Hahnemann not only honored very high potencies but invented some of the most dilute scales in the history of physical science to address the depth of miasmatic illness.

Hahnemann's miasmatic analysis had carried him well past his original proposition of constitutional disturbances curable through activation of the vital force. When he came down, like Moses from the mountain with new commandments, he found his disciples worshipping the idols. He wrote angrily in a newspaper:

I have heard for a long time and with displeasure, that some in Leipsic, who pretend to be Homeopaths, allow their patients to choose whether they shall be treated homeopathically or allopathically. . . . Let them . . . not require of me that I should recognise them as my true disciples. . . .

Blood-letting, the application of leeches and Spanish flies, the use of fontanels and setons, mustard plasters and medicated bags, embrocations with salves and aromatic spirits, emetics, purgatives, various sorts of warm baths, pernicious doses of calomel, quinine, opium and musk, are some of the quackeries by which, when used in conjunction with homeopathic prescriptions, we are able to recognise the crypto-homeopath, trying to make himself popular. . . . They swagger in the cradle of homeopathic science (as they choose to call Leipsic) where its founder first stepped forward as a teacher. But behold! I have never yet acknowledged you; away from me, ye medical—![26] [The newspaper chose not to print the final word.]

Later miasmatic layers have been diagnosed by esoteric homeopaths since Hahnemann's time. By now we may be more miasmic than human as rap, artificial intelligence, abstract expressionism, avant-garde dance, and revenge porn replace the melancholy chords of Beethoven and expressive colorizations of J. M. W. Turner in our long waves.

Medical Theocracy

Many homeopathic movements sprang up in the early nineteenth century, not only in Leipzig where seeds were sown, but throughout Europe and America. Hahnemann's fame spread, in part because of his successful cures during the European cholera epidemic of 1831–32. In a perception that predates microbiology, he described minute but discrete disease entities. He defined the "cholera miasm" as an "organism of lower order" and later spoke of an "invisible cloud of perhaps millions of such miasmatic living organisms, which, first brought to life on the broad and marshy shores of the tepid Ganges, are continually seeking out man to his destruction."[27]

In the last years of his life, Hahnemann renounced many of the doctors and hospitals he had initially blessed and helped found. As his reputation grew and spread, he charged heretofore unheard of sums of money for his services while continuing to work on later editions of the *Organon*. He had moved from empiricism to medical theocracy. Then an unexpected event whisked him away from his disciples and practice.

Hahnemann's wife of forty-nine years died in the spring of 1830, and in 1834, a French woman, thirty-two years of age, having been inspired by the *Organon*, arrived in Köthen, ostensibly to meet the author in person and seek his aid. Handley writes:

It is clear that what started out as a professional consultation took an unforeseen turn. Within three days of their meeting Hahnemann had proposed to Mélanie, and she had accepted. She had at last found a man she could admire as well as love, and he found himself kissing and embracing her in not quite the "paternal" manner he had originally intended. Over the following three months Mélanie sent a number of letters to him which show how immediate and powerful was the attraction between them. In only her second letter she wrote: "You have told me: 'I have never loved anyone so much as you, we shall love each other till eternity.' You have said: 'I cannot live any longer without you, stay with me for ever; we must be married.'" She had responded: "I can no longer live now without your good opinion and love;" and "you will always be my husband in my thoughts; no other man will ever lay a profane hand on me, no mouth other than yours will kiss my mouth. I give you my faith, and I swear to you eternal love and fidelity."[28]

They were married in June 1835. He was eighty. He had always praised and even prescribed marriage, on one occasion before remarrying calling it "a general specific for body and soul."[29] With Marie Mélanie Hahnemann, he moved to Paris, where she presented him to the French homeopathic community. It was as though, on a journey to the land of the dead, she had returned with Hippocrates himself.

Hahnemann lived in Paris until his eighty-ninth year, practicing medicine, continuing to revise his books, and preaching against the ravages of allopathy and what he called "homeopathic half-breeds." He was cared for, admired, and pampered. The gossip that surrounded his departure from Leipzig, however, expanded in his absence. Visitors to Paris claimed that his wife had taken over his practice, that no one could see Hahnemann except through her, and that she alone did the diagnosis and prescribing while he sat, impassive and observing. It was also reported that he prescribed two remedies at one time, a violation of the single cure. In any case, the combination of his charisma and fame as a miracle physician and the notoriety of his marriage to a woman well-known in French intellectual and artistic circles brought no end of wealthy and notable patients and curiosity-seekers to the Hahnemanns' lodge.

Madame Hahnemann did, in fact, assume her husband's prescribing, but no simple conclusion can be drawn from this, and certainly not that the old man was bewitched or addled. He chose a form of retirement and discipleship through her. Perhaps he saw in her a medical brilliance and strength, for she did later become a homeopathic physician of talent and renown after his death. Aware of the delicacy of the situation, she wrote of Hahnemann's daughters: "They treat me like an adventuress who has probably come to seduce you, and you (the author of the *Organon*) like a feeble and libertine old man."[30]

This was not the case. From his Paris outpost, Hahnemann continued to participate in the spread and advancement of homeopathy. His instruction of an English physician from India led to the emergence of homoeopathy on that subcontinent. Yet he dropped out of touch with former associates and abandoned his children in Saxony, even in his will. His death, on July 2, 1843, went unannounced for many weeks, and his interment was private—no friends or family from either France or Saxony. Marie Mélanie Hahnemann buried her husband at a grave site occupied by two other spouses she had already outlived by the age of thirty-two—and she kept the sixth revision of the *Organon* unavailable during her lifetime, likely because its requirements for editing and publication overwhelmed her.

Hahnemann was, all his life, an avowed Christian, even in his departures. Obsessed with robust health, he mixed exercise with scholarship. He was a stern father and unyielding teacher and master, blind to any other psychological or spiritual system. Born at midnight, the legendary cusp of prophecy and revelation, he had the sort of mind and attention that bore through diversions and distractions to the center of things. But he never turned that analysis back on himself, on his own emotional life or behavior. Like many sages and gurus, he was a mystic more by ideology than by practice.

So homeopathy comes to us as a system of tags and epigrams in an unexamined cosmology. That hasn't affected its practice, growth, or seeming veridicality, but veridical to what? Hahnemann's original loyalty may have been to physical science, botany, and laboratory chemistry, but by the time his dominos were in place, spirit had replaced matter. From there, he created and practiced as an artist with homeopathy his medium. There are plants, animals, minerals, and radiations and, of course flesh-and-blood people and their pathologies, but beneath these is a pattern of energies, vibrations, and frequencies. Hahnemann's puritanical stubbornness led him to keep calling his mishmash regular old medicine or mainstream science and to attempt to deliver it to the world as orthodoxy, though he had made the clinical practice of occult or quantum chemistry. Even today, as poet William Blake augured, physics is a dream from which we have yet to awake.

The only way back into matter for Hahnemann would have been through mind—psychosomatic or somatoemotional transduction— but he never admitted mind into his system, either as psyche or episteme, hence homeopathy's nonintersecting, parallel course with

psychiatry. Jung later called spirit back into matter through individuation of personal and collective psyches. His marriage of spirit and
matter yielded archetypes: geometric shapes, myths, and morphologies concomitant to Similars in flowers, crystals, starfish, cuttlefish,
and galaxies, as we saw in Whitmont's interpretations of homeopathic
remedies. The "archetypes" are the mind or intelligence behind matter that minded matter recognizes in itself.

Early physical science had divorced itself from magic's "wireless"
divinations, replacing dodecahedrons and zodiacs with apples and
orbits. By installments, it developed its own instrumentality. Kepler
and Newton were fence-sitters who didn't know there was a fence.
Paracelsus, Giordano Bruno, Edward Kelley, John Dee, Robert Fludd,
Francis Bacon, John Donne, Michael Maier, Thomas Digges, and
Galileo Galilei fell on either side of the invisible picket.

Nowadays historians assign Copernicus, Newton, Galileo, and
Bacon to the scientific half, but in their time they were members of
a sorcerers' lodge too. Crossover hermeticism was practiced by Plato,
Ptolemy, Paracelsus, Fludd, Dee, and Agrippa. They were receptive to
both *magikos* (enchantment, sorcery) and *experior* (experience, experiment), rendering respectively unto God and Caesar.

British historian Frances Yates documents a Rosicrucian movement that stretched from Greco-Roman, Egyptian, and pseudo-
Egyptian sources through Europe's sixteenth and seventeenth
centuries. In benchmark texts—*Giordano Bruno and the Hermetic
Tradition, The Rosicrucian Enlightenment, Theatre of the World*, and
The Art of Memory—she depicted "the roots of the change that came
over man when his life was no longer integrated into the divine life
of the universe," adding, "In the company of 'Hermes Trismegistus,'
one treads the borderlands between magic and religion, magic and
science, magic and art or poetry and music. It was in those elusive
realms that the man of the Renaissance dwelt."[31]

It may have been a midsummer night's dream, but it wasn't a fallow slumber. Technology has launched air travel and built skyscrapers but, with its side effects of climate change, pollution, and extinction, marks the dream's shift into nightmare. It may take another century or two to resolve it definitively.

After scientists succeeded in separating crafts and objective experiments from charms of magicians, they valorized the empirically oriented works of Newton, Darwin, James Maxwell, and crew, while discounting and excluding their concomitant alchemy, astrology, and magic as defects of clouded intellects. Newton the alchemist and Darwin the theologian were dismissed.

But science ended up, two centuries later, back in the "hermetic" lodge, confronting the Sphinx and Oracle in new guises: light waves, relativity, quantum entanglement, nanodose effects. Max Planck, Werner Heisenberg, Erwin Schrödinger, Niels Bohr, and Albert Einstein had no choice but to become magic moles. The subatomic universe was, if not telekinetic, consciousness-infested.

Concluding her discussion of Rosicrucianism and Freemasonry, Yates described a current in which scientist-magicians swam, "a reservoir of spiritual and intellectual power, of moral and reforming vision." She noted:

The great mathematical and scientific thinkers of the seventeenth century have at the back of their minds Renaissance traditions of esoteric thinking, of mystical continuity from Hebraic or 'Egyptian' wisdom, of that conflation of Moses with 'Hermes Trismegistus' that fascinated the Renaissance. . . . Below, or beyond, their normal religious affiliations they would see the Great Architect of the Universe as an all-embracing religious conception which included, and encouraged, the scientific urge to explore the Architect's work.[32]

And, finally, the urge to decode, deconstruct, and replicate. That is where we are today: a magic driven by science's stake in matter and its struggle to hold off its own shadow and blowback. Microdoses are as much its ghost and gadfly as UFOs and krakens.

Hahnemann's "archetypes" were spirit-like quantum energies imprinted on balls of sugar and alcohol—each pellet chemically inert, but each containing a song that could manifest through a living organism. By ignoring mind as mind, Hahnemann translated intelligence directly out of matter itself.

Then he fell before the attractions of the anima and was lured from family and disciples into a foreign country by a nixie adept in such trysts, who withheld his final work and buried him unnamed in a tomb with her earlier lovers.

Yet this last escapade was a heroic statement of homeopathic vitality, to adventure amorously rather than to stay in Leipzig and squabble with foes until his death. One Saxon journalist accused him of trying "to prove to the world how his system has been glorified in him. . . . The young man is still vigorous and strong, and challenges all Allopaths: imitate me if you can!"[33] Hahnemann had long ago cast his lot in strange lands with unknown voices, and in his eighties, with his scholarship completed, he vanished into exile again and returned his system to the pagan forces whose offspring it was.

Homeopathy had been his destiny and crowning achievement, but it took him a lifetime to get there, and then he transformed it back into a cipher: one remedy, many remedies; material medicine, spiritual medicine; overt disease, covert disease; curable ailments, miasmatic complexes. No wonder homeopathy has sought a clarification and second coming since.

6

The Homeopathic Tradition in North America

The Rise, Fall, and Reprise of American Homeopathy: A Précis

Homeopathy had its heyday in the early nineteenth century as America's first great medical fad. It was both heralded and vilified as the "New School." By the Civil War, homeopaths were more numerous than allopaths and maintained a network of prestigious medical schools and hospitals. Hahnemann's protocols of hygiene had helped modernize general medicine, and he was still one of the "good guys." Only after the mainstream establishment adopted a series of reforms, many suggested by him, did it dismiss his signature method of treatment.

In 1844, three years before the advent of the American Medical Association (AMA), the American Institute of Homeopathy was founded in order to license homeopathic physicians and maintain standards of practice. The body also served as a clearinghouse for provings of North American native plants and other new remedies.

The AMA was formed, in part, as a competing guild to protect the interests of allopathic physicians; it was to become many things thereafter, but it was *never* a neutral scientific body.

The winds of enthusiasm that made homeopathy a major American medicine at the time of the Civil War and in the decades after changed trajectory in the early twentieth century. In a very short period, homeopathy went from a progressive modern medicine to a museum piece per the principles chemists and biologists chose to agree on and, as lawmakers of the scientific community, imposed on all systems purporting to be science. Until then, medical science was like the cartoon cat that, having crawled beyond the branch onto which it had first climbed, forgot to look down. It finally did—and saw nothing.

Subsequently homeopathy succumbed to a no-holds-barred attack by the AMA, supported later by pharmaceutical companies. In its restandardization of medicine and goal of consistency and accountability, the AMA either did away with or adapted every alternative method and technique—homeopathic, osteopathic, naturopathic—to its own paradigm. That is where matters stand. Most Americans today know nothing of either homeopathy or allopathy: there are only doctors, diseases, and treatments.

Most early twentieth-century homeopaths in America acceded to the verdict and joined the mainstream. Many jumped ship because they no longer understood the distinction between homeopathy and allopathy or between vitalism and materialism. They did not want to be deemed quacks or lose their lien on the cutting edge of science. Also, earning both AMA credentials for practicing medicine itself (the M.D. license) and a separate homeopathy license was expensive and time-consuming. It was not long before a homeopathic certificate had roughly the standing of a Ph.D. in alchemy. Yet a bare beat of history had passed since homeopathy's renaissance.

In the late twentieth century, homeopathy was revived as an

alternative medicine, but its restored version did not entirely match Hahnemannian homeopathy, which had evolved in an eighteenth- and nineteenth-century framework. Similarly, modern shamanism, acupuncture, and osteopathy do not exactly replicate their forerun- ners. New applications and syntheses bring together historically diver- gent systems and create novel modalities from their fusions. Consider the broader modern mix of flower remedies, herbal tinctures, entheo- gens, homeopathic nanodoses, and nonhomeopathic microdosing.

Early American allopathy, with its leeches and mercury medi- cines, likewise bore little resemblance to current allopathy, which is a mixture of traditional Western medical theory, breakthroughs made during and since the late nineteenth century, and an ongoing tradi- tion of empirical experimentation.

Since the mid-twentieth century, medical science has progressed to genomic research and CRISPR technology. The present goal is to cut and splice the life code itself and extirpate inherited diseases at their DNA basis, even to drive our genome's evolution—and not just the human genome. Homeopathy addresses the vital basis of those same helices without contacting or cutting and patching them or turning the life code into a data card. How biotech and homeopathy can be reconciled and find common goals is a task for a future medi- cal science.

Nineteenth-Century American Medicine

New World homeopaths began to practice in the mid-1820s. Most were immigrant European doctors, though a few American-born physi- cians learned the system by correspondence with colleagues or on visits abroad. A graduate of Germany's Wurtzburg University, Constantine Hering, founded the first American school of homeopathy, the Nordamerikanisch Akademie der Homeopathischen Heilkunst, in Allentown, Pennsylvania, in 1835, with instruction in German. The academy trained doctors for six years. Seven years after its closing, Hering revived it as the Homeopathic Medical College in Philadelphia, with instruction in English. Graduates of his college diffused primarily to Middle Atlantic and southern states, while fresh homeopaths arriving from Germany put out their shingles across the East Coast and Midwest.

During the nineteenth century, the North American medical profession was a mélange of modalities beyond a dialectic of homeopathy and allopathy. As plants indigenous to North America were studied by generations of European-trained herbalists, they were freely incorporated by newcomers. Midwives, Indigenous American–trained doctors, and lay herbal practitioners thrived in cooperation with one another, leading to a hybrid of traditional European botanicals with naturopathic remedies developed in the New World. New systems of manipulation and palpation like osteopathy and chiropractic were systematized, then taught and disseminated through their own medical colleges (see below). The system of steam baths and herbal treatments of the New Hampshire farmer Samuel Thomson was especially popular, and his followers operated their own hospitals, drug manufacturing plants, and drugstores. In 1839, when the whole population of the United States was estimated to be seventeen million, Thomsonism had three million patients.

An age-old suspicion of doctors still lurked. People suffered from ailments caused by calomel, as mercury poisoning became its own quiet epidemic. Mothers clutched their children in the presence of the family doctor and would not let them be treated during outbreaks of malaria, croup, and other respiratory and intestinal diseases.

While homeopathy appealed to patrons of naturopaths and Thomsonians, it also reassured the mainstream public by providing physicians trained in medical schools who gave pleasant-tasting sugar pills by contrast to high doses of foul-tasting mercury. Homeopaths also heard out a person's full complaints before proceeding; they took life histories.

The outward simplicity of homeopathy enhanced its popularity. It was intellectually arcane but functionally accessible. A lay practitioner need know nothing about advanced physiology or chemistry. Pills could be dispensed by clergymen, lawyers, housewives, and babysitters. Hering put out a kit with instructions for common maladies. Pills were identified only by numbers. A certain condition might require number 8, but if the fever was higher, number 3 was used, or number 12 if the ailment was primarily on the right side, or number 18 if it turned into a rash. It was not uncommon for the wives and children of allopaths to treat their families homeopathically in secret while the head of the household failed to notice or care any more than he might worry about a box of exotic chocolates.

The cholera epidemic of 1849 was a major boon for the homeopathic brand. The allopathic establishment had no cure for the scourge. Though bleeding was of little use, it remained the allopathic Hail Mary. Hahnemann had tried *Camphor* for cholera, with the remedy's symptoms of alternating diarrhea and constipation "similar" to those of the disease, and it soon became the main homeopathic remedy. In Cincinnati, homeopaths claimed a 97 percent cure rate in over a thousand cases and published a daily list of patients in the newspaper with names and addresses of those who were cured and those who died under both allopathic and homeopathic care.

It is no wonder that an allopaths-only medical organization was established soon after. It was a counterpunch. The strictures of the American Medical Association, founded in 1847, enforced later by Abraham Flexner's report titled *Medical Education in the United States and Canada* (1910), marginalized homeopathy by turning it into a poster child for charlatanism and quackery.

Mid-nineteenth-century allopaths had a hard time accepting the cholera results. Alternate hypotheses were advanced: late-acting allopathic remedies, medical hypnotism, placebo, even the flaws of their own techniques, hence the advantage of *no* treatment at all (which is what they considered homeopathy). A common interpretation of the unusually high cure rate of homeopathic hospitals was that it came not from their medicines but from their hygiene and diet. By prescribing "nothing," they followed the Hippocratic rule: "first do no harm." Nature did their work for them.

Copying Hahnemann's methods changed allopathy from within, shifting it toward homeopathy's priorities of sanitation and nutrition without turning it into homeopathy. But allopaths could not allow the validity of microdoses or power of Similars.

The model of the "irritable mechanism," developed by William Cullen and John Brown in England, was the prevailing fashion in early American medical-school biology. The body was portrayed as a machine made out of protoplasm, with membranous pipes, pulleys, levers, and strainers, its hydraulics maintained by breath and heart pumps. Doctors prescribed to either provoke or relax spasms. For an overactive system, vomiting was induced or blood drawn off and cold baths administered. Even though bleeding with leeches was deemed a relaxant, some doctors bled to stimulate, using an epicycle-like model to explain the contradictory effect and save their own appearances. Opium, liquors, hot baths, garlic, mercury, and wine by the gallon were used for phlegmatic ailments as stimulants. This rationale lingers today in laxative formulas and "coffee breaks" to disperse stalled matter in the bowels, the magnesias, alkaline milks, and vegetable antacids dumped into an overactive gut, and triple-antibiotic ointments. An "allopathic" glass of wine can be taken as either a relaxant or a stimulant at dinner.

Eighteenth-century oversimplification, reinforced by fad, had settled on one mercurous chloride medicine, originally a stimulant, as the absolute cure-all. Called "calomel," after the Greek for "beautiful black," though its final form was a white powder, it was used in high doses for every imaginable illness and as a general preventive for future ailments. Benjamin Rush, the most respected American physician of the late eighteenth and early nineteenth centuries, was a strong advocate of mercury and bloodletting. Harris Coulter described a scene from the 1793 yellow fever epidemic in Philadelphia:

> Rush was surrounded one day . . . by a crowd in Kensington, north of Philadelphia. All implored him to come and treat their families.
>
> There were several hundred. Rush, without stepping down, threw back the top of his curricle, and addressed the multitude "with a few conciliatory remarks." Then he cried in a loud voice, "I treat my patients successfully by bloodletting and copious purging with calomel and jalap—and I advise you, my good friends, to use the same remedies."
>
> "What?" called a voice from the crowd, "bleed and purge every one?"
>
> "Yes!" said the doctor. "Bleed and purge all Kensington! Drive on, Ben!"[1]

Some historians of medicine still use the alibi that early American homeopaths were successful primarily because they did *not* use mercury or draw blood.

Initially Americans did not have a clear sense of homeopathy. Some patients and doctors assumed it was a sect of German medicine. Others lumped it with Indigenous medicines as another botanical apothecary. Its difference from allopathy was so poorly understood that many doctors considered them compatible systems, varying only as one physician varies from another.

The late nineteenth century was a transitional time overall in America, marked by a border war between Missouri and Kansas, bank and train robberies by outlaws Frank and Jesse James, and coal-mine strikes in Idaho during which anarchist miners dynamited trainloads of scabs, their own mines, and then the governor himself. Exotic Christian cults flourished. Millenary churches featuring clairvoyance, clairaudience, and automatic writing encompassed branches of Freemasonry, theosophical covenants, Swedenborgian churches, John Ballou Newbrough's 1882 *Oahspe* Jehovan Bible, and Mary Baker Eddy's Christian Science. Blending elements eclectically, the Church of Jesus Christ of the Latter-Day Saints (LDS) with its telekinetic golden tablets proved to be the superstar and main survivor of early American millenarianism.

In the early twentieth century, unfederated metaphysics was a popular passion, as evidenced by *The Urantia Book*, two-thousand-plus pages of extraterrestrial dictation to a group of otherwise skeptical intellectuals in 1920s Chicago. Religious in orientation, *Urantia* was Christianized science fiction, with chapters such as "The Central and Superuniverses," "The Local Universe," and "Earth (Urantia)." It concluded with seventy-seven papers on "The Life and Teachings of Jesus," a set of apocrypha surpassing the New Testament itself, with details on Christ's childhood, teenage years, and preaching tours.

In a Barnum & Bailey, Ripley's Believe It or Not, Houdini landscape, homeopathy flourished without a second glance, its true gist unnoticed. How much of a freak is a microdose beside a four-legged girl, a bird-eating tarantula, and underwater escapes from padlocked chains?

As homeopathic works were translated into English and homeopathic doctors became more prevalent, allopaths began to realize this was more than another branch of science; it was an attack on their own models of organismic irritability, proposing to supersede them with a superior etiology; that made it an existential threat to their livelihoods. They began depicting homeopathy as a Euro-scam based on illusional properties contrived to hoodwink backwoods Americans. "Sane men," doctors declared, "should not be fooled by such patent bunkum." Wrote one: "[The] whole art is reduced to the precision of a game of ninepins."[2] Another described it as "the entire range of diseases, the entire range of therapeutics, converted into Chinese puzzles; the phenomena of diseases and the effects of drugs upon them treated as algebraical equations."[3]

These critiques, which are as salient today, missed the forest for the trees. Homeopathy is not a reduction to ninepins; it is a shift from gross anatomy—the walnut and its many shells—to the vital force, which is overdetermined along multiple pathways. Notions of "free energy" are *always* anathema to materialists. Yet though they still hunt for the grail of nuclear fusion, they ignore nanodoses and psi phenomena.

The Zenith of Homeopathy in America and the Dawn of Its Demise

Though vulnerabilities in their pharmaceutical model were being exposed, homeopaths generally ignored them. Through the 1870s and 1880s, and into the early twentieth century regionally in the United States, they were enjoying unprecedented success, doing three to seven times the business of allopaths with the backing of politicians and commercial interests, the editorial support of the *Detroit Daily Tribune* and the *New York Times*, and a conservative lobby much like today's gun lobby in the Republican Party (without ideological concomitance). During the yellow fever epidemic of the 1870s in the South, homeopaths not only used microdoses successfully but succeeded in legislating sanitary reforms in the canals, sewage systems, dry wells, and bogs around Savannah and New Orleans. Elsewhere, homeopaths were appointed to state medical boards and federal pension examination panels. They were supported by government funds and covered by insurance companies. In the late nineteenth century, hundreds of homeopathic hospitals, clinics, insane asylums (or "sane asylums," as medical historian Jerry Kantor likes to call them), nursing homes, orphanages, and schools dotted the United States and were as unchallenged as gas stations, public schools, and supermarket chains today.

The first serious countershot was fired unnoticed in 1842 when the New York State Medical Society ruled that homeopathy was not science but a form of quackery and "a departure from the principles of a well-defined system of medical ethics."[4] Committee members contended that Hahnemannian medicine should *not* be granted immunity as an independent medical system with its own licensing because it dealt in sugar tablets under the guise of pharmacy. Four years later, when the National Medical Convention met in New York to review their homeopathic dilemma, the members agreed that, since homeopathic pills were placebos, the public success of homeopathy was likely a result of their own poor marketing and public relations.

Since many of the allopaths' own medical schools at the time were unscrupulous or spurious, issuing bogus degrees (risible QDs: doctorates of quackery), it was difficult for the public to tell the difference between a fake certificate and an affidavit from a real training program. In preparation for their trademark battle against alternative practitioners, allopaths set out to police their own ranks. If they could define who they were and what they did, they would be able to interdict everyone not practicing sound science according to their rules. Homeopaths, naturopaths and other so-called "medical illusionists" could be marginalized as quacks. The AMA's long-term goal, they averred, was the improvement of medical education for the good of all. That was likely true for a majority of allopaths, but the short-term goal of the firebrands was the ostracism of homeopaths, naturopaths, and, later, unrepentant osteopaths.

In its original charter, the AMA withheld membership from state and local medical organizations until they assured the national organization that no homeopaths belonged. Only Massachusetts balked. In 1856 the AMA banned any discussion of homeopathic medical theory in its journals and threatened the expulsion of any member doctor who consulted with a homeopath. Allopaths married to homeopaths were also expelled!

A version of allopathy's historic battle with homeopathy was repeated during the twenty-first-century COVID-19 pandemic when previously well-regarded physicians who questioned gene-transfer vaccines or prescribed ivermectin and hydroxychloroquine for the virus had their medical licenses revoked irrespective of their success in treating patients and absent any complaints. Hard-won certificates were cancelled by the whims of politicians who had spent not half a second in medical school.

In the fall of 2022, 187,000 people worldwide watched a livestream of Dr. Meryl Nass's hearing before six attorneys general in Maine as she defended herself against a medical board (two regulation-minded doctors, two commercial pharmacists, and a real-estate agent) that had suspended her right to practice. Nass was not just a successful lifelong family and hospital physician with countless satisfied patients and no black marks, but also an expert in anthrax, Lyme, Ebola, and vaccines in general and had been employed by the government to resolve bioterrorism issues. She also used homeopathic and herbal remedies when indicated and practiced Buddhist meditation.

Like now, the early-twentieth-century allopathic establishment argued that its stance was against *all* quackery in an attempt to police the medical profession. But homeopathy was its original target, and medical monopoly its ultimate goal.

Initially the strategy failed. The public was offended by a rule that seemed arbitrary and excluded cherished doctors, in fact sometimes the only physician in a town or region. Most people viewed medical philosophy as a side issue and consulted their preferred local physicians regardless of affinity. Doctors were also used to cooperating with each other and taking each others' patients in emergencies. It seemed like politics rather than medicine.

While the majority of medical schools eventually ceded to the new regime, some, the University of Michigan in particular, retained a homeopathic curriculum and eventually forced a compromise on the AMA. In Michigan, many members of the board of regents were patients of homeopaths, and local elected officials were inclined to favor their own doctors over a trade association.

More significant, ultimately, was the inevitable if inadvertent merger of the two systems. The average homeopath already practiced some allopathy as a conversion to "modern" medicine. Innovative equipment and procedures were, in a sense, nondenominational, adopted by virtually all practicing physicians. The current hard distinction between homeopathy and allopathy was still abeyant. So even as homeopathy survived a frontal allopathic assault, the number of pure traditional homeopaths declined by attrition, by crossover, and because it was a difficult system to understand, explain, and justify biochemically. They lapsed into "homeopathic allopaths."

Without a scientific rationale that could be analyzed and updated, homeopathy fragmented from within. Some homeopathic physicians viewed themselves simply as doctors and considered "homeopathy" and "allopathy" obsolete labeling. To them, the Law of Similars was just one rubric of nature and curative principle. They adopted new protocols and drugs and upheld technological progress and an ideal of universal medicine without a corresponding commitment to Similars. They preferred low potencies because these still had some physical substance in them and were compatible with vogue American pharmacy and science. Their arguments against *totally* nonmaterial doses paralleled ones that allopaths had been making for decades. They strayed from Hahnemann's laws without knowing it and without certainty as to what homeopathy even was. It was easier to follow the futurist parade.

Mainstream medicine took notes from homeopathy's book, giving the appearance of compromise and integration. While allopaths did not switch to "spiritual" pills, they recognized that their own heroic doses were counterproductive and dangerous—that sheer mass of medicine did not equate to power or degree of healing. Acceptance of specifics returned, and the standard medicine chest was updated and restocked. Calomel, quinine, and jalap quietly passed out of fashion and, with them, bleeding. Doctors experimented with different natural remedies and compounds innovated by emerging drug companies. Those who did not accept microdoses could prescribe the same substances in material form. If a physician valued a remedy from the homeopathic materia medica but did not accept the Law of Similars, he could explain its action mechanically, e.g., that *Kali nitricum*, or St. Ignatius's bean, had the power to stimulate the system. Since much of the homeopathic pharmacopoeia came from classical, medieval, and Arabic sources, the allopathic drugstore could reclaim its shared heritage with a supply chain going back to Paracelsus and earlier.

The blurring of pharmaceutical distinctions made it easier for ordinary homeopaths to stray from Hahnemannian purity. The AMA didn't defeat homeopathy outright. Allopathy became palatable enough for most homeopaths to embrace it even as numerous allopaths were endorsing Similars in macrodose form.

One prominent allopath, William Holcombe, wrote of his guilt and sleeplessness the day he administered his first homeopathic remedies out of frustration when nothing else worked: "The spirit of Allopathy, terrible as a nightmare, came down fiercely upon me and would not let me rest. What right had I to dose that poor fellow with Hahnemann's medicinal moonshine?"[5]

Demographic factors played an overlooked role. In the medical census at the end of the nineteenth century, the ranks of homeopathy had swelled with newcomers and converts from the yellow fever and cholera epidemics. These doctors were poorly, if at all, trained in repertorizing and the materia medica, so they were practicing allopathy with a slightly "Similar" bent. Opportunistically attempting to follow more lucrative currents, they too were swept into general medicine.

Homeopathy was buoyed by the mid-nineteenth-century lifestyle, while allopathy benefited from twentieth-century demographic shifts. Local homeopaths had been used to continued contact with not only single patients but families, communities, and generations. Social continuity supported their detailed symptom assessment and ensured a stable clientele. Through the transportation revolution of the twentieth century, the homeopathic clientele began to fission. People did not move their medical philosophies across the country, so they came to count on standardization from locale to locale. A shifting populace reinforced what seemed most expedient and "scientific." Marooned by economic and social forces beyond their control, many homeopaths resorted to any remedies that would get quick results. Specialization became as popular and essential in medicine as in other facets of an industrializing society. In this general sweep, homeopaths were absorbed into allopathy, priests who forgot their own ceremonies.

Osteopathy

Homeopathy was not the only American alternative medicine that came into conflict with the allopathic establishment. Osteopathy was developed by Andrew Taylor Still in the 1870s in Kansas. Like homeopathy, it began as a physical science and turned into an energy medicine only after experiments and actual practice revealed other layers. The founders of osteopathy (Still) and, at the turn of the twentieth century, cranial osteopathy (William Sutherland) started as loyal mechanists and ended up as vitalists based on their empirical discoveries. In much the same way, Hahnemann started out as a pharmacist and ended up as an alchemist or nanochemist.

Osteopathy evolved from a solidist model of the body as an "irritable" mechanism. Andrew Taylor Still was an engineer seeking a method for curing ailments by working the body's pipes, pulleys, levers, strainers, and hydraulics, filling and draining its channels (veins and arteries) and ponds (bladders). As a materialist, he believed that he was palpating tissues, organs, and bones—God's machinery—not cellular resonances, let alone subcellular frequencies and chakralike control centers. Yet he opened the door to anatomical vitalism—a science still not exhumed over a century later.

Still's disciple, William Sutherland, discovered a deeper subtle-energy field by experimenting on himself with a helmet designed to restrict the movements of the bones of his cranium. His "craniosacral provings" led to an array of exotic maladies in his body, a distortion of mental and emotional states, and a set of techniques for treating them by palpation based on the flow of cerebrospinal fluid, the texture of tissues, and the fractal compression of bones and other anatomical shear forces. Contemporary cranial-osteopathy practitioners continue to find new governance centers, with homunculi dispatching epigenetic information and pulses that radiate throughout the fascia, musculoskeletal webs, and viscera.

Daniel David Palmer, the founder of chiropractic in the 1890s, was not a solidist; he began with magnetic healing and subluxations (for electromagnetic and mechanical misalignments of the spine). In the development of chiropractic healing, bones become tuning forks, living grids that share information with other organs. Patients feel as though they are being globally recalibrated and then put back together.

Palmer ultimately merged with many of Still's theories and practices, so these modalities coalesced. They are now practiced with homeopathy in the same holistic clinics.

The Birth of the Modern
Pharmaceutical Industry

A pharmaceutical revolution also played a role in the transformation of nineteenth- and early twentieth-century medicine. When
calomel-style drugs passed into disuse, they were replaced by a mixture of Indigenous medicines, substances originating in homeopathic
materia medicas, and new laboratory compounds. Coulter's survey
of contemporary pharmaceuticals derived from homeopathy during the late nineteenth century includes *Apis mellifica* (bee poison
for rheumatism), *Bryonia, Cactus* (as a heart medicine), *Cannabis*
(for gonorrhea), *Cocculus indicus, Conium* (for cancer and paralysis),
Drosera rotundifolia (for whooping cough), *Hellebore, Pulsatilla
nigricans,* and *Rhus toxicodendron* (poison ivy).[6]

The common use of other medicines was extended by homeopathic provings. Camphor for cholera was one instance. Homeopathy
introduced *Thuja occidentalis* (arbor vitae) for secondary illness
caused by vaccination and gonorrhea. Poison nut and red pepper came
to be prescribed in paralysis and hemorrhoids, respectively; *Ailanthus
glandulosa* for scarlet fever and coffee for headaches were also homeopathic extensions.[7] They, along with all the other indigenous herbal
medicines, were jumbled, displaced, and obscured in the synthetic
melee of modern pharmacy, but they lie at its base, along with medicines from rainforests and outbacks. Newly powerful drug factories
came to render all doctors obsolete. Coulter wrote:

> Sharpe and Dohme, E. R. Squibb, and Frederick Stearns got
> their start during the Civil War and were later joined by William
> R. Warner (1866), Parke-Davis (1867), Mallinckrodt Chemica
> Works (1867), Eli Lilly (1876), William S. Merrell, H. M. Merrell,
> E. Merck, Abbott Laboratories, and others. For the first decade
> these firms competed in terms of the traditional medicines used

by the profession. In the 1870s, however, it became clear that this was too narrow a channel for disposing of the commodities of an ever-growing industry, and the outcome was an invasion by these "ethical" drug companies of the patent-medicine field.[8]

That is, drug companies, after appropriating and then patenting copyright-commons medicines from both First Nations and colonists, pyramided from the production of simple recipes whose ingredients were familiar to physicians and whose uses were established by tradition to the invention and marketing of complex synthetic compounds whose basic chemistry was unfamiliar and whose uses had to be extrapolated almost entirely by the principle of Contraries or antidoting. The ingredients of new formulas known as "proprietaries" were trade secrets of the drug companies producing them, and their application was little more than a designation on the label. They could be marketed directly through pharmacies to clients, who would be "informed" by advertising rather than provings or cause-and-effect backup. Even though doctors stood between a drug company and a pharmacy, they would be as ignorant as the patient since they did not know either the makeup or effects of the compounds they prescribed.

At the time, as Harris Coulter documented, honest physicians expressed outrage, but they had no idea how corrupt and irretrievable the situation would become:

The first stupendous error, one which is so vast in its influence that it hangs like a withering blight over the individuality of every man in the profession, is the dictation of innumerable pharmaceutical companies, the self-constituted advisers in the treatment of diseases about which they know nothing, to the entire profession. . . . They are so solicitous that they flood your office with blatant literature, full of bombastic claims and cure-alls, and I am sorry to say, too frequently with certificates or articles used by permission from physicians who call themselves reputable.[9]

In 1900 the American allopathic medical profession was at open war with every system that threatened it, and Squibb, Parke-Davis, and others were as much threats as the disciples of Hahnemann. Then the axis of conflict was calculatingly seized by both industries. Drug companies and doctors recognized each other as allies, sensing that homeopaths and naturopaths were a common enemy in terms of both medical-chemical commodities and commercial agendas (and their version of "ethics" only by default or as public relations). They collaborated in a "public be damned" conspiracy of silence that has become the hallmark of post-moral corporations ever since. They will do it every time they feel they have to protect their market share. Moderna is no different in that regard from Microsoft, the company formerly known as Twitter, or Boeing.

Parke-Davis and Squibb soon began publishing their own medical literature. Never openly propagandist, seemingly historical and scientific in intent, their pamphlets and periodicals rewrote history in favor of the proprietary medicines, congratulating the medical profession for being in the vanguard of new science. Parke-Davis alone was responsible for a startling number of ostensibly respectable journals: *New Preparations, Detroit Medical Journal, American Lancet, Therapeutic Gazette, Medical Age, Druggists' Bulletin*, and *Medicine*.[10] In some cases, they purchased existing journals and renamed them; in other cases, they expanded house organs into quasi-scientific publications, with the addition to their staff of professors of medicine and well-known doctors. Many physicians advanced professionally by their letterhead association with the journals.

Patronage did not stop with the development and takeover of publications. Virtually all other medical journals, at least all the major ones, including the *Journal of the American Medical*

Association (*JAMA*), were supported through the advertising of proprietary medicines. Doctors could be solicited as successfully and ingenuously as the public had been. And the journals, which gave the drug manufacturers their legitimacy, at the same time anointed the AMA from the status of another economic interest group to a scientific and professional body representing the whole legitimate medical profession. Gradually, the resistance to proprietary medicines quieted, and the drug companies, under protection of the trademarked secrecy of their products in a market economy, were held only to the most perfunctory disclosure of the contents of drugs advertised in medical journals.

Tactics of biased favoritism have—no surprise—accelerated. In 2021, Twitter blacklisted an entire European medical journal that discussed treating COVID-19 with ivermectin; that is, they blacklisted *everything* from that journal, including unrelated health topics.

The Twilight of Hahnemannian Homeopathy

As "allopathy" and "homeopathy" became archaisms, a new system arose, with controlled experiments, sophisticated machinery, modern laboratories, and a microbiological pharmacy. A fellowship of science was proclaimed: "We are all now professionals," the argument went. "No more schools and sectarian positions, only general universal objective medicine." It was a compelling plea. But since homeopathic and allopathic principles are opposed, the new system had to work by one principle rather than another, and it was clearly allopathic (or sometimes isopathic) in its allegiance.

From 1899 to 1911 George H. Simmons was general secretary of the American Medical Association and editor of the *JAMA*. He remained editor until 1924. Notably, he was once a homeopath (in Nebraska), and, according to Coulter, an ardent one. After his conversion to allopathy, he was well qualified to handle the thorny sectarian issue. Instead of continuing the long-standing attack, he went against precedent (and against much of the AMA membership) in inviting not only homeopaths but all alternative practitioners into the AMA (as long as the former stopped calling themselves "homeopaths" and stopped using homeopathic medicines). They were welcomed in celebration of the end of sectarianism. A great number of homeopaths accepted, especially low-potency practitioners who felt more cut off from their fastidious Hahnemannian colleagues than from their mainstream competitors. Homeopathic pharmacies were converted into standard American drugstores, carrying proprietaries and patent medicines because the public, uninvolved in the philosophical issues, demanded them. These drugs were widely advertised and prescribed. Most stores also continued to carry homeopathic remedies until they were no longer in demand— allopathic addition by subtraction.

The continued passage of so many homeopathic doctors into general nonhomeopathic practice weakened the Hahnemannian movement. Mainstream allopathy advanced the position that the aim of medicine was to effect cures of the sick and not to hold to rigid positions at the expense of healing, so the *JAMA* declared:

> It is a favorable sign to find a faithful follower of Hahnemann who acknowledges the natural tendency of which most medical men are aware, and it causes us to renew our hope that the time is not so very distant when the believers in the efficacy of dilutions will cease to shut themselves up in a "school" and will become a part of the regular medical profession, the members of which are ready and anxious to employ any and every means which can be scientifically shown to have a favorable influence upon the course of disease.[11]

Most homeopathic medical schools, as noted, were converted to allopathy, initially with elective courses in homeopathy. No one wanted to waste a working facility. Lower-potency prescribers felt at home with courses in anatomy, physiology, and pathology. Those who taught materia medica were kept on in acknowledgment of school charters but became "historians" of medicine; materia medicas were turned into grimoires. Hahnemann was prescient when he challenged half-homeopathy. Half-homeopathy is nonhomeopathy. He viewed these hybrids as "worse than allopaths . . . amphibians, who are most of them still creeping in the mud of the allopathic marsh and who only rarely venture to raise their heads in freedom towards the ethereal truth."[12]

Once a significant proportion of homeopaths accepted general nonsectarian medicine—many of them innocently, thinking it was an inroad for homeopathy to be heard and even scientifically tested in wider circles—the basis for separate homeopathic training evaporated.

Mainstream medicine, with its organizing body, the AMA, and its academic corroboration, the *JAMA*, had exclusive access to medical schools. Having taken the sectarians into their mainstream, allopaths now claimed their right to a say in *all* medical education, even homeopathy (though they were ignorant of prescribing by Similars). Representing a new syncretism, they sought to develop universal standards and criteria for practice.

A field secretary hired by the American Institute of Homeopathy could do nothing to turn the tide. He wrote in his final report:

He who sits comfortably in his easy chair in his smoking jacket enjoying a genuine Havana bought with silver earned by means of a successful homeopathic prescription, grunting a "Cui bono?" when called upon to do his share toward the perpetuation of the homeopathic doctrine, and he who vainly asserts that "Similia is a mighty truth and cannot die, no matter whether I get busy on its behalf or not!" letting it go at that, are likely to awaken some wintry morn to find themselves undeceived.[13]

In fact, that day had already come. In association with the Carnegie Foundation for the Advancement of Teaching, the American Medical Association prepared a working paper on medical education in America and Canada. This study, issued in 1910 under the name of Abraham Flexner, the Carnegie representative, gave the AMA a basis for refusing licenses to the graduates of low-ranking institutions. The AMA was coronated by the Flexner Report, as it came to be known, and it helped the AMA vanquish naturopathic, homeopathic, and osteopathic rivals and limit consumer options to essentially two: drugs or surgery.

Ostensibly a neutral, even-handed survey, the Flexner Report, rightly or wrongly, became the basis on which medical education was reorganized. Its balanced curriculum became a web from which homeopathy could not extricate itself as long as it advanced the methodology handed down by Hahnemann. Modern medicine was recognized as the collection of the methods and theories that had proven effective *and* scientific. Other sectarian schools were not immediately forced out of business, but they were identified as something other than medical institutions. Their attendance declined, and during a period when orthodox medicine received substantial foundation funding and government support, they were left to their own resources. Over the years since, the financial gap has increased. Mainstream medicine has been lavishly funded; sectarian and integrative schools have dwindled and, for a time, all but disappeared. The Flexner Report said:

> Now that allopathy has surrendered to modern medicine, is not homeopathy borne on the same current into the same harbor?

For everything of proved value in homeopathy belongs of right to scientific medicine and is at this moment incorporate in it; nothing else has any footing at all, whether it be of allopathic or homeopathic lineage.[14]

Who could argue with such reasonable terms of cease-fire?

Homeopaths had once caused less pain than the allopaths, but with palliative first-aid drugs, allopathy had drawn even—and without the patient sometimes having to suffer a period of trial and error or a "healing crisis." Suppression become a more popular commodity than health.

The bubble of homeopathy's economy burst. Since homeopaths needed more case-taking time with patients, they charged a higher sum for an initial visit. That wasn't a disincentive when allopaths offered similarly expensive first visits. As the zeitgeist shifted, family homeopaths were suddenly in competition with cut-rate mass medicine and homogenized care. Homeopaths became as old-fashioned as they had once seemed modern.

Seven homeopathic medical schools were left at the end of 1918, but they soon converted. The Hahnemann Medical College of Philadelphia lasted only until the 1920s, when it changed its orientation to allopathy. In Quebec, where homeopathy benefited from a general acceptance throughout the British Commonwealth, the Montreal Homeopathic Hospital didn't change its name and vocation to the Queen Elizabeth Hospital until 1951 (an ironic choice, as many of the royals continued to use homeopathy). Yet homeopathic experimentation, lacking a scientific way to pose the effectiveness of microdoses, became as irrelevant as alchemical transmutation of metals.

The decline of homeopathy inadvertently changed the popular perception of medicine. Emphasis switched from chronic conditions, which were often untreatable allopathically, onto severe illnesses and ultimately a unified front of HMOs, industrial hospital complexes, and Medicare. Chronic diseases were either passed on to specialists or declared undiagnosable and managed symptomatically by palliatives and Contraries. The kinds of fees doctors expect after years of medical training do not come from treating headaches, restless legs, and digestive disorders. Most doctors are also specialists in their domain of anatomy and don't want to try to solve complicated conditions and cofactors. These are often passed on to psychoanalysts, who link them with neuroses or other personality disorders for which the default intervention is psychotropic. Only by becoming classified as mental illnesses do many chronic diseases get attention. Even then, they are held hostage by fashions of the drug industry. Meanwhile, functional holistic medicine operates pretty much under the radar without many practitioners or referrals.

Lost are mental aspects of disease itself as well as the inner physician and its psychosomatic and homeostatic terms of cure, never mind the energetic basis of health and remediation. If there were anything significant in Hahnemann's progression of symptoms or emotional-physical planes of disease, modern medicine is in no position to discover it. In fact, we have *regressed* from Galen's day. Humors were as functionally biochemical as anything conceived by Pfizer, Purdue, or Bristol-Myers Squibb. In an Obamacare juggernaut for which the Republican remedy is worse, the patient is the lowest common commodity of pharmaceutical and insurance industries. Capitalism seeks quick turnover of assets.

The Eclipse and Resurgence of American Homeopathy

From 1910 until the late 1960s, few new homeopaths entered the ranks in the United States and Canada. As the last classes of homeopaths graduated from American medical schools in the 1920s and 1930s, only physicians trained abroad replaced them. Homeopathy remained a viable medicine throughout western Europe, in the countries once part of the British Empire, and in Chile and Argentina, where many German and Swiss immigrated. As James Gorman wrote in 1992, "32 percent of family physicians in France and 20 percent in Germany prescribe homeopathic medicines, while in Great Britain 42 percent sometimes refer patients to homeopaths. In France, where the best-selling flu remedy, Oscillococinum, is homeopathic, the national health-care system covers homeopathic prescriptions from traditional physicians."[15]

North American homeopathy entered the 1970s as a dwindling cluster of private practices. It is hard to believe that something once so fervent and popular could have ended so abruptly and completely—or that it would soon start up again in phoenix-like fashion.

Nowadays people shrug and smile if anyone suggests that homeopathy ever represented enough of a threat to spawn a powerful lobby like the AMA. How quickly stages of history and impregnable brands and institutions vanish: wall-mounted phones, Woolworths, Esso stations, Studebakers, Pan Am, propellor planes, Rheingold beer, Milkshake bars. Each new generation is born into a refurbished landscape.

Yet nineteenth-century homeopathy is a mere blink of the eye away, seen in fading names on buildings, once chiseled in stone and then covered by a wooden sign announcing a new clinic or a multimillion-dollar health facility. Remains of an old homeopathic "empire" are scattered throughout the United States, especially in its eastern half, like the earth mounds of the Southeastern Ceremonial Complex of pre-Columbian nations. Hospitals, clinics, and even Hahnemann's name have been repurposed by allopaths. Homeopathy collections were moved out of the science section of libraries into storage or historic archives. That's where I discovered homeopathy in 1968, in a corner of the University of Michigan medical stacks. Volumes were later dispersed at library sales with failed fiction, old dictionaries, and James Fenimore Cooper hardcovers.

Loyal patients patronized the last of the old-breed doctors, until they retired as minions of an antiquarian cult with no one to take over their practices. As the last wave of homeopathic doctors died out, their legacies died with them. My original anthropology field-work project, "The Nature of the Cure," was to study these and other naturopathic practices in 1969 in Maine, but politics in the anthropology department at the University of Michigan made that project impractical. My proposal, funded by NIMH (the National Institutes of Mental Health), holds my original writing for this book.

Classical homeopathy was doomed from its inception. In the absence of a chemico-physical explanation, it required a commitment to purism that few doctors could maintain, especially in the face of rationalist critiques. While Hahnemann's early students were purists, their successors more and more used homeopathy as simply another tool. If a homeopathic procedure failed, there were many other systems of medicine to fall back on, including treatment by opposites.

As long as homeopathy opposed the notion that a disease could be known, it was in opposition to both evidence-based science and post-Newtonian empiricism; it became a quasi-laboratory branch of spiritualism and "Christian" science. For the miasmic believer, research into cause of disease was equated with inquiry into the evolution of man or genesis of life. These were Adamic sins with a psoric impulse as their cause. The disease source remained in the mind of God.

Maintaining Hahnemann's fundamentalism and politics, purists allied with other conservative elements in American life, often taking positions that reflected the cultural conventions of Hahnemann's time more than of their own. Progressive ideas were slandered as "disease complexes." Psychoanalysis and social work were dismissed. A miasmatic interpretation of "unclean sexuality" had little traction in socially liberal circles or during San Francisco's Summer of Love that paradoxically gave rise, soon after, to turbaned and white-robed homeopaths in sandals. One homeopathic journal of the late 1960s even mixed professional papers with appeals for the immediate bombing of Hanoi.

The rise of the 1970s counterculture—a Vietnam-based anti-war movement, a shift in diet toward natural foods, a back-to-land mindset, and a growing attention to ecology and environmental pollution—turned the tables on allopathic medicine too. If you are what you eat, as the motto went, you are also what you take as medicine. Allopathy's failures with chronic and psychosomatic ailments and its sky-rocketing costs, along with the takeover of the medical profession by insurance companies and nonmedical bureaucrats, played its own part in a revival of alternative medicine in the 1970s.

Planet Medicine, a previous book of mine and the origin of much of the writing in this book, was coterminous with the overall holistic-health movement and shares its inspiration, idealistic proselytization, and millenarian hyperbole. As my thesis advisor in the 1970s, Roy Rappaport, an ecological anthropologist, said on the book's back cover, "The author deliberately violates the canons of scientific objectivity in a sustained attempt to understand systems of medicine and therapeutic logic that lie outside of contemporary respectability and rationality in both their own and perennial universal terms. . . . He discusses the crisis of mainline medical practice in terms of commoditization, power, and meaninglessness." By offering this blurb to the publisher, he managed to support my effort while maintaining academic cachet. He had been unable to do the same with my fieldwork (I ended up studying fishing cultures, a more ecologically justifiable project, instead).

The same "alibi" covers my overall critique of technocracy and scientism: I am violating precedent and syllogism in order to get at a deeper truth—the current crisis of commoditization, power, and meaninglessness. Homeopathic etiology describes the "self-cure" contained in every healing crisis and medicinal act, and the symbolic and sociocultural basis of all healing. Read by a generation of students, *Planet Medicine* was a small contributor to the revival of alternative medicine in the West, helping to redefine medical anthropology and return it to an ethnomedicine basis.

In April 1978, as I was completing *Planet Medicine*, a homeopathic conference in San Francisco seemed to herald its fruition. It brought together practitioners from around the United States, mainly west of the Rockies. Homeopathy's then current superstar, George Vithoulkas, flew from Athens, Greece, to deliver fifteen hours of lectures to five hundred students and potential students at the California Academy of Sciences. At the end of event, the International Foundation for the Promotion of Homeopathy was formed with the intention of raising standards of homeopathic practice throughout the world. The founding directives included "strict scientific research on homeopathic potencies and their clinical application" and the establishment of full-time four-year homeopathic schools in Greece and California.

The appearance of an internationally renowned homeopath stirred many of the ambiguities of American homeopathy. His audience was made up of local Bay Area students and practitioners of homeopathy, a few older homeopaths from throughout the United States, and hundreds of doctors, lay prescribers, nurses, and patients, many of them practicing incognito. After Vithoulkas gave a lecture at, of all places, the University of California Hospital in San Francisco, he received a five-minute standing ovation from the medical personnel despite the fact that his words had demolished everything the building and its medical practices stood for.

At the Academy of Sciences, he was interrupted with applause and laughter, sometimes for anecdotes about outdueling an allopath in a difficult case or the demise of a specific allopathic patient. A woven banner on the curtains behind the podium with the homeopathic motto of SIMILIA SIMILIBUS CURENTUR stitched between two bright yellow calendula flowers heralded a medical lecture and revival meeting. At crescendos, Vithoulkas was serenaded with "right on." People stood and shook fists and gave V signs.

For the older homeopaths, this display must have been equal parts disturbing and elating, deconstructing their own strategy of fifty years. They had feared that an outpouring of this sort would bring down the wrath of the AMA and U.S. Food and Drug Administration (FDA), which, to that point, has been content to let homeopathy harmlessly die out. Since 1938, when a homeopath in the United States Senate, Royal Copeland (Democrat from New York), added the drugs in the *Homeopathic Pharmacopoeia* to the list recognized by the FDA, microdoses had been legally protected, though the FDA never tested their efficacy.

The attitude of the audience in 1978 San Francisco was "Bring it on!"

Even as Vithoulkas was cheered, he warned the audience about their cultish attitude. "Faddism," he said, "will give the momentary illusion of success, but it will lead even more swiftly to the end of this wonderful science than any amount of isolation."

In the years since that conference, homeopathy has thrown off much of its cultlike history and esoteric reputation and repackaged itself in computerized offices with new reference texts and trained personnel. In its second coming, it has learned to collaborate with mainstream medicine as well as with other New Age therapies and businesses, cross-pollinating within a larger holistic health and complementary medicine market. It is practiced in the company of Asian medicines, craniosacral therapy, Feldenkrais bodywork, rebirthing, acupuncture, polarity, qigong, and conscious diets as well as at consumer-oriented clinics with Pilates or CrossFit training. Its medicines have become indistinguishable from Chinese herbs, Bach flower remedies (which are also spiritualized tiers of energy), and modern vitamin compounds. The sort of integrative holism—allopathy, naturopathy, osteopathy, homeopathy, herbalism, even prayer, color healing, sound baths, and Reiki—that the Flexner Report censured has spread into the medical mainstream and continues to spread.

Homeopathy has also been revitalized by new physics, parapsychology, and the deconstructionist and hermeneutic philosophies of Jacques Derrida and Jacques Lacan, themselves derived from the unconscious mind and psychosomatics of Sigmund Freud. Homeopathy also benefited from branches of physics that discovered quantum-entangled particles and fractal series in nature.

At the same time, a combination of M.D.-like specialized training programs have sprouted up in naturopathically oriented colleges and schools, and classy marketing has given homeopathy a digital-age image. Software has put repertorization on personal laptops. Financial firms have recommended homeopathic pharmacies for socially conscious portfolios. Within ecological and holistic subcultures, cylindrical vials labeled "Aconite" or "Arnica" have become as recognizable as Tom's Toothpaste and kombuchas, pickles, brines, mushroom teas, and herbal tinctures—the medicine of choice in not only natural groceries and Whole Foods but shopping malls' concession to "green" pharmacy. Homeopathy's Hollywood, rock 'n' roll clientele is a far cry from Hahnemann's Parisian madrasa.

Many people know of homeopathy these days through the advertised formulas that blend many microdoses into one remedy. These are obviously not individualized but are sold for anyone's PMS, headaches, flu, back pain, allergies, digestive problems, and the like, much as allopathic drugs are. Most modern homeopaths accept that either synergy or catchall effects are triggered when, for instance, the ingredients for treating five different conditions are combined. In any case, this may be the only way the general public gets to try out homeopathic remedies.

To say that combination remedies oversimplify homeopathic diagnosis and treatment overlooks the enigma that until we know with confidence how homeopathic remedies work, we cannot limit or define their range of preparation and application. As long as a variety of alternative pharmacies and energy medicines are available, people are going to test the boundaries of systems exemplifying psychic and quantum as well as physical and cultural factors. At my first class with him in 1975, Dana Ullman opened by saying, "[Your] minds are about to be blown. Homeopathy, in case you don't know yet, is quantum physics, UFOs, and Jefferson Airplane combined!" Later in the hour he proclaimed, "Now we hit warp speed. We are going to turn nothing back into something!"

Our global, multicultural marketplace provides syntheses far beyond the imagination of nineteenth-century physicians. We have lived long enough past Newton, Darwin, Lamarck, and Cullen to realize the truth in each of their works, while noting contradictions, gaps, and errors.

Now that practitioners generally accept (even if they do not fully understand) that microdoses do not and cannot work according to a standard biochemical model, they can move outside homeopathic literalism and begin to explore actual efficacies, including those from other energy medicines. We are finally as free to use homeopathy on a "patent pending" basis as we are to explore new paradigms of physics and biology. The era of worshipping technological synthesis as a "miracle drug" factory will someday end. A new era of microdoses, meridians, chakras, and natural sources of immunity will emerge.

The emergent paradigm shift was relevant enough by 1992 that the *New York Times Magazine* accepted James Gorman's article on homeopathy, "Take a Little Deadly Nightshade and You'll Feel Better." In keeping with his educated but cynical audience, Gorman opened with a description of a revival that must have seemed to some readers like a rebirth of witchcraft on the New York Stock Exchange. While most of his milieu, including himself, had been asleep, homeopathy "jus' grew." Upon investigation, Gorman noted, he found the following:

Almost everyone I knew either had used a homeopathic remedy or knew someone who did. Drugstores that a few years ago were carrying only mainstream products like Nyquil and Sudafed were displaying homeopathic lines in their windows. And not in amber bottles, but in small, colorful cardboard containers with the pills comfortably ensconced in blister packs. There was Quietude—"the homeopathic insomnia remedy" in a white box with blue and pink pastel borders. And Alpha CF, for colds and flu, in an icy-blue package with a snowflake design. . . .

The homeopathic pharmaceutical companies . . . are already undergoing a renaissance. Old companies are reviving, and new companies are getting into the field, which in the late 1970s and early 1980s made a miraculous recovery from near death. According to the Food and Drug Administration, sales of some homeopathic drug companies increased 1,000 percent. Growth has continued apace ever since, with the American market for homeopathic drugs now estimated at [$150] million. . . .

Imagine—medicines that have no side effects, so safe that a child could swallow an entire bottle of pills, yet able to cure picky ailments like fatigue, insomnia and allergy that have baffled modern medicine. How could such medicines be produced? What went into them? . . .

Boericke & Tafel's brand-new headquarters seemed the best place to look on the new face of homeopathy, so I flew to San

Francisco and then drove north to Santa Rosa. The plant was spanking clean, just the way you want a pharmaceutical plant to be. In the laboratory-like production rooms, everyone (including me) wore white coats, surgical masks and gloves and disposable caps. . . . The workers also put on special white shoes, which they wore only while in these areas. Visitors and all other personnel were given covers for theirs. (The last time I had seen people dressed this way was at my son's birth.) In one area a tablet-making machine was busy making tablets. In another, the tincture storage room, there were scores of amber bottles on stainless-steel racks, all very pharmaceutical. But there was no amoxycillin or Prozac, no Xanax or AZT. Instead there were tinctures of Rhus radicans (poison ivy), Berberis vulgaris (barberry) and Calcarea silicata (silicate of lime). In another area, Calendula officinalis (marigold) was macerating in what seemed to be large stainless-steel stockpots.

Next we entered the "single remedy room," where medicines were actually being produced. First the technician weighed out a gram's worth of drops from one bottle of Natrum muriaticum 25X. Otherwise known as sodium chloride or table salt, the Natrum muriaticum had been diluted 25 times at a ratio of 1 to 10, leaving 1 part salt to 10 to the 25th power parts of alcohol and water. . . . After each dilution the solution was shaken 10 times by hand and banged against a rubber pad, a process known in homeopathy as "succussion." In homeopathy this process of diluting, shaking and banging is known as "potentizing." In homeopathic speak the solution was at 25X potency.

To this already ethereal solution the technician added more liquid to dilute it 1 to 10 once again. She then succussed the solution by shaking it 10 times by hand (up and down) and banging it against a rubber pad on each down stroke. The solution was now Natrum muriaticum 26X. She repeated the same procedure again to produce a 27X solution. The final steps (done later) would be to repeat the dilution and succussion process three more times to achieve Natrum muriaticum 30X. Then drops of this solution of 1 part salt to 10 to the 30th power parts liquid would be added to sugar tablets, resulting in a product reputedly useful for allergy, anemia, cardiovascular problems and grieving states.

As I watched this process I heard within me the whimper of offended reason. By all known laws of physics and chemistry, the initial preparation had been diluted so many times that it was highly unlikely that a measurable trace of salt remained, not a molecule. And this was before the five succeeding dilutions, and the final dosing of the sugar pellets. What was being created, it seemed, was not a drug, but the idea of a drug, what an artist friend of mine calls "conceptual medicine." I thought, Welcome to homeopathy.[16]

From 1981 to 1996, approximately a thousand new M.D.s took up homeopathic practice. In 1996 a survey of AMA primary-care physicians showed a surprising 49 percent interested in homeopathic training; that figure was 69 percent in a separate Maryland census. Almost two thousand conventionally trained M.D.s actually practiced some form of homeopathic prescribing; another three thousand to five thousand health professionals, including dentists and nurses, used homeopathy in their treatments. Add to these some five thousand chiropractors and an untold number of lay practitioners and consumers who repertorize medicines from books and kits with only informal or indirect training. Homeopathic training programs, only four in 1990, were at around thirty in 1996 and have dramatically increased since then.

Additionally, 34 percent of all medical schools have training in alternative medicine in one form or another. As Mark Twain prophesized, "You may honestly feel grateful that homoeopathy survived the attempts of the allopathists to destroy it."[17]

Meanwhile, research into perhaps an undiscovered parascience has continued. Dana Ullman continued to cite experiments and statistics. In 1998 he summarized several promising studies:

[In 1991] the *British Medical Journal* published an eight-page review of 25 years of clinical trials in homeopathy. This meta-analysis was completed by three Dutch epidemiologists who were commissioned by their government as the result of an earlier study which indicated that 45 percent of Dutch physicians consider homeopathic medicines to be effective. It uncovered a total of 107 controlled clinical trials, 81 of which showed the efficacy of homeopathic medicines. The researchers carefully evaluated each of these experiments and determined that 22 studies were of a particularly high quality in terms of their research design and the number of subjects used. Fifteen of these 22 studies showed the efficacy of the homeopathic medicines. These trials indicated the range of successes that homeopaths commonly observe, including the effective treatment of arthritis, migraine headaches, allergies and hay fever, influenza, respiratory infections, postoperative infections, injuries, and childbirth.

The researchers concluded that "the amount of positive evidence even among the best studies came as a surprise to us. . . . The evidence presented in this review would probably be sufficient for establishing homeopathy as a regular treatment for certain conditions."

In a well-controlled, double-blind study of patients with hay fever which was published in the *Lancet* [in 1986], Reilly et al. showed that the 30c of a mixture of 12 common pollens in the Glasgow area was very successful in reducing symptoms of hay fever.

In 1980, the *British Journal of Clinical Pharmacology* published a double-blind study of patients with rheumatoid arthritis. The study showed that 82 percent of those who had been given an individually chosen homeopathic remedy experienced some relief of symptoms, while only 21 percent of those who had been given a placebo experienced a similar degree of improvement.

In addition to these and numerous clinical trials, there are also dozens of laboratory experiments. A study, published in *Human Toxicology*, replicated earlier work and showed that homeopathic doses of arsenic helped rats excrete through their urine and feces the crude doses they earlier had been given. This study also used radioactive tracers to evaluate efficacy of the microdose. Ultimately, the 7c and 14x were found to have the greatest benefit. The implications of this work are quite significant when one considers the environmental exposures that humans and animals commonly experience today.

Those skeptics who many years ago said that homeopathy had no research basis were unfamiliar with a double-blind study in 1944 funded by the British government which evaluated the homeopathic treatment of mustard gas burns. This research showed that *Rhus Tox* 30c, *Mustard Gas* 30c, and *Kali Bichromicum* 30c each provided benefit when compared with placebo treatment. If a placebo, homeopathic pills were a more effective placebo.

Other early well-controlled studies include some 1942 research by the Scottish physician W. E. Boyd and his work using enzyme diastase in starch hydrolysis. He showed that hydrolysis was accelerated using the enzyme inhibitor mercuric chloride at 61x, while hydrolysis was inhibited at lower potencies. This work was done so meticulously that it was strongly praised by an associate dean of an American medical school.

Singh and Gupta demonstrated antiviral action in eight of ten homeopathic medicines tested on chicken embryo virus. Between 50 [and] 100 percent inhibition was common for these drugs. A similar test of four medicines on Similike Forest Virus (a virus that causes paralysis in mice) showed that none had any observable effect as compared with the control.

Several studies have shown that homeopathic medicines can control fungal and viral diseases in plants.[18]

Could this all be placebo or mass delusion?

In the next chapter, I will take homeopathy outside medical rubrics and consider Similars, microdoses, and succussion in broader contexts of energy medicine, the subtle body, particularization of substance into information, and the morphogenetic potential of living fields. I won't be writing about homeopathy as much as trying to find other contexts for it. That means, first, reviewing how my understanding of homeopathy has evolved.

7

Homeopathic Parallels: Other Similars and Microdose Effects

Pill-less Potentized Microdoses: The Sequence of My Homeopathic Education

I first heard of homeopathy in 1968 while collecting work for *Io Magazine*, a journal that my wife and I had begun publishing three years earlier as college undergraduates. In 1967, while I was in graduate school studying anthropology in Ann Arbor, Michigan, we compiled our first issue around a specific topic and released it with its own title: "Alchemy." It drew a bunch of new subscribers, so we followed up with another thematic issue: "Doctrine of Signatures." With the help of a friend who translated a section of Michel Foucault's *Les Mots et Les Choses* from French for me, I summarized my understanding:

Signatures are hermetic marks in nature, seals of the macrocosm in the microcosm. Foucault found them in shapes of flowers and crystals, behaviors of animals, star constellations, and properties of herbs. The walnut inside its shell was a signature of the brain, and hence secreted a medicine for mental disorders; hepatic-shaped liverwort similarly cleansed the liver. Among Plains Indians, the turtle was a signature of the sun, for the varying number of serrations and squares on its shell represented the numerology of solar rays.[1]

Poet Theodore Enslin, a contributor to the "Alchemy" issue, wrote us that there was a parallel Doctrine of Similars with greater medical significance. I was only vaguely aware of homeopathy then; it had vanished from the mainstream cultural landscape and had not yet been revived by the counterculture. Ted, who practiced as a lay homeopath in Temple, Maine, asked me to go across town to the University of Michigan library and try to find several "lost" volumes for him. Most were still catalogued and shelved in the medical section. I read parts of them, and after just a month I was able to write:

"Similars" linked signatures—substances in nature—to ailments and constitutions. Patients were diagnosed as Sulphur, Lycopodium, Arsencium, Sepia, Calendula, or some other animal, vegetable, or mineral based on which extract imbibed caused the same symptoms in healthy people. They were then treated by a microdose of the same tincture.

Homeopathic pills were alchemical, not pharmacological, for they were prepared by an unknown molecular transmutation. After a source batch was made from a purified substance, it was shaken and diluted hundreds or thousands of times in water or alcohol until no molecules of the original tincture were left. This process, called succussion, somehow transferred a therapeutic signature from the substance into a medicinal nectar that, with each dilution, increased in potency. Similars were activated totems or charms.[2]

When I interviewed Ted in person in Town Hill, Maine, in 1969, he enlarged my perspective still further as he talked about homeopathy as a way of thinking about nature in general. He identified other "microdoses," such as an inspiring thought, a nostalgic song, or a startling synchronicity; he called these "homeopathic cures," meaning therapeutic transfers of information. An avant-garde musician and a bard, Ted also cited the words of William Carlos Williams, a conventional medical doctor as well as a poet, from his signature poem "Asphodel": "It is difficult / to get the news from poems / yet men die miserably every day / for lack / of what is found there."[3] Williams had intended, Ted joked, poetry's microdose effect—he was a homeopathic poet if not a homeopathic doctor: essences of "succussed" language or art bring enchantment and a change in body-mind states.

Encountering Pill-less Potencies Directly

I met homeopath Dana Ullman six years later in California and received my first formal homeopathic training and pill. I recounted the scene at the time:

> The next afternoon at a Euclid Street café over carrot cake and smoothies, Ullman offered to take my case. Before I could consent, he began shooting questions like whether I was mostly hot or cold, what foods I liked or disliked, and whether I tended more toward sorrow or anger, recording each response on a preprinted pad designed for repertorizing. After about thirty or so such queries, he said he had figured out my remedy.
>
> "Aren't you being a bit simplistic?"
>
> "You're typical of East Coast people. Everything has to be complicated. They spend years going to psychiatrists, but James Tyler Kent said the causes of our ailments are unknowable. You don't waste time looking for a cause, you look for a Similar; you change the energy field. And, then, guess what?—you can be cured in an instant by a single dose."
>
> I had read as much in books, but I didn't believe it.

Back at his study, Dana lifted down a giant brown jar of homeopathic Sulphur and poured a cluster of tiny sugar balls into a folded sheet of paper. "Here. Just roll those under your tongue!"

It was potentized sulfur, I told myself, a form that Renaissance alchemists hadn't considered when they used the mineral as a reagent of mercury to turn common salt into metamorphic brine.

"Homeopathy," I said, stalling on putting a strange substance from a stranger in my mouth, "is alchemy reborn, but then, I guess, so is nuclear physics." Staring at pellets that held only spirit, no sulfur, I continued my skit, "The Jungian archetypes manifested!"

"In California, we're not so intellectual."

Sunlight on leather tomes—materia medicas and repertories— lent majesty to the moment as I scanned the scene briefly like a director capturing a transitional moment. I tipped my head back, aimed the trough under my tongue, and braced for an LSD-like rush.

A burning sensation shot from the center of my back to my chest. I couldn't tell if I was hallucinating or having a sonic transmission.

"Wow," Dana clucked, "look at that microdose go! You really lit up."

"Lit up?" I said. "I almost passed out."

"That's because you're not used to vital energy."[4]

A year later, Dana proposed—and I agreed—that we publish a joint imprint of homeopathy books. By then Lindy and I had converted our journal into a publishing company called North Atlantic Books. The second title on Dana's list (after we reprinted James Tyler Kent's *Lectures on Homoeopathic Philosophy*) was Edward Whitmont's analyses of constitutional remedies like *Silica, Sulphur, Phosphorus*, and *Lycopodium*, using both homeopathic and Jungian rubrics. The essays were in journals and uncollected. Dana assigned me the task of gettting Whitmont's consent to an anthology when I returned to the East Coast. He had been unable to rouse a response via the era's best option: snail mail.

I wrote Whitmont and asked if I could pay him a visit to discuss the project. He agreed. The day before my appointment, I found myself still struggling with a flu-like ailment that had been with me for weeks. Using a self-help kit I got from Dana, I selected *Phosphorus* as a remedy in the hope of improving enough to travel. The next day, I went to my scheduled meeting from Plainfield, Vermont (where I was teaching college), to Yonkers, New York— about 260 miles.

> On a warm autumn morning, I drove six hours to Yonkers in a mild stupor.
>
> A slight, wiry older chap with a German accent, Dr. Whitmont gave a quick blessing to our book. Without my asking, he said that he had a few minutes before the next patient and he would take my case if I wanted. I told my symptoms and story, including the fact that I had just recently learned that neither my stepfather nor my legal father was my genetic father.
>
> "Ailments like yours are fence-sitters," he said, "neither purely physical nor purely mental. Phosphorus was a good guess but no longer relevant. You need to find your birth father—not in person necessarily, for who knows how that will turn out—but as a psychic force. Learning his identity will be your homeopathic remedy."[5]

I proceeded into New York City and, with fresh resolve, tracked down his identity. With his name (Brandt), my condition cleared up, whether it was from a surname's microdose effect, the similitude effect of a laxative I took for a stool sample, *Phosphorus*, or the body's natural medicine. If healing is overdetermined, even the "wrong" train can get you to the right station.

The following spring, I invited Ted Enslin to address a class at Goddard College. After his talk on homeopathy, my student Jessie pursued a series of questions about whether the wish to get well wasn't more of a homeopathic cure than any potentized pill. After Ted agreed that the wish to get well was indeed a high potency, Jessie asked whether resistance to getting well wasn't itself a disease. He wanted to know which came first—potency or will. Their Socratic dialogue, starting with Jessie, concluded with a homeopathic jolt from Ted:

> *"Would a person wanting to get well stand a better chance of cure than a person taking a homeopathic remedy?"*
>
> *"There is a direction to your repeated question," Ted declared. "You're hammering at this one particular thing. But if you really want to know, don't want to know!"*
>
> *"How do you make yourself not want to know?"*
>
> *"We think," Ted rejoined, "we think we are masters. We forget that we aren't any more important than a raccoon. If only we could drop this delusion, maybe we wouldn't have to go through this backward trip through the labyrinth to get to where we could really function."*
>
> *"We could theorize—" Jess corrected.*
>
> *"Don't theorize," the exasperated poet broke in. "Do it! Of course it's impossible; therefore do it!"*[6]

After Dr. Whitmont met me at his office in 1976, we got together periodically to discuss topics of mutual interest. Sixteen years later, he told me that he had experimented with alternate ways of transmitting homeopathic remedies (as if they weren't paraphysical enough!), sometimes writing down the name and giving the piece of paper to the patient instead of a packet of pills, sometimes speaking the name or even just thinking it. He confessed that he got the same curative effect in all cases.

I pondered this conundrum through subsequent decades, raising it with healers of multiple persuasions. Was Whitmont implying that he could telepathically or telekinetically send the remedy, or was some sort of synchronicity or placebo effect at work?

I came to no definitive answer, but from my own and others' insights on the matter, I concluded that speaking or writing (or thinking) the remedy *couldn't* work as consistently as giving a microdose—otherwise the whole of Hahnemannian pharmacy was a ruse. But the fact that it *worked at all* pointed to a complex set of relationships among thought, intention, energy, and potentization.

Osteopath John Upledger called a related form of transmission "cell talk" and used therapeutic palpation to activate it. The fact that biological systems don't speak English, or any language, overlooks the fact that all languages arise from collaborations of tissues—belly, heart, and lungs to throat, tongue, palate, teeth, and lips. Organs are evolved confederations of sea creatures, while DNA is their original phonemic transmission. This is the life code behind healing energy.

Modalities of Energy

In holistic medicine, a broad spectrum of signals can trigger a cure: the concentrated scent of a flower (aromatherapy), dew collected from its petals (Bach flower remedies), puffs of liquid droplets during shamanic or Vedic ceremonies, massage of the aura without touching the body (Reiki), icaros and other mantras, prayers (see M.D. Larry Dossey's research on therapeutic praying), Zen koans, psychoanalytic transference, tarot and oracle readings, spirit and animal guidance, movements and postures (asanas) in yoga, Breema bodywork, qigong, mineral baths, stories and myths embedded in sand paintings, and abreaction from medicine bundles, masks, and ritual performances. Each in its way embodies the three central homeopathic rubrics: matching by similitude, potentization, and specification. Each provides a shock to an apathetic or deranged system.

There is a distinction between a telekinetic or quantum transmission and a pharmaceutical. Overdetermination aside, minded, directed energies (meditations) and machine-focused transmissions from laboratories function quite differently in living systems. In the former, the innate aliveness of the sender transmits a wave, which can also be activated by plant and animal "meanings." For practitioners of manual medicine, Sting's "Love Is the Seventh Wave" is an unsung anthem: "There is a deeper world than this / tugging at your hand . . ."

Various shamanic, osteopathic, and homeopathic healing systems succeed because they activate the self-organizing homeostasis of living systems, tap energy and specificity of information at micro and nano levels, and activate the link between cell consciousness (molecular code) and minded consciousness. However—and this is key when it comes to distinguishing between homeopathically prepared microdoses and pill-less potencies—not just anyone can transfer healing by thought, sign, or cell talk; it takes a trained healer, a sensei or sorcerer, to potentize and specify active essences. Thoughtforms, when potentized, can transmit something like prana and chi to tissues and cells—and that is the case even when a hummingbird or dolphin conducts them subliminally.

In the 1990s, John Upledger proposed that dolphins practice intentioned healing. When captured and put in tanks with patients, they overlooked the indignity and loss of freedom and sent therapeutic information by sonar. They nuzzled activation points for lesions and aimed their sonar through blockages—or, in Upledger's nomenclature, "energy cysts."

The sea "physicians" knew how to transmit active love, even though they don't specifically "love" us. Their love was "heart chakra" transmission—radiant energy transferred from one domain into another with the charge of eros but transpersonal and nonlibidinal. Free and in the ocean, they likely dispatch it to other dolphins, perhaps also to whales, fishes, cephalopods, and Gaia at large.

Other healers have reported similar transmissions from owls, ravens, parrots, butterflies, octopuses, elephants, manatees, dogs, cats, and horses. According to spiritualist researcher David Barreto, cats detect subtle energy shifts and disharmonic balances of electrons and positrons and conduct etheric filtration in households while they sleep. As pigeons cluster, they mentally clear egregores (collective thoughtforms) in nearby humans and crowds. He adds:

> The center of a dog's electromagnetic field is one of the largest in the animal kingdom, thus the purification of degrading and depressing emotions in the environment are efficiently dispersed by the strong currents coming from the canine heart chakras. Their powerful vortex influences humans on the grounds of interpersonal energies. . . .
>
> Ants emanate an energetic plasma that simulates a pheromone of pleasure and sweetness. These waves radiating from ants or anthill strings in the house are a sign of where such a plasma is missing. In the same way that ants exhale this pheromone of sweetness, they absorb the antagonists of sweetness.[7]

Consider this the next time you start to spray an ant invasion! A meditation on the swarm might have a better microdose effect.

French anthropologist-priest Pierre Teilhard de Chardin spoke of an inertial power equivalent to gravity and with more power than any weapon or technology. "Someday," he wrote, "after mastering the winds, the waves, the tides, and gravity, we will harness for God the energies of love. And then, for the second time in the history of the world, humankind will have discovered fire."[8]

I am not proposing that the above instances depict or represent a mostly unexplored energy and its agency; I am proposing them as a way to begin thinking about them and to understand microdose healing in a broader context.

Medical Hexing

When I interviewed Freudian parapsychologist Jule Eisenbud in 1972, he proposed an unconscious voodoo field also in play, the antithesis of focused love but from the same microdose physics. He said:

> Thoughts alone can kill; bare naked thoughts; isn't all this armor of war, this machinery, these bombs, aren't they all grotesque exaggerations? We don't even need them. To put it schematically, and simplistically, and almost absurdly, because we don't wish to realize that we can just kill with our minds, we go through this whole enormous play of killing with such—, of overkilling with such overimplementation; it gets greater and greater and greater, as if . . . it's a caricature of saying: how can I do it with my mind? I need tanks; I need B-52 bombers; I need napalm, and so on, and so on.

Substitute "heal" for "kill" and make the equivalent swaps throughout his screed, and you have a first axiom of energy medicine. In a concluding flourish, Eisenbud honored his mentor Sigmund Freud:

> All science has produced cover stories for the deaths we create; it's streptococci; it's accidents, and so on. But what I'm trying to say is, there must be, I feel, a relationship between this truth, which we will not see, and this absurd burlesque of aggression that goes on all around us, as if we're trying to deny that the other is possible.[9]

The response from the 'hood in an imaginal future—after crime clans, drug cartels, and street gangs have graduated into healing societies and shamanic lodges—is "Right on, late brother!"

In my ongoing discussion with Whitmont, he adduced a more discrete form of unconscious transference that is practiced, he proposed, mostly unknowingly by all healers: sometimes cures, sometimes

curses. An insincere physician, from innate narcissism, medical mega-
lomania (thinking that their M.D. skills provide a free pass), or their
own unresolved traumas, can drive or metastasize deeper diseases in
patients *despite* those skills otherwise. The doctor reifies the pathology by overmaterialized beliefs and treatments. This catch-22 is characterized by a line from my college friend Sid Schwab about his own
profession: "A surgeon can kill you, and you'll sleep right through it."
An unhappy or poorly sublimated surgeon, that is.

Universalizing the language of homeopathy, Whitmont suggested
that the state of awareness and active compassion of doctors (or shamans, medicine people, healers, and so on) potentizes their *own* therapeutic potential and transmits this information from their "being"
directly to the patient along with whatever drug, surgical intercession,
or other modality they are conferring. They stand in a therapeutic
or hexing role, either wittingly or unwittingly; their sheer presence
either enhances the power of a sick organism to heal or, if they are
incompetent or subconsciously hexing, undermines the patient and
dampens both the patient's and their own energy fields and healing
potential. Again, this is in *addition* to the actual treatment—and the
entire concept mirrors the homeopathic maxim that the healer is the
first remedy.

In his *Alchemy of Healing*, Whitmont explored the role of unconscious projections in doctor-patient relationships. He defined medical hexing as a form of pathological transference from a doctor to a
patient with occasional countertransference from patient to physician.
He pointed to the high number of cases of suicides and dementia
among allopaths after their retirement and suggested that potenti-
ated disease and cure states were transferred back and forth. In this
paradigm, doctor and shaman can converge in iatrogenic as well as
therapeutic projections.

Sincere, empathic physicians, even allopathic surgeons or prescribers of pharmaceuticals, instill beneficial psychic energy in their

treatment, no matter if the overt tool is a knife or drug. This is why doctors' life experience, emotional depth, and sacred wounds play a part in all treatments. Doctors project their state of subconscious clarity into a pathology and patient. Patients sense this, regardless of modality. Well-trained physicians may lack a spiritual quality necessary for transference, yet because this is a material world, their exterior skills still function satisfactorily at the level of disease manifestation. Both modalities can work in their own ways: material and psychic, conscious and unconscious.

Some Indigenous healers acknowledge that they use sleight of hand, stage magic, and other tricks in their practices. It is a way to shift fixed beliefs or stuck thoughtforms that have externalized in tissue pathology. "Western doctors open people up like car mechanics," one explained to a friend of mine, "and they try to fix them by changing their parts. We heal them by changing their belief systems."

Quesalid, an elderly Koskimo (Kwakuitl) shaman from the Pacific Northwest interviewed by anthropologist Franz Boas, admitted that the bloody down he pulled out of a sick person's body was crumpled feathers darkened from biting his own tongue. After having been removed from his family to study at a government school, he planned to expose the local shamans as chicanerers. However, he was called into premature practice by his appearance in a sick woman's vision. After a miracle cure followed by others, he arrived at a more nuanced understanding. Healing is *transformational theater*. Killer whale and toad are the real shaman makers, as are their masks and symbols; ultimate rectitude rests with them. Each of his patients assimilated a totem object and converted it into parasympathetic energy.[10]

Even while knowing the bloody down is a sham, a shaman calls on a fellow medicine man to treat him when he becomes sick. Some Indigenous physicians even return to their native villages as M.D.s and seek out the local "witch doctor." They want a hit of that old-time energy medicine too.

In 2021, when I was wondering whether to get a vaccine for COVID-19 in the middle of the pandemic, Vatsala Sperling emailed me this microdose affirmation: "If you must have the vaccine, have it with an open, optimistic, and happy heart, fully trusting that it will not harm you. Make friends with the virus and the injection—both will be kind to you."

Rewriting my old homeopathy book to produce this new edition has been a microdose too. Forty-six years after I discovered and first wrote about homeopathy, I realize that I can more deeply breathe and assimilate vital energy by the way I have come to understand it. Darker energies too. Even hexing can be healing if received with neutrality and gratitude.

Astrology

A routine critique of astrology is: How can tiny, highly dilute bodies like Chiron or Pluto have impacts equal to or greater than those of vastly more massive planets like Jupiter or Saturn or stars like the sun, let alone how can planets and stars have *any* effect at all at their immense distances, and how can constellations generate life patterns when they are formed by stars at different light-year distances of three-dimensional space?

The first answer is that astrological influences, however they might originate, are transmitted in nanodoses, not heroic doses, succussed by their source bodies' movements, spin, orbits, and collective fields. Specified at conception and again in the womb by macrocosm-microcosm relationships, zodiacs are said by some astrologers to be imprinted like runes in the fluids of human embryos and, according to anthroposophist Rudolf Steiner, on the soft-forming jellies of the brain and skull.

Anything specified enough to incur a mass also holds a point in a gravitational or symbolic field; its position and path generate correspondences—synchronicities. A dwarf planet as small as Quaoar, a planetoid as meager as Ursula or Hermione, even a centaur as incidental as Asbolus carries and transmits a load. The physical influences are infinitesimal but not zero, certainly not in a universe that ostensibly chundered from a single particle (or portal) and remains quantum-entangled.

The barycenter of Pluto and its moons (Charon, Hydra, and Nix down to tiny unnamed moonlets), when commuted through living and symbolic systems, cascades astrologically as global effects, in some ways more intense than those of the heavier loads of Uranus and Neptune. Pluto's microdose, specified first by telescopes in 1930, became repotentized in a web of etymologies and gods.

Even Jupiter and Neptune are not so much masses distributing astrobiological forces as they are weightless gears in a nonlocal mechanism and a relativistic field. But again, I don't mean to imply that planets send energy, or that anything physical *does*, simply that planets designate where effects arise in a field of energies and meanings: breakups of inertial structures and dynamic totalities.

Astrosophist (anthroposophical astrologer) Willi Sucher proposed that, just as "the process of potentisation and trituration develops a spiritual curative agency, . . . our tiny Solar system is a dynamically integral entity in the tremendous choir of Greater Universes. Is it not possible that there exist other systems which also exert on the whole a dynamic influence rather than make an impression by sheer quantity and size?" He attributed "the principles of relationships between the Greater Universe and our Solar system" to a "relationship [between] the cosmos and the Spiritual world beyond it [and] the union between the human microcosmos, endowed with Selfhood, and the Macrocosmos."[11]

That Whitmont achieved the same curative dynamics by

"intending" or writing a remedy as by having patients put a micro-dose under their tongue took his prescribing, in effect, from a medicinal to an astrological context. It suggested that planets like-wise don't "send" anything; they just hold their places in a herme-neutic field. To repertorize without giving a pill is, in effect, writing a "horoscope." A microdose at one frequency is an acausal equiva-lence at another, a birth chart at another. While explaining why he believed that the deepest cures are symbolic (field-based and unconscious) rather than material—causal in the esoteric meaning of the word (see psychic homeopathy below)—Whitmont invoked a greater archetypal field:

> The breaking-up of the physical form manifestation of a substance, as it occurs in homeopathic potentization, operates as a dynam-ization in that it activates the "pure essence" behind the formal manifestation. An analogous procedure is the arousal of key points of the Qi meridians through acupuncture needles or the manipula-tion of the relevant spinal vertebrae or bones of the skull. . . .
>
> If we are to deal with our complexes in a fashion that could turn them into healing factors, we must abstain from either con-cretely acting them out or identifying with them. Instead we may enact them in their "potentized" form symbolically, psychodra-matically or in fantasy, painting, meditation, etc. By analogy to the acupuncture needle's penetration into the critical points of the body's meridians or the homeopathic medicine's radiating field, we assimilate the creative possibilities of their archetypal essence.[12]

Martial artist Robert Pittman made a personal study of astrology and Siberian shamanism in which he came to similar conclusions as Whitmont. He shared the following with me from his unpublished manuscript *The Chiron Text*:

*The planets themselves do not radiate these powers or vibrations—
it is just that these vibrations have become associated with these
planets because it is the location or direction in space from which
these vibrations come. Each of these planetary vibrations also creates
a particular state of mind. They combine to form what astrologers
call an individual astrological chart. In other words, we are born, live,
and breathe inside a series of twelve moving fields that constantly
shift in relation to one another according to planetary movement.*[13]

Vortices that emanate as galaxies at one level form genetic helices at another, atoms at another, quarks at another, microdoses at
another, lines on palms at another, and so on. We and our lives—in
fact all acts and events—unfold relative to them, meaning relative not
as mass but as what they actually are.

Psychic and Dream Homeopathy

There are countless psychic delivery systems, both conscious and
unconscious. A nightmare can function as a high-potency "homeopathic" medicine inside dream consciousness. A rivet of terror is slid
oneirically into a narrative as a way of dissolving its own fear "picture."

A remedy can also be generated by the dreamer within the
"dreamwork." For instance, even as homeopathic *Arsenicum* is not
chemical arsenic, arsenic in a nightmare is not a poison but an activated symbol. An *"Arsenicum"* value can be dreamed as a rabid dog
or as rat poison, plutonium, or some other lethal substance that your
oneiric self finds itself consuming, to its observer's horror. The formation energy of the dream becomes curative. Dreams, in fact, are
the original arena of self-healing, as noted at the end of chapter 4.

Visualized flowers, pills, and animals, once imaginally generated,
are no longer ordinary objects or even enhanced mental states but
semistable charms. Their powers are certified among tribal peoples in

amulets, totems, and altars. I say "semistable" because, after you create them, in order to sustain or replenish them you have to reinvent them from scratch, certainly for every use but also, to a degree, with every breath. As such, they are unconscious homeopathic projections.

Even outside dreams (as we have seen in Whitmont's remedy projections), *Aurum metallicum, Cadmium sulphuricum, Arsenicum*, and the others are unconscious objectifications.

Note: Homeopaths do not as such employ dream symbology, psychology, or Freudian and Jungian analyses of dreams in repertorizing. They take dream personae and landscapes at face value and decipher only what remedy they indicate. Their rubrics are summarized in the sections marked "Sleep, Dream" and "Mind, Dream" in James Tyler Kent's repertory and others.

The map known as the Seven Planes of Consciousness gives us a model for how the universe might be arranged in tiers or dimensions at different frequencies. They could as easily be called Seven Planes of Matter or Seven Planes of Manifestation. I learned my version from psychic teacher John Friedlander, who adapted it from theosophy and Vedic philosophy. I believe that the recognition of seven originary or creationary chords is universal. When I taught the Seven Planes system in eastern Maine in 2011, a visiting Penobscot healer told our group that his teachers imparted a similar grid with different divisions and, of course, Indigenous names.

The system basically depicts seven tiers of energy in our overall human range, though only the lower (denser) portions of the denser three of them are perceptible. These make up our everyday reality.

The planes don't climb so much as deepen and change pitch, though they do not project concrete energies like those of physics. They are literally planes (or atlases) of fields because their states of subjective apperception are inseparable from their objective manifestations. The hierarchy operates at the intersection of energy, mind, and form such that each plane is also tantamount to a whole reality equal to or vaster than this one.

The validity of these planes cannot be demonstrated in the way that one might attest to a sand dune or riverbed. They are attempts by psychic explorers to identify modes of energy and dimensional jumps they encounter, taking into account that our ordinary consciousness is limited to our nervous system while the universe is not. However, this is a model, and you don't have to take it literally; you can adapt it to your use.

The seven planes of our particular reality have acquired traditional names. In a theosophical roster, moving from subtler to denser, they are called Adi, Monadic, Atmic, Buddhic, Mental-Causal, Astral, and Physical-Etheric. "Subtler to denser" does not capture the planes' full nature, for they are not independently configured spaces generating sovereign phenomena; every landscape in our universe incorporates all seven just to manifest as a landscape. The higher a plane (or subplane within a plane), the more links and relationships it has—the more complex its consciousness and rich its dimensionality.

In this system, acupuncture takes place in the densest plane, the Physical-Etheric, but within its finer (Etheric) range. According to Friedlander, any unfinished business of a particular lifetime that doesn't get assimilated into its soul lingers as "permanent seeds" in the next incarnation's Etheric body. Because that business was unfinished, it couldn't be assimilated into the soul, so it got left behind and became the agenda for another lifetime. The acupuncturist's needles tap the seeds' plasma as it flows through the body's nadis and meridians just above a material frequency as pulsations—a kind of lymphatic electricity.

Just above or interior to the Etheric frequency is the densest portion of the Astral plane, where our emotions travel energetically from the last incarnation's seeds. It is here, according to homeopaths who use this map, that homeopathy, a diagnostic system that emphasizes the Mentals—meaning emotional vibrations—acquires its diagnostic and healing qualities. Unfinished emotional business hangs around in the Astral plane and becomes its own "permanent seed" to sprout and cultivate during the same incarnation. As the soul reenters the physical realm, it imbues these seeds and they become the basis of its expression and orientation, as well as its ailments and predispositions to disease.[14]

Potentized microdoses resonate with the Astral plane's polarities. As their substances are succussed in denser subplanes, they take on therapeutic aspects by aligning with Astral vibrations senior to Physical-Etheric ones. Specification attunes the vibration of a patient and their ailment to the frequency of a remedy. Higher potencies activate more karmic treatments, and lower ones more temporal healing.

The homeopathic repertory uses the Mentals for diagnosis and treatment of physical diseases because each remedy matches its ailment's Astral note at an emotional frequency. This model might explain why homeopathic microdoses retain only imprints of original vital substance in them. As they shift into the nonmaterial Astral plane, they forfeit Physical-Etheric density in order to acquire Astral virtues. Unsuccussed herbs and tinctures are predominantly Physical–Etheric. It is not a case of better or worse. Some ailments respond best to an Astral signal, and others to an Etheric or Physical one.

Microdoses based on Similars do not just convey Astral signals; they turn their properties into patterns and templates, which infuse their molecular forms with healing properties in potentized forms of iron, tin, zinc, lead, mercury, silver, gold, and the like, but also potentized forms of plants like foxglove, tansy, clematis, arnica, and rock rose and animal products like beeswax, snake venom, hawk feathers, dog milk, and cuttlefish ink. Light and radiation can also be raised to the Astral plane. Returned to the physical plane, they imprint Astral qualities in proteins, personalities, and constitutions.

According to many practitioners of the Seven Planes and systems like it, the plane or subplane immediately above the physical realm, whatever it is called, is the source of *every* physical core ailment and miasm, the core disease that Hahnemann and Kent deemed imperceptible. These conditions form in the subtle body like seeds growing into beanstalks and suggesting the pods of Jack Finney's 1950s' sci-fi novel and movie *Invasion of the Body Snatchers.* His panspermia beans became clones of humans they replaced but without psyches or souls; this might have been a creatively Gothic intuition of our situation in developing body-minds—we are clones of our subtle bodies *but not without souls.* As our permanent seed, our Etheric form picks up both ancestral and environmental illness before our physical body does and transfers them to it for reconciliation and healing.

Near-death experiences may be Etheric and Astral visitations of an oversoul (a truer name might be proxy-death experiences).

During Seven Planes journeys with my Maine psychic group in 2011, I recommended that, instead of trying to treat ourselves with direct elemental energy from Astral or higher planes, we take a cue from homeopathy and "succuss" an imaginal Astral pill, setting it to the vibrational field of a chosen ailment. The pill would be a visualization like a grounding cord or Buddhist lotus blossom. As in pharmaceutical homeopathy, it doesn't matter if there is more than one ailment to treat because the "pill" is holistic; it activates the vital force behind the organism. In addition, all physical pathologies have emotional and psychosomatic components.

Once the psychically potentized microdose is created like thoughtform at an Astral frequency, it is matched to a physical ailment.

Try it. Either repertorize your condition and choose a remedy from a materia medica (*Phosphorus, Lachesis, Pulsatilla,* et al.) or project your constitutional field and its disturbance directly into a visualization, a thoughtform or "tulpa" of a rose, stone, or energetic pattern. The thoughtform functions as an independent sentient object created by a concentration of thought and endowed with its own autonomy. It is not merely a pill-like sigil; it is a *living* entity. It can become multidimensional—resonating, rotating, and spiraling as it travels within the subtle body, altering its shape and nature as the energy composing it stabilizes.

Convert the visualization at an Astral frequency. Let the psychic pill match your ailment. Alternatively, swallow the lozenge and let its energy imbue your cellular matrix as mind or breath. Move your visualization and breathing to sites of ailments or blocks. You may want to illuminate—enhance—the pill with orange, yellow, indigo, or infrared light. You could also shrink it and insert it via the third eye.

The higher the Astral subplane of your potentization, the more powerful your medicine. But you have to match frequencies, not just shoot for the max, or you miss attunement.

You can also try potentizing a remedy at Causal-Mental, Buddhic, Atmic, and Monadic frequencies. An Atmic pill is effective for more serious diseases like Parkinson's, multiple sclerosis, or cancer because the laws of the Physical-Etheric realm are generated Atmically. The intergalactic, interdimensional Monadic matches the superconscious and superpositional aspects of different energy medicines. Anywhere becomes everywhere, though Monadic power is difficult for humans to modulate and specify.

The difference between alchemical nanopharmacy and telepathic nanopharmacy is situational. Either way, the next step is for the healee to assimilate the "pill." Using active imagination or subtle energy, you can in this way support the initial inklings of change.

You can even potentize an allopathic medicine psychically for extra virtue or antidoting side effects. According to this model, many pharmaceutical concoctions have Etheric and Astral side effects, some more curative (or harmful) than their clinical ones. While formulas based on herbs and other natural substances are more reliably salutary, even synthetic pharmaceuticals retain a scintilla of subtle energy, or else they couldn't transfer energy on this plane.

Herbal essences like burdock, tansy, blue cohosh, echinacea, and schizandra have less immediate wallop than most drugs but carry long-term information. Homeopathic remedies are *solely* informational. Either, again, can be psychically potentized.

You may also refer back to the section on microdose preparation in chapter 3 and make use of the specific techniques, though you probably won't want to go through the whole process of high-potency succussion imaginally. You might, though, potentize objects psychically that you wouldn't molecularly. For instance, the violence in the culture that has attached to your aura might be partly healed by triturating—grinding up—a visualized bullet and then diluting and succussing its powder. If those who commit gun violence were trained in this exercise, there might be less murders and mass shootings. The violence and the guns are collectivized both psychically and miasmatically, so each person can reduce their energy in their own aura, heal some aspect of the miasm in themselves, and lower the vibration of the projections and weaponized placeholders. Bullets can be triturated into fine power; then the powder can be diluted, succussed, and stored in pills. Sustaining the meditation and its sequence of images is itself curative. It is as much a form of pill-less homeopathy as Dzogchen meditation is a form of making and enhancing mental and physical stability.

You can also try preparing psychic homeopathic doses of standard pharmaceuticals and psychotropic drugs, either while still taking them or *instead of* taking them. It is a way to test the power of your own thoughtforms and the innate placebo effect.

Think of other miasmatically pathologized cultural totems for psychic homeopathy. Use your imagination; money and polarized political symbols are a good start. You may be surprised at how a seemingly fugitive seedling—a "mere" thought—develops a root system and expands its field throughout your psyche and cells.

In another form of psychic homeopathy, osteopath Steve Curtin recommends filling an imaginal balloon with water, placing it in a larger body of water, and meditating on it as it sinks underwater and its membrane dissolves, making the two waters electrically and magnetically one. This technique is meant to distribute imaginal water to areas of the body parched with too much heat (earth and air); it ameliorates conditions like digestive spasming, bloating, vertigo, and migraine. Curtin recently changed the sign outside his Ellsworth, Maine office from osteopathy to alchemy.

John Friedlander proposed that some of our worst fears as well as our habits of self-sabotage and self-shaming may be someone else's energy drawn into our aura when we match it subconsciously. Frozen there into knots and pictures, it feels like our own energy and imposes its same personal obligation. While reminding students that other people's cords can be removed by using psychic tools and creative visualizations—tweezers, acid, or fire—or by placing and dissolving them in psychic roses, he offered an old Berkeley Psychic Institute exercise in which one replaces a disease (or fear) picture with a facsimile that is not energetically attached to the aura—you visualize a neutral photocopy or Similar of the disease.

Here's my version of how John's psychic homeopathy works: Imaginally copy an emotional or physical malaise or an unwanted energy—make a replica of its feeling or tone. Then substitute—literally insert—the objectified proxy into your visualization in the place of the original, supplanting it.

I have found that fashioning a conscious psychic proxy is like freezing a still from a movie or taking an imaginal MRI of one's energy field—then inserting its card, a radionic replica with the same circuitry but *without* an emotive (or electric) charge, into its slot. The alias can be plugged directly where fear or another emotion has been running. Once it is inserted like a credit card in a reader, the mind-body "sees" it—sees itself in relation to it—and is startled out of the imposter motif.

Picture an astronaut on a tether with a handheld jet. Psychic homeopathy is swifter, in fact instantaneous, for the jet is imaginal, and hence capable of interstellar and interdimensional transit.

Decoys are not cure-alls—for one, you have to fill the crevice created by the old stuff's ejection with something other than more of the same gunk. This is not a simple proposition, for a stunned system doesn't recognize gunk as gunk, so it may not experience its removal as a real removal or its return as a return. That is why you have to keep revisualizing ("blowing") your image. Like a homeopathic medicine's succession of remedy pictures, the psychic remedy will continue to shift energetically and call for a next phase.

Nothing can be anywhere without something holding it in place: that's the basis of thoughtform generation, whether Buddhist, Gnostic, or a Sioux war dance. All artifacts annex energy, energy that has been shaped by something, just as all thoughts are made of energy—Physical, Etheric, Astral, or higher. Objects and symbols naturally align with and decompose into that energy, feeding unconscious renditions, the body-mind, and the universe. That is how subtle essence *is*. It disseminates in gossamer packets per nanosecond like a haunted mist. John Friedlander summarized dissolution of karma this way:

> Karma appears in your aura as a disk. The way you clear karma is with psychic homeopathy. You start by taking from your own aura some of the energy of the person with whom you have karma. If you have karma with any person, you will always have some of their energy in your space—so you don't have to go out and grab it from them, it will be there in your space. You don't need to know the person with whom you have the karma, you may never have

met them, they may not even be incarnated now. By feel, you can get a sense of them, and that sense is enough to find their energy. Most of this process is done by feeling or seeing; intellectual understanding may or may not come but is entirely unnecessary. To have karma with someone, you have to be holding onto some of their energy and have some experience that your soul hasn't assimilated. You just drop the energy—a little piece of energy of the person with whom you have the karma—into that karma disk like homeopathy. And the disk just breaks it up, it implodes. Now it might not entirely implode, but some of it will implode. If some of the karma remains, you can try again, check if some of the karma is with a different person. You can keep the disk inside your aura or place it outside. Most psychic clearing works better if you put what you're clearing outside your aura because it's a cleaner space. If it's inside your aura, there are all sorts of other things going on.[15]

Psychic homeopathy is a way of understanding the psychic—immaterial, subtle energy—basis of Hahnemannian homeopathy. The placebo effect is like psychic homeopathy condensed into unconscious thoughtforms.

When I first studied embryology, I was horrified to realize that my well-being and existence depended on a collaboration of trillions of tiny, independent organisms. I felt as though I might come apart at any moment.

It wasn't the revelation it should have been: that we are held together in our physical manifestation by not only evolving networks of atoms, molecules, cells, and codes but something else bracketing them—an Etheric field or vital force. It organizes them, or they would never congeal in the first place. That "something" can become a bridge from old-fashioned biology to a new concept of identity and organism.

"Thou Cannot Know": A Case Study

The paradox of homeopathy as well as its magic was illustrated by a case that developed in my own family in the early 1980s. My wife, Lindy, and I went through a baffling ailment with our daughter Miranda, starting when she was barely nine years old. We lived in Berkeley, California, at the time.

Miranda's illness surfaced in September of 1983 with a boil (sty) on her left eye following a cold. It took two weeks of soaking to break it open. A typical "pink eye" infection followed, spreading to both eyes. When the infection persisted for another week, we took her to our general practitioner, a doctor sympathetic to homeopathy and alternative medicines. He prescribed an antibiotic (erythromycin), after which the pink eye improved. However, her eyes never really felt right to her; they itched and were very red in the morning. She had times, especially at school, when she wanted to close them and keep them shut, so that we periodically had to fetch her home. Since her school was a new and difficult academy for which she wasn't fully prepared, we and the GP presumed a psychosomatic influence.

She has large, light blue eyes that have always attracted attention and provide a lightning rod for projections, hers and others'.

One Sunday morning in February, Miranda developed shooting pains in both eyes. They grew so uncomfortable that she rolled on the floor. We made an emergency phone call and met a substitute for our GP at his office. He could find no visible sign of infection, but in testing her vision, he found that it had deteriorated significantly since the past September, when it had been better than 20/20. He sent us to the only ophthalmologist in town available on a Sunday.

We ended up at a clinic filled with young children and elderly people. After a several-hour wait, the doctor examined her with eye charts and slit lamps. Based on her poor vision at the time, he was mainly interested in prescribing glasses. He did see signs of an infection, but he downplayed it as secondary to her poor vision and prescribed a stronger antibiotic with a steroid. He assured us the infection would be gone in two weeks.

Although Miranda had no further attacks after the treatment, her eyes still bothered her. She described it as a sensation of something being caught in them. She did not want to open them in bright light. Often when we were outdoors, she would pretend to be blind and ask to be led—a game that amused her and frightened us.

We kept our two-week appointment, at which the ophthalmologist declared the infection healed; he then of course wanted to proceed with glasses. Since her sight before the infection had been fine, we decided to wait. Meanwhile, the physician mother of one of Miranda's friends told us that we should be concerned about a systemic disease. On that tip we called a relative, a gynecologist in San Francisco. He recommended an ophthalmologist who, he said, was the best children's eye doctor in the Bay Area; he even set up our first appointment within a week.

This ophthalmologist was both compassionate and knowledgeable. He said almost immediately, "This is a very uncomfortable little girl and for good reason." After a thorough exam, he told us that the original doctor didn't know what he was talking about; Miranda had an extensive infection that had left disease products in both her eyes and mottled their corneas. He prescribed a stronger antibiotic with cortisone and regular cleansing of the vicinity around the eyes with a Q-tip and a particular shampoo. The brand name was No Tears, though Miranda came to call it More Tears.

To this point we had made no attempt to find an alternative physician. The disease was in a sensitive area and had begun as a seemingly common infection for children. We were not naive about deeper or more systemic causes, but much of life is spent *not* following through on creative agendas or seeking the underlying origins of situations, especially when acting as young parents in crisis mode. It is striking how many homeopathic sympathizers either overlook or abandon homeopathy at *just* the moments of crisis when it is most legendarily successful. But Miranda was already having trouble keeping up in school, and there seemed little room to experiment, especially with an organ as nonnegotiable as eyes. We were operating on what I have come to call "the technocratically sponsored fear channel"; it has a nonstop medical station that not only broadcasts widely but advertises 24/7 in the background of our civilization.

These days, most health care is sought and dispensed a bit like going to the nearest fast-food outlet when you're hungry because there is only an hour before you're due back at work. It's why many people postpone holistic self-inquiry. One is inattentive until their dilemma is so importunate or unresponsive to the range of allopathic treatments available that they are forced into radical attention and action.

When "systemic illness" rather than "infectious eye disease" entered my awareness, my first thought was homeopathy. However, when the heralded ophthalmologist dispelled the possibility of a more severe disease—and later confirmed his dismissal by lab tests— I returned to my former myopia (pun unintended), eschewing notions of psora and suppression of disease layers. To continue an antibiotic, now supplemented with cortisone, was disconcerting by homeopathic standards, but we planned to use it for as brief a period as we could. The credentials of our ophthalmologist led us to believe that the disease would be resolved quickly on at least a symptomatic level. Then we could explore a constitutional, if we chose, from a safer plateau.

Miranda began a daily regimen of cleaning with shampoo and a Q-tip and applying the antibiotic. Her improvement—if any—was minor, but at least she did not have recurrences of acute attacks. When summer came, she complained about her eyes sweating and the effect of traffic fumes and people's perfume on them, which, she said, caused her eyes to "go crazy." She demonstrated with frenzied jigs. She was still hypersensitive to light and avoided sunlight. We made another eye appointment in August. The ophthalmologist reexamined her thoroughly and said, despite her complaints, that he saw no further indication of infection. It was only a matter of time, he felt certain, before all effects of the disease disappeared. He told her to continue scrubbing scrupulously.

During the first weeks of school in the fall, Miranda's condition escalated. On several occasions, she ended up sitting along the classroom wall with her eyes closed, and either Lindy or I were called to rescue her. We finally took her directly from school to the ophthalmologist.

The once-charming physician was frayed; he accused us of not following through on his treatments because we believed in alternative medicines, and he insisted that her relapse was our fault. He did, however, agree that the infection was still raging. He referred us immediately to a San Francisco clinic specializing in infectious diseases of the eye.

Miranda's examination and culture there cost $200 (more like $600 by a 2023 value). We were told that she was having an allergic reaction to an underlying infection. There was no cure for the complex, the doctor said, but it could be treated hygienically. This meant continuing the shampoo treatments but extending them to the nostrils and sides of her nose. He emphasized that all of our previous methods had been either in error or incomplete. The early erythromycin was the only antibiotic to which her bacteria were susceptible, he said, and the later antibiotics prescribed by both ophthalmologists were wrong and, in the case of the cortisone, contraindicated and sight-threatening. The cleaning would work only if she cleaned *all* the infected zones, which meant her entire face and scalp too. Otherwise, bacteria would simply spread again from the neglected pockets.

Stung by the earlier doctor's insinuations, we implemented the treatment rigorously for three and a half months into December. The ailment improved enough that Miranda was able to stay at school and keep her eyes open, but she was unable to participate in outdoor sports in direct light (thus sat on the side in shade) and still had very red eyes each morning and a good deal of difficulty getting them open.

At this point we assumed that allopathy could make no further headway, and we had Dana Ullman take her case. He prescribed *Pulsatilla* on a constitutional basis. He also asked us to discontinue the topical antibiotic for at least ten days, advising us that she might experience an immediate aggravation. She did develop a heavy cold, but her eyes neither improved nor got worse.

Later in the month we were in rural northern California and visited a macrobiotic naturopath we knew through a friend. He suggested eliminating all dairy products, plus carrying out a mild saltwater bathing of the eyes twice daily. This included snorting the solution through her nostrils. He felt that Miranda's sodium balance was off, and he prescribed a complete mineral salt to improve it as well as to make up for what he called "trace element deficiencies." He said that homeopathy, for using just one substance at a time, could never fill the range of needs in her system. It was a misunderstanding of homeopathy, but even complementary vitalistic systems can be irreconcilable without being incompatible. Nonlinear effects synergize the oppositional aspects of rival modalities. Nonetheless, holistic contradictions lead to skepticism, loss of faith, and polypharmacy.

After two weeks Miranda's eyes were itchy and red again, and it was time for her to return to school. Clinically we were back at the starting gate. We did not want to antidote the homeopathic treatment, but we needed to lower her discomfort level, so we returned to the San Francisco clinic, which recommended more erythromycin while continuing the scrubbing; we also continued her restrictive diet. A few days later the right eye was clear, but the left was swollen almost shut. We called the clinic and they said there was nothing we could do but persist in the treatment. We called the prior ophthalmologist, and he said that the swelling was probably an infection in the gland and to continue soaking it. At this point we were at another impasse, so I phoned Edward Whitmont and related Miranda's history in detail.

After expressing his reservations about remote prescribing, he mailed us *Tuberculinum* 30C and included a cover letter in which he described her condition as a deep-seated psoric miasm and warned that use of the remedy with the antibiotic would cause aggravation. Within days after we gave her the remedy, the sty went down, but a second sty formed on her upper eyelid and swelled to the size of a small marble. We continued to soak it, but there was no improvement and she couldn't go to school.

We returned to our GP. He felt that, despite whatever else was true, he had to prescribe an oral antibiotic to deal with the immediate infection. She took tetracycline, and the sty eventually broke, although two months later a much smaller replica formed and lingered. During those months she continued the hygienic treatment and occasionally used topical erythromycin. Whitmont later attributed the failure of the remedy to the fact that she mistakenly took it twice—in his mind a dangerous gaffe. "It's lucky," he said, "it was her eye and not her heart"—homeopathic hyperbole, I hoped.

In early March the situation escalated. Running down a hallway, Miranda bumped into her older brother Robin and struck her eye. She screamed for almost five minutes and said she wanted to die. I called my gynecologist cousin and reviewed the alternatives. The next morning, he rang me back, having gotten us an appointment with a research ophthalmologist who did not ordinarily see patients but nonetheless would meet us in his laboratory that afternoon.

Chandler Dawson was a wise, grandfatherly gentleman, near retirement; he was gentler with Miranda than any ophthalmologist had been. With a graduate student, he ran her through a battery of slit lamps, dyes, and cultures and then heard out the whole history, including naturopathy and homeopathy. He said he knew her condition and could understand our series of blind circles. The disease was essentially—as the clinic had explained—a special reaction to ordinary bacteria. But he was more precise: It wasn't an infection of the eye in the usual sense and certainly should not have been treated as conjunctivitis. It was possibly the result of a preadolescent acne so slight as to be almost imperceptible except for an oiliness and slight scaling around her nose. The bacterial by-products of the skin got into the eyelids, into the lashes, and onto the cornea itself, causing the scarring. Through his magnifying lenses I could see the stained surface of Miranda's cornea with pits and streamers of irritation. "Deep-seated psoric miasm indeed," he mused. "The language is not contemporary, but the diagnosis is essentially correct. I wouldn't say anything when my student was here because he'd have my head. Graduate students are so narrow these days. But she has inherited a complex to which she is unable to generate a normal immune response."

We went back to our regimen of washing and using a topical ointment. Miranda visited the laboratory every other week; her vision was tested, the surface of her eyes mapped, her face photographed, and a culture taken. "I'm the star," she remarked. "There's no cure. I'm going to be like this forever. He'll have a photo album of my whole life."

Later, as a young adult in a comedy-club vignette touching on her ailment, Miranda acted out her ophthalmological crisis, then stood on a chair, threw out her arms theatrically, and asked, "Shooting star or movie star?" Even later, in *Love Diamond*, a one-woman theatrical piece that she developed in Portland, Oregon, and performed internationally, she reenacted her ophthalmic history as a series of J. B. Rhine–like parapsychology exercises in which a blindfolded patient conflates a test of her telepathy with an eye exam. As the piece went on, she transformed a preteen's sight-threatening corneal disease into an avant-garde artist's intimation of "alien abduction," impersonating Zeta Reticulan–like ophthalmologists who cut tiny holes in her cornea.

In the arc of *Love Diamond*, "seeing" and "being seen" kept changing places, and the line between sex and science broke down along with the line between violation and treatment. Porn-store fantasy booth replaced medical office. To seduce and examine became acts of the same impassive, mostly male authority.

Creative transfiguration continued to play a role in the ultimate deconstruction and healing of her ailment decades later, though the onion was never completely peeled.

After many childhood visits and reevaluations, Miranda's discomfort level and the scarring at the surface of her cornea improved. Photophobia and irritation remained, but her vision stabilized.

Three months into the cleansing regime she developed full-blown acne rosaceae. We were now trapped between systems of medicine. A new Berkeley homeopath said that we had to let the acne run its course because it was the externalization of the disease into less vital organs. Dawson said, "Hogwash! The acne is the *source* of the infection, and it is now rampant. Unless we treat this immediately with an internal antibiotic her sight will be permanently affected."

We agreed to let her go on tetracycline. For his part, Dawson promised the smallest possible amount—"a homeopathic dose," he joked. At the same time, we went to see the only homeopath in our area known for working with patients using allopathic drugs. On the day Miranda started the tetracycline, he took her entire case and prescribed *Mercurius*, at a very low potency—6C—and had her take it three times daily. He also prescribed homeopathically pre-pared microdoses of tetracycline to reduce negative side effects from the drug. I asked the obvious questions: Wasn't the skin ailment an outward, healthy transposition of the disease? Won't the antibiotic and potency still aggravate each other? Isn't giving repeated homeo-pathic doses dangerous?

He said: "I'm not an ideologue. I am interested in treating Miranda as she is. Her sight is threatened, so she should be taking an antibiotic. A good homeopathic treatment isn't bound by rules. I'm involved only in restoring her vital force, which is stronger than any pharmaceutical. I've never had problems with antibiotics or mul-tiple doses, and I consider such a view of homeopathy hogwash or superstition."

During a month of family travel on the East Coast, Miranda took all three remedies—a pharmaceutical and two sugar pills containing spiritualized essence—and she continued to scrub. She experienced the most dramatic improvement yet. Her skin cleared completely, and she was able to be outside in bright sunlight for the first time in years. When we returned to California, her bacteria level tested way down and her cornea was less aggravated. Dawson thought the tetracycline did it but admitted he didn't know how. "I gave it to her in subthera-peutic doses, and she missed a number of days at that. It's really a black box. Maybe homeopathic mercury is the answer, but I won't write that down anywhere. Who cares, as long as she's better?"

When I remarked that it was too bad that we couldn't know for sure, he said with a smile, "Oh, Son of Man, thou cannot know."

That spring Dawson expressed disappointment that, despite other improvement, Miranda's cornea was still pitted and her vision hadn't improved. Independently (at least by an allopathic model), she developed plantar warts, and they had spread along her feet and become quite painful. With the reduction of sensitivity in her eyes, she had begun ballet, and the warts made movement difficult. Lindy wanted to have a dermatologist treat them, as was done in her own childhood; I felt that they were somehow connected to the antibiotic and the eyes and I wanted the homeopath to see her first.

We compromised. Miranda went first to a dermatologist, who said that the warts were deep-seated and would be difficult to remove without surgery—best to leave them. The next day she went to the homeopath. In taking her case anew he repetorized a remedy that covered both scarring of the cornea and plantar warts (*Silica*). He reasoned that *Mercurius* was no longer relevant; it had been selected primarily for photophobia, which had been handled.

Within twenty-four hours the plantar warts had turned black and begun to fall off. A week later Dawson found her cornea remarkably cleared, and on the eye chart she shot right through the 20/20 line and kept on going until he said, with a smile, it was good enough.

Since we have no information about how either subtherapeutic tetracycline or microdoses of *Mercurius* and *Silica* work, or how Miranda's preadolescent metabolism and individuating psyche affected any of this, we can resolve nothing vis-à-vis competing systems, nor did we have any guarantee the cure would be sustained. *Thou cannot know.*

In fact, her ailment came back a decade later, somewhat less acutely, at age twenty-one, and proved difficult to treat in ensuing years. *Silica* and *Mercurius* had no follow-up success. Craniosacral therapy, notably adjustments freeing the movement of the sphenoid bone behind the eyes, was beneficial in relieving an associated headache and a feeling of tightness in her skull, but it did not affect her eyes. Acupuncture, applied kinesiology, and Chinese herbs, each in turn, seemed to improve mental and circulatory aspects without a beneficial ophthalmological response. If anyone says that they found the absolute system for curing everything for everyone, you know that they are fabulizing or have missed the point of holism and integration.

A Comparison of Homeopathy to Other Modalities

In summary, homeopathy resembles a number of other healing practices; these are ways in which it is similar to and distinct from each of them.

Homeopathy resembles **herbal medicine** and **Bach flower remedies** in that it is botanical and ethnopharmaceutical. It differs insofar as it uses spiritualized doses in place of substances, tinctures, or dews.

Homeopathy resembles **ayurvedic pharmacy** in that it employs animal, vegetable, and mineral substances according to constitutional principles and prescribes remedies by characterology. It differs from ayurveda in its emphasis on minute doses and algebraic preparations and also in its development of a repertory of symptoms and constitutional types according to a Western system of taxonomy of a few centuries rather than several millennia.

Homeopathy resembles **Chinese acupuncture and moxibustion** (and to some degree, Chinese herbs) in its constitutional theory and emphasis on a dynamic vitalized field. It differs in its basis of self-complete symptom pictures rather than humors or humoral cycles in need of rebalancing, in its pharmacy made by dilution and succussion rather than mortar and pestle or blade, and in its dynamic basis one frequency subtler in the Astral rather than the Etheric plane.

This does not preclude that both traditional Chinese medicine and ayurveda use homeopathic frequencies in their treatments; they are very old medicines encompassing many principles of healing not part of their overt protocols.

Homeopathy resembles **osteopathy** (including **chiropractic, cranial osteopathy,** and **craniosacral therapy**) in its indirect morphogenetic activation. Osteopaths almost never go to the site of a symptom but approach it indirectly on lines of compression and tractioning, often using fascial tissue to close ground between entry point and lesion. They may gently first hold—often cranially or sacrally—gears driven by tidal rhythms of the cerebrospinal pulse until the system achieves neutrality, a blend of body dowsing and geomancy.

By moving "homeopathically" toward rather than away from strain patterns, osteopaths release them like removing Chinese finger cuffs. After initially meeting tissue resistance, they withhold further pressure. This light palpation activates and enhances organ rotations—called inspir and expir—by which liver, kidneys, lungs, and so on, like interdependent relics of ancient independent invertebrates, flush out toxins in their environs and revitalize themselves, much as their oyster ancestors in a mineral sea.

By holding stillpoints and following lines of tension as they naturally unwind, osteopaths support pulses and rotations, releasing new energy through nerves and tissues while bringing the spine alternately into flexion and extension (or folding and unfolding). The message is: Go *into* tension in order to release it. Don't pull; do what's counterintuitive—tighten, then let go. That's homeopathic in principle: curing by Similars.

Some osteopaths believe that cerebrospinal fluid potentized by subtle touch functions as a homeopathic microdose. Likewise, the osteopathic stillpoint transmits information in a way that resembles high potencies. It energetically recapitulates the moment at which the embryonic primitive streak turns into a notochord and sets the basis for tissue layers.

Some people respond to both homeopathy and osteopathy; others respond only to palpations or only to potentized pills.

Homeopathy differs from all osteopathic medicines in its use of a pill rather than palpation, the use of character types instead of visceral "energy cysts," and an emphasis on succussed information transmission rather than energetic palpation.

If homeopathy is played on a theremin, osteopathy resembles a synthesizer.[1]

Homeopathy resembles **allopathy** in their shared history going back to Arabs, Greeks, and Romans, encompassing lineages of empirical medical schools that taught both allopathy and homeopathy until relatively recently; homeopathy's use of statistical science; its formal doctor-patient dyads; and its use of a biophysical rationale. Homeopathy differs from allopathy in its priority of individual constitutions over disease definitions, its spiritualized pharmacy, its distinction between a disease's core and its symptom layers, its treatment by Similars rather than Contraries, and its miasmatic theory of disease and civilization.

Homeopathy resembles **psychoanalysis** in its recognition of the psychosomatic components of all diseases and the importance of treating them emotionally and mentally as well as physically, as well as in its transference-like elicitation of symptoms and use of abreaction to jolt apathetic systems. It differs from psychiatry in not deconstructing neuroses, interpreting symbols, or finding affective causes for

personal behaviors. Stated otherwise, homeopathy uses psychological elements in its diagnosis but not in its treatment. Like Chinese
medicine, ayurveda, shamanism, osteopathy, and other holistic and
energetic modalities, it presumes that body, mind, and spirit integrate
dynamically at the moment of the correct treatment. Words are superfluous. In this insight, most non-Western medicines bypass Western
psychoanalysis, for as Indigenous healers around the world propose,
any disease can be cured by the form of energy that caused it.

One of my first energy teachers, Paul Pitchford, told me in 1975,
"Psychology is another obsession of this culture. It might be this
thing that happened or that. It might be present loss. It might be
from another lifetime. Who knows? Right now, there is only the
energy at our disposal. It doesn't matter where it comes from—genes,
chi, the stars. We get to use it all the same."

Homeopathy resembles **shamanism** in its use of totemic substances
and symbolic aliases and its magical relationship between a remedy,
healer, and healee. Homeopathic succussion miniaturizes some of the
dynamizing features of chanting, drumming, and evocative masks in
microdoses and jolts to systemic apathy. In that sense, homeopathy is
a modernized, clinical version of shamanic alchemy.

Homeopathy resembles **alchemy** in its apparent transduction and
transmutation of substances, which are pharmaceutically rather
than minerally potentized. Homeopathy encompasses but does not
reify alchemical sequences like those from mercury, sulfur, arsenic,
and antimony to silver and gold. It also differs from alchemy in that
it uses a decimal-based, microcosmic, nonhumoral paradigm and is
based on a miasmatic theory of disease rather than a gnosis of spirit
evolving through matter. Homeopathy represents a partial rebirth of
alchemy after the scientific revolution, for it is alchemy carried out in
submolecular alembics and athanors.

Radionics is like homeopathy in introducing a potentized energy, a form of radiance and illuminescence, and an interdimensional "telecom." While WiFi, the internet, cell phones, and degrees of broadband were discovered and developed *in this dimension,* they have analogous wiring for *inter*dimensional communication. Instead of being run like phone lines, printed circuits, and motherboards, radionic networks are drawn like sacred geometry in two dimensions and then hieroglyphically potentized to intercept and transmit clairsentience. Radionic devices use these sigil-like grids for transmission, replacing metals and transistors with runes. They send and receive other-dimensional energy, not electrons. Radionic bracelets, rings, coins, and medallions look like the guts of an old portable radio, but the stations they receive are clairaudient.[2]

If we were to imagine the signatures or crystalline transmissions of homeopathic microdoses enlarged to visibility, they might look like snowflakes, radionic circuits, or molecular hydroglyphs.

Homeopathic Resources

Americans for Homeopathy Choice
PO Box 203
Shelley, ID 83274
www.homeopathychoice.org

American Institute of Homeopathy
909 Summit View Lane
Charlottesville, VA 22903
www.homeopathyusa.org
A leading organization for licensed clinicians

Homeopathic Educational Services
812 Camelia Street
Berkeley, CA 94710
510-649-0294
www.homeopathic.com
A source for books, medicines, medicine kits, software, e-courses

National Center for Homeopathy
PO Box 1856
Clarksburg, MD 20871-1856
info@homeopathycenter.org
www.homeopathycenter.org

North American Society of Homeopaths
www.homeopathy.org
Organization of professional homeopaths

Vatsala Sperling
Rochester Homeopathy
One Park Street
Rochester, VT 05767
www.rochesterhomeopathy.com

For Further Reading

Certain areas touched on in this book are covered in greater depth in my other writings. Morphogenesis is examined throughout my two embryology books, *Embryogenesis: Species, Gender, and Identity* (2000) and *Embryos, Galaxies, and Sentient Beings: How the Universe Makes Life* (2003). Alchemical medicine is described in my essay "Alchemy: Pre-Egyptian Legacy, Millennial Promise," which appears in an anthology I edited, *The Alchemical Tradition in the Late Twentieth Century* (1991). My discussion of homeopathy for optical migraines appears in *Migraine Auras: When the Visual World Fails* (2006, see pages 167–169 and 186–207).

The relation of homeopathy to other alternative medicines is explored throughout editions of my two-volume work on the history and philosophy of medicine: *Planet Medicine: Origins* (2001) and *Planet Medicine: Modalities* (2003).

Acknowledgments

My thanks to Dana Ullman (the 1990s) and Vatsala Sperling (2023) for providing core material for different editions of this book. They are the true homeopaths; I am more of an ethnographer and riddler. Thanks to Elizabeth Perry and Nancy Ringer for helping me make a patchwork text into a true book. It took brilliant, far-seeing editing on their parts. Thanks to Aaron Davis for a beautiful cover.

Notes

Chapter 1. What Is Homeopathy?

1. James Gorman, "Take a Little Deadly Nightshade and You'll Feel Better," *New York Times Magazine*, August 30, 1992, 26.
2. Dana Ullman, "Homeopathic Medicine: A Modern View," *Whole Earth Review* (Fall 1993). The material I quote here comes from an expanded prepublication version of this article.
3. Theodore Enslin, speaking at a seminar at Goddard College, Plainfield, Vermont, May 1977.

Chapter 2. The Origins of Homeopathic Medicine

1. *Hippocrates*, translated by W. H. S. Jones (Cambridge: University of Harvard Press, 1923), quoted in Harris L. Coulter, *Divided Legacy: A History of the Schism in Medical Thought*, vol. 1, The Patterns Emerge: Hippocrates to Paracelsus (Washington, DC: Wehawken Book Co., 1975), 77.
2. Coulter, *Divided Legacy*, vol. 1, The Patterns Emerge, 76.
3. Coulter, *Divided Legacy*, vol. 1, The Patterns Emerge, 89.
4. Coulter, *Divided Legacy*, vol. 1, The Patterns Emerge, 35.
5. *Hippocrates*, translated by W. H. S. Jones, quoted in Coulter, *Divided Legacy*, vol. 1, The Patterns Emerge, 26.
6. *Hippocrates*, translated by W. H. S. Jones, quoted in Coulter, *Divided Legacy*, vol. 1, The Patterns Emerge, 79.
7. Coulter, *Divided Legacy*, vol. 1, The Patterns Emerge, 196.
8. Aulus Cornelius Celsus, *De Medicina* (ca. 47 CE), quoted in Coulter, *Divided Legacy*, vol. 1, The Patterns Emerge, 274.

9. Aulus Cornelius Celsus, *Prooemium to De Medicina*, quoted in Coulter, *Divided Legacy*, vol. 1, The Patterns Emerge, 252.

10. Aulus Cornelius Celsus, Aphorisms from *De Medicina*, quoted in Coulter, *Divided Legacy*, vol. 1, The Patterns Emerge, 256.

11. Aulus Cornelius Celsus, *De Medicina*, quoted in Coulter, *Divided Legacy*, vol. 1, The Patterns Emerge, 258.

12. Galen, quoted in Coulter, *Divided Legacy*, vol. 1, The Patterns Emerge, 308.

13. Paracelsus, *Das Erste Buch der Grossen Wundarznei* (1539), quoted in Coulter, *Divided Legacy*, vol. 1, The Patterns Emerge, 346.

14. Paracelsus, *Intimatio, basileae* (1527), quoted in Coulter, *Divided Legacy*, vol. 1, The Patterns Emerge, 347.

15. Paracelsus, *Entwuerfe zu den vier Buecher des Opus Paramirum* (1562), quoted in Coulter, *Divided Legacy*, vol. 1, The Patterns Emerge, 380.

16. Paracelsus, Das Buch Paragranum (1565), quoted in Coulter, *Divided Legacy*, vol. 1, The Patterns Emerge, 425.

17. Coulter, *Divided Legacy*, vol. 1, The Patterns Emerge, 384.

18. Paracelsus, *Liber de podagricis et suis speciebus*, quoted in Coulter, *Divided Legacy*, vol. 1, The Patterns Emerge, 417.

19. Paracelsus, *Drei Buecher der Wundarznei* (1536), quoted in Coulter, *Divided Legacy*, vol. 1, The Patterns Emerge, 426.

20. Albertus, *The Alchemist of the Rocky Mountains* (Salt Lake City: Paracelsus Research Society, 1976).

21. Paracelsus, quoted in "Doctrine of Signatures," *Io Magazine* 5 (epigraph for special issue, 1968): 4. The original source of the quote is Oswald Croll and Paracelsus, *Philosophy Reformed And Improved: In Four Profound Tractates*, trans. Henry Pinnell (London: Lodowick Lloyd, 1657).

22. Paracelsus, *Von Oeffnung der Haut*, quoted in Coulter, *Divided Legacy*, vol. 1, The Patterns Emerge, 443.

23. Oswald Croll, quoted in "Doctrine of Signatures," *Io Magazine* 5 (epigraph for special issue, 1968): 31–32. The original source of the quote is Croll and Paracelsus, *Philosophy Reformed And Improved*.

24. Harris L. Coulter, *Divided Legacy: A History of the Schism in Medical Thought*, vol. 2, Progress and Regress: J. B. Van Helmont to Claude Bernard (Berkeley, CA: North Atlantic Books, 1988), 110–11.

25. Jan Baptista van Helmont, *Oriatrike, or Physick Refined* (1662), quoted in Coulter, Divided Legacy, vol. 2, Progress and Regress, 15.

26. Jan Baptista van Helmont, *Oriatrike, or Physick Refined*, quoted in Coulter, *Divided Legacy*, vol. 2, Progress and Regress, 33.

27. Jan Baptista van Helmont, *Oriatrike, or Physick Refined*, quoted in Coulter, *Divided Legacy*, vol. 2, Progress and Regress, 56.

28. William Harvey, *The Works of William Harvey* (1847), quoted in Coulter, *Divided Legacy*, vol. 2, Progress and Regress, 129.

29. Thomas Steele Hall, *Rene Descartes: Treatise of Man* (Cambridge: Harvard, 1972), 5–6.

30. Hermann Boerhaave, *Dr. Boerhaave's Academical Lectures on the Theory of Physic, Being a Genuine Translation of his Institutes and Explanatory Comment* (1742–1746), quoted in Coulter, *Divided Legacy*, vol. 2, Progress and Regress, 130.

31. Coulter, *Divided Legacy*, vol. 2, Progress and Regress, 171.

32. Giorgio Baglivi, *De Praxi Medica ad Priscam Observandi Rationem Revocanda Libri Duo* (1696), quoted in Coulter, *Divided Legacy*, vol. 2, Progress and Regress, 185.

33. Thomas Sydenham, *The Works of Thomas Sydenham* (1848–1850), quoted in Coulter, *Divided Legacy*, vol. 2, Progress and Regress, 187.

34. Thomas Sydenham, *The Works of Thomas Sydenham*, quoted in Coulter, *Divided Legacy*, vol. 2, Progress and Regress, 191.

35. Théophile de Bordeu, *Oeuvres* (1818), quoted in Coulter, *Divided Legacy*, vol. 2, Progress and Regress, 241–42.

Chapter 3. The Tenets and Rubrics
of Homeopathic Medicine

1. Samuel Hahnemann, *The Lesser Writings*, quoted in Coulter, *Divided Legacy*, vol. 2, Progress and Regress, 375.

2. I originally wrote this anecdote for my (as yet) unpublished manuscript *Episodes in Disguise of a Marriage*.

3. M. L. Tyler, *Homoeopathic Drug Pictures* (Holsworthy Devon, U.K.: Health Science Press, 1942).

4. Tine, Edward P. Sr., "Repertory of the Homoeopathic Materia Medica," *Journal of the American Institute of Homeopathy* 58, no. 1–2 (Jan.–Feb. 1965).

5. Samuel Hahnemann, *The Organon of Medicine*, quoted in Coulter, *Divided Legacy*, vol. 2, Progress and Regress, 350.

6. Claude Lévi-Strauss, *Totemism*, trans. Rodney Needham (Boston: Beacon Press, 1963).

7. Rajan Sankaran, *Homeopathy for Today's World: Discovering Your Animal, Mineral, or Plant Nature* (Rochester, VT: Healing Arts Press, 2011), 87.

8. Sankaran, *Homeopathy for Today's World*, 11.

9. Sankaran, *Homeopathy for Today's World*, 32.

10. Sperling, *Colubrid Snake Remedies & Their Indications in Homeopathy Practice* (Kandern, Germany: Narayana Verlag, 2023).

11. Didier Grandgeorge, *The Spirit of Homeopathic Medicines: Essential Insights to 300 Remedies*, trans. Juliana Barnard (Berkeley, CA: North Atlantic Books, 1998), 205.

12. Tyler, *Homoeopathic Drug Pictures*, 707–16; Grandgeorge, *The Spirit of Homeopathic Medicines*, 165.

13. Tyler, *Homoeopathic Drug Pictures*, 143–52; Grandgeorge, *The Spirit of Homeopathic Medicines*, 47.

14. Samuel Hahnemann, quoted in Tyler, *Homoeopathic Drug Pictures*, 147.

15. Tyler, *Homoeopathic Drug Pictures*, 798–801; Grandgeorge, *The Spirit of Homeopathic Medicines*, 187–88.

16. Tyler, *Homoeopathic Drug Pictures*, 289–99.

17. Grandgeorge, *The Spirit of Homeopathic Medicines*, 67.

18. Tyler, *Homoeopathic Drug Pictures*, 586–93; Grandgeorge, *The Spirit of Homeopathic Medicines*, 138–39.

19. Tine, "Repertory of the Homoeopathic Materia Medica."

20. Tyler, *Homoeopathic Drug Pictures*, 666–70; Grandgeorge, *The Spirit of Homeopathic Medicines*, 156–57.

21. W. A. Boyson, "Repertory of the Homoeopathic Materia Medica," *Journal of the American Institute of Homeopathy* 58, no. 1–2 (Jan.–Feb. 1965).

22. Philip M. Bailey, *Homeopathic Psychology: Personality Profiles of the Major Constitutional Remedies* (Berkeley, CA: North Atlantic Books, 1995), 279–84; Tyler, *Homoeopathic Drug Pictures*, 681–87; Grandgeorge, *The Spirit of Homeopathic Medicines*, 159–61.

23. Bailey, *Homeopathic Psychology*, 279–84; Tyler, *Homoeopathic Drug Pictures*, 681–87; Grandgeorge, The *Spirit of Homeopathic Medicines*, 159–61.

24. Tyler, *Homoeopathic Drug Pictures*, 683.

25. Jerry Kantor, "Donald Trump's Homeopathic Remedy," Hpathy.com, August 17, 2016.

26. Jerry Kantor, personal communication, February 3, 2023.

27. Jerry Kantor, "Hillary Clinton's Homeopathic Remedy: Cross Me and You Have Crossed a Rattler," Right Whale Press website, July 26, 2016.

28. Jerry Kantor, "Hillary Clinton's Homeopathic Remedy."

29. Bailey, *Homeopathic Psychology*, 386–97.

30. Grandgeorge, *The Spirit of Homeopathic Medicines*, 192; Tyler, *Homoeopathic Drug Pictures*, 830–42; Bailey, *Homeopathic Psychology*, 386–88.

31. Grandgeorge, *The Spirit of Homeopathic Medicines*, 194.

32. Samuel Hahnemann, *Materia medica pura*, vol. 1 (New York: William Radde, 1846), 408.

33. Jonathan Shore, "After the Remedy," undated sheet given to patients at his office in Corte Madera, California, in the early 1990s. He was director of the Wholistic Health and Nutrition Institute in San Rafael.

34. Theodore Enslin, speaking at a seminar at Goddard College, Plainfield, Vermont, May 1977.

35. Kent, Lectures, 253–65.

36. Edward Whitmont, *The Alchemy of Healing: Psyche and Soma* (Berkeley, CA: North Atlantic Books, 1993), ix.

37. See Harris L. Coulter, *Vaccination, Social Violence, and Criminality: The Medical Assault on the American Brain* (Berkeley, CA: North Atlantic Books, 1990).

38. Alessio Fasano and Susan Flaherty, *Gut Feelings: The Microbiome and Our Health* (Cambridge, MA: MIT Press, 2021).

39. Zack Bush, "Zack Bush on COVID-19, Glyphosate, and the Nature of Viruses," interview by Jeffrey Smith for the Institute for Responsible Technology, June 30, 2020.

40. Hahnemann, *The Lesser Writings*, quoted in Coulter, *Divided Legacy*, vol. 2, Progress and Regress, 389.

41. "Methods of Preparation of Homeopathic Remedies," Preparation, Hahnemann Labs website, accessed December 21, 2023.

42. Whitmont, *The Alchemy of Healing*, 75.

43. Whitmont, *The Alchemy of Healing*, 10. In Whitmont's book, the paragraph that follows this quotation is also a part of the quotation. I wrote this second paragraph for Whitmont while editing his book, and he accepted it. I am reclaiming and editing it here to remake a useful distinction given his strong influence otherwise on my own belief system.

44. G. P. Barnard and James H. Stephenson, "Microdose Paradox: A New Biophysical Concept," *Journal of the American Institute of Homeopathy* (Sept.–Oct. 1967): 278.

45. Barnard and Stephenson, "Microdose Paradox," 278.

46. Whitmont, *The Alchemy of Healing*, 6.

47. Gorman, "Take a Little Deadly Nightshade," 73.

48. Jonathan Shore, personal communication, 1998.

49. Whitmont, *The Alchemy of Healing*, 7.

50. Whitmont, *The Alchemy of Healing*, 139–40.

51. Remennikova drafted this anecdote as part of the manuscript for an (as yet) unpublished book, *Activating Our 12-Stranded DNA*.

52. Gorman, "Take a Little Deadly Nightshade," 28.

53. Ullman, "Homeopathic Medicine."

54. Robert Poole, "More Squabbling Over Unbelievable Results," *Science* 241 (August 15, 1988): 658.

55. Thomas H. Maugh II, "Journal Probe of Lab Test Results Sparks Furor," *Los Angeles Times*, July 27, 1988.

56. Ullman, "Homeopathic Medicine."

57. Kent, *Lectures*, 96.

58. Theodore Enslin, speaking at a seminar at Goddard College, Plainfield, Vermont, May 1977.

59. Wyrth P. Baker, Allen C. Neiswander, and W. W. Young, *Introduction to Homoeotherapeutics* (Washington, DC: American Institute of Homeopathy, 1974).

60. Gorman, "Take a Little Deadly Nightshade," 28.

61. Dana Ullman, "Extremely Dilute Solutions Create Unique Stable Ice Crystals in Room-Temperature Water," press release, *Homeopathic Educational Services* (Berkeley, California), December 29, 1997.

62. Dana Ullman, "Extremely Dilute Solutions."

63. Dana Ullman, "Extremely Dilute Solutions." See also Shui-Yin Lo, "Physical Properties of Water with IE Structures," *Modern Physics Letters B* 10, no. 19 (1996): 921–30.

64. Brandon Specktor, "Frozen Tardigrade Becomes First 'Quantum Entangled' Animal in History," *Live Science*, December 20, 2021.

65. Richard Grossinger, *Bottoming Out the Universe* (Rochester, VT: Park Street Press, 2020), 254.

66. Grossinger, *Bottoming Out the Universe*, 89–90.

67. Iris R. Bell and Mary Koithan, "A Model for Homeopathic Remedy Effects: Low Dose Nanoparticles, Allostatic Cross-Adaptation, and Time-Dependent Sensitization in a Complex Adaptive System," *BMC Complementary and Alternative Medicine* 12 (October 22, 2012): 191.

68. Chandran Nabiar, "Nanoparticle Model of Iris Bell and Mary Koithan for Homeopathy—Skyscraper on a Flimsy Foundation," Redefining Homeopathy (blog), December 11, 2015.

69. Bell and Koithan, "A Model for Homeopathic Remedy Effects."

70. Bell and Koithan, "A Model for Homeopathic Remedy Effects."

71. Edward Whitmont, "Toward a Basic Law of Psychic and Somatic Interrelationship," *Homeopathic Recorder* (February 1949), 206; republished in Whitmont, *Psyche and Substance: Essays on Homeopathy in the Light of Jungian Psychology* (Berkeley, CA: North Atlantic Books, 1992).

72. Carl Jung, *Psychology and Alchemy*, trans. R. F. C. Hull (London: Routledge & Kegan Paul, 1953), 132.

73. Whitmont, *The Alchemy of Healing*, 216.

74. Edward Whitmont, "The Analysis of a Dynamic Totality: Sepia," *Homeopathic Recorder* (March 1950), 232; republished in Whitmont, *Psyche and Substance*.

75. Whitmont, "The Analysis of a Dynamic Totality: Sepia," 233.

76. Edward Whitmont, "Natrum Muriaticum," *Homeopathic Recorder* (1948), 119; republished in Whitmont, *Psyche and Substance*.

77. Edward Whitmont, "Phosphor," *Homeopathic Recorder* (April 1949), 265; republished in Whitmont, *Psyche and Substance*.

78. Rudolf Hauschka, *The Nature of Substance*, trans. Mary T. Richards and Marjorie Spock (London: Stuart and Watkins, 1968), 136–37.

79. Edward Whitmont, "Lycopodium: A Psychosomatic Study," *Homeopathic Recorder* (1948), 264–65; republished in Whitmont, *Psyche and Substance*.

80. Edward Whitmont, "Psycho-physiological Reflections on Lachesis," *British Homeopathic Recorder* (January 1975); republished in Whitmont, *Psyche and Substance*.

81. Edward Whitmont, "Non-causality as a Unifying Principle of Psychosomatics—Sulphur," in *Psyche and Substance*, 147–55.

82. Stanley Keleman, personal communication, 1978.
83. David E. Young, *The Mouse Woman of Gabriola: Brain, Mind, and Icon Interactions in Spontaneous Healing* (Coastal Tides Press, 2013), 9.
84. Young, *The Mouse Woman of Gabriola*, 34.
85. Young, *The Mouse Woman of Gabriola*, 8.

Chapter 4. Homeopathy and Modern Medicine

1. Kent, *Lectures*, 39.
2. Whitmont, *The Alchemy of Healing*, 105.
3. Ullman, "Homeopathic Medicine."
4. Hahnemann, *The Organon of Medicine*, quoted in Coulter, *Divided Legacy*, vol. 2, Progress and Regress, 385–86.
5. Theodore Enslin, "On Homeopathy," interview by Richard Grossinger, Cape Elizabeth, Maine, 1969, published in "Dreams," *Io Magazine* 8 (special issue, 1971), 319–320.
6. Andrew Solomon, *The Noonday Demon: An Atlas of Depression* (New York: Scribner, 2001), 292.
7. Solomon, *The Noonday Demon*, 400.
8. Solomon, *The Noonday Demon*, 400.
9. Foucault, *Madness and Civilization: A History of Insanity in the Age of Reason*, trans. Richard Howard (New York: New American Library, 1967).
10. Jerry Kantor, *Sane Asylums: The Success of Homeopathy before Psychiatry Lost Its Mind* (Rochester, VT: Healing Arts Press, 2022).
11. Richard Klein, Amherst Class of 1966 ListServ, January 2, 2023.
12. Sid Schwab, Amherst Class of 1966 ListServ, January 3, 2023.
13. Daniel Pinchbeck, "From Vacillation to Vaccination: Why, Despite Uncertainty, I Got the Johnson Shot," Daniel Pinchbeck's Newsletter, Substack, August 21, 2021.
14. R. E. Dudgeon, ed., *The Lesser Writings of Samuel Hahnemann* (New York: William Radde, 1852), quoted in Coulter, *Divided Legacy*, vol. 2, Progress and Regress, 319.
15. George Vithoulkas, *The Science of Homeopathy: A Modern Textbook*, vol. 1 (Athens, Greece: A.S.O.H.M., 1978), 134–35.
16. See Harris L. Coulter, *AIDS and Syphilis: The Hidden Link* (Berkeley, CA: North Atlantic Books, 1987).

Chapter 5. Samuel Hahnemann and the Fundamentalist Basis of Homeopathy

1. Richard Haehl, *Samuel Hahnemann, His Life and Work*, vol. 1 (London: Homeopathic Publishing Company, 1922), 10.

2. Haehl, *Samuel Hahnemann*, 11.

3. Haehl, *Samuel Hahnemann*, 36.

4. Haehl, *Samuel Hahnemann*, 35.

5. Haehl, *Samuel Hahnemann*, 58.

6. Haehl, *Samuel Hahnemann*, 63.

7. Haehl, *Samuel Hahnemann*, 64.

8. Samuel Hahnemann, aphorism 18 in *Organon of the Rational Art of Healing*, trans. C. E. Wheeler (London, 1913; orig. 1810), quoted in Handley, *A Homeopathic Love Story: The Story of Samuel and Mélanie Hahnemann* (Berkeley, CA: North Atlantic Books, 1990), 70.

9. Hahnemann, *Organon of the Rational Art of Healing*, quoted in Handley, *A Homeopathic Love Story*, 20.

10. Hahnemann, *Organon of the Rational Art of Healing*, quoted in Handley, *A Homeopathic Love Story*, 322.

11. Handley, *A Homeopathic Love Story*, 90–91.

12. Dudgeon, ed., *The Lesser Writings of Samuel Hahnemann*, quoted in Handley, *A Homeopathic Love Story*, 91.

13. Barnard and Stephenson, "Microdose Paradox," 278–79.

14. Haehl, *Samuel Hahnemann*, 126.

15. Coulter, *Divided Legacy*, vol. 2, Progress and Regress, 170.

16. Coulter, *Divided Legacy*, vol. 2, Progress and Regress, 171.

17. Gorman, "Take a Little Deadly Nightshade," 28.

18. Quoted in Haehl, *Samuel Hahnemann*, 100.

19. Handley, *A Homeopathic Love Story*, 76–77.

20. Handley, *A Homeopathic Love Story*, 77–78.

21. Handley, *A Homeopathic Love Story*, 77–78.

22. Samuel Hahnemann, *The Chronic Diseases, Their Peculiar Nature, and Their Homoeopathic Cure* (Philadelphia: Boericke & Tafel, 1904), 12.

23. Hahnemann, *The Chronic Diseases*, 12.

24. Hahnemann, *The Chronic Diseases*, 38.

25. Hahnemann, *The Chronic Diseases*, 38.

26. Haehl, *Samuel Hahnemann*, 179.
27. Haehl, *Samuel Hahnemann*, 179.
28. Handley, *A Homeopathic Love Story*, 5–6.
29. Haehl, *Samuel Hahnemann*, 222.
30. Handley, *A Homeopathic Love Story*, 6.
31. Frances Yates, *Giordano Bruno and the Hermetic Tradition* (Oxfordshire, U.K.: Routledge and Keegan Paul, 1964), 455.
32. Frances Yates, *The Rosicrucian Enlightenment* (Oxfordshire, U.K.: Routledge and Keegan Paul, 1972), 219.
33. Richard Haehl, *Samuel Hahnemann, His Life and Work*, vol. 2 (London: Homeopathic Publishing Company, 1922), quoted in Handley, *A Homeopathic Love Story*, 12.

Chapter 6. The Homeopathic Tradition in North America

1. Harris L. Coulter, *Divided Legacy: A History of the Schism in Medical Thought*, vol. 3, The Conflict between Homeopathy and the American Medical Association (Berkeley, CA: North Atlantic Books, 1982), 62–63.
2. Coulter, *Divided Legacy*, vol. 3, The Conflict between Homeopathy and the American Medical Association, 168.
3. Coulter, *Divided Legacy*, vol. 3, The Conflict between Homeopathy and the American Medical Association, 168.
4. Coulter, *Divided Legacy*, vol. 3, The Conflict between Homeopathy and the American Medical Association, 180.
5. Coulter, *Divided Legacy*, vol. 3, The Conflict between Homeopathy and the American Medical Association, 106.
6. Coulter, *Divided Legacy*, vol. 3, The Conflict between Homeopathy and the American Medical Association, 264–65.
7. Coulter, *Divided Legacy*, vol. 3, The Conflict between Homeopathy and the American Medical Association, 269–70.
8. Coulter, *Divided Legacy*, vol. 3, The Conflict between Homeopathy and the American Medical Association, 403.
9. Coulter, *Divided Legacy*, vol. 3, The Conflict between Homeopathy and the American Medical Association, 411.

10. Coulter, *Divided Legacy*, vol. 3, The Conflict between Homeopathy and the American Medical Association, 414.
11. Coulter, *Divided Legacy*, vol. 3, The Conflict between Homeopathy and the American Medical Association, 438.
12. Haehl, *Samuel Hahnemann*, 187.
13. Coulter, *Divided Legacy*, vol. 3, The Conflict between Homeopathy and the American Medical Association, 441.
14. Coulter, *Divided Legacy*, vol. 3, The Conflict between Homeopathy and the American Medical Association, 447–48.
15. Gorman, "Take a Little Deadly Nightshade," 26.
16. Gorman, "Take a Little Deadly Nightshade," 23.
17. Mark Twain, "A Majestic Literary Fossil," *Harper's Magazine*, February 1890, 444.
18. Dana Ullman, *Evidence Based Homeopathic Family Medicine* (Homeopathic Educational Services, 1998). Ullman updates and expands this reference guide every year.

Chapter 7. Homeopathic Parallels: Other Similars and Microdose Effects

Some parts of the first section of this chapter, "Pill-less Potentized Microdoses," were adapted from "On Healing" in my book *The Bardo of Waking Life*, pages 177–78.

Some parts of the second section, "Astrology," were adapted from my books *The Return of the Tower of Babel: Birth Pangs of the Aquarian World* and *The Night Sky: Soul and Cosmos*, pages 551–54.

Some parts of the third section, "Psychic and Dream Homeopathy," were adapted from my books *Bottoming Out the Universe*, pages 81–82; *Dark Pool of Light: Reality and Consciousness*, vol. 2; *Consciousness in Psychospiritual and Psychic Ranges*, pages 172–74; *Dark Pool of Light: Reality and Consciousness*, vol. 3; *The Crisis and Future of Consciousness*, pages 51 and 54–55; and my preface to *Other Dimensional Entities*, self-published in Cork, Ireland, by Christopher Freeland in 2022.

1. I originally drafted this text for my (as yet) unpublished manuscript *Episodes in Disguise of a Marriage*.

2. I originally drafted this text for my (as yet) unpublished manuscript *Episodes in Disguise of a Marriage*.

3. William Carlos Williams, "Asphodel, That Greeny Flower," from *Pictures from Brueghel and Other Poems* (New York: New Directions, 1962).

4. I originally drafted this text for my (as yet) unpublished manuscript *Episodes in Disguise of a Marriage*.

5. I originally drafted this text for my (as yet) unpublished manuscript *Out of Babylon, Book Two: The James Brothers*.

6. I originally drafted this text for my (as yet) unpublished manuscript *Episodes in Disguise of a Marriage*.

7. David Barreto, *Karma and Reincarnation in the Animal Kingdom: The Spiritual Origin of Species* (Rochester, VT: Destiny Books, 2023), 50 (ant), 67 (dog).

8. Pierre Teilhard de Chardin, "The Evolution of Chastity," in *Toward the Future*, trans. René Hague (San Francisco: HarperOne, 2002), 86–87.

9. Jule Eisenbud, "Interview with Jule Eisenbud," January 8, 1972, in Richard Grossinger, ed., *Ecology and Consciousness: Traditional Wisdom on the Environment* (Berkeley, CA: North Atlantic Books, 1992), 152.

10. Claude Lévi-Strauss, "The Sorcerer and His Magic" in *Structural Anthropology*, (New York: Doubleday, 1967), 161–180, discussed in Richard Grossinger, *Planet Medicine: Origins* (Berkeley, CA: North Atlantic Books, 2001), 169–182.

11. Willi Sucher, "The Zodiac of the Constellations," in *Star Rhythms: Readings in a Living Astrology*, ed. William Lonsdale (Richmond, CA: North Atlantic Books, 1979), 75 and 102 (rearranged for my context).

12. Whitmont, *The Alchemy of Healing*, 158 and 184.

13. Robert Allen Pittman, *The Chiron Text*, unpublished manuscript.

14. John Friedlander, *Recentering Seth: Teachings from a Multidimensional Entity on Living Gracefully and Skillfully in a World You Create but Do Not Control* (Rochester, VT: Bear & Company, 2022), 372–73.

15. Friedlander, *Recentering Seth*, 275.

Appendix II. A Comparison of Homeopathy
to Other Modalities

1. I first wrote this description of our craniosacral training for my (as yet) unpublished manuscript *Episodes in Disguise of a Marriage.*

2. Christopher Freeland, *Other Dimensional Entities: Their Recognition & Release* (self-published, 2022).

Bibliography

Albertus, Frater. *The Alchemist of the Rocky Mountains*. Salt Lake City: Paracelsus Research Society, 1976.

Bailey, Philip M., *Homeopathic Psychology: Personality Profiles of the Major Constitutional Remedies*. Berkeley, CA: North Atlantic Books, 1995.

Baker, Wyrth P., Allen C. Neiswander, and W. W. Young. *Introduction to Homoeotherapeutics*. Washington, DC: American Institute of Homeopathy, 1974.

Barnard, G. P., and James H. Stephenson. "Microdose Paradox: A New Biophysical Concept." *Journal of the American Institute of Homeopathy* (Sept.–Oct. 1967): 278–79.

Barreto, David. *Karma and Reincarnation in the Animal Kingdom: The Spiritual Origin of Species*. Rochester, VT: Destiny Books, 2023.

Bell, Iris R. and Koithan, Mary. "A Model for Homeopathic Remedy Effects: Low Dose Nanoparticles, Allostatic Cross-Adaptation, and Time-Dependent Sensitization in a Complex Adaptive System." *BMC Complementary and Alternative Medicine* 12 (October 22, 2012): 191.

Boyson, W. A. "Repertory of the Homoeopathic Materia Medica." *Journal of the American Institute of Homeopathy* 58, no. 1–2, (Jan.–Feb. 1965).

Bush, Zack. "Zack Bush on COVID-19, Glyphosate, and the Nature of Viruses." Interview by Jeffrey Smith. Institute for Responsible Technology, June 30, 2020.

Coulter, Harris L. *AIDS and Syphilis: The Hidden Link*. Berkeley, CA: North Atlantic Books, 1987.

———. *Divided Legacy: A History of the Schism in Medical Thought*. Vol. 1, *The*

Patterns Emerge: Hippocrates to Paracelsus. Washington, DC: Wehawken Book Company, 1975.

———. *Divided Legacy: A History of the Schism in Medical Thought.* Vol. 2, *Progress and Regress: J. B. van Helmont to Claude Bernard.* Berkeley, CA: North Atlantic Books, 1988.

———. *Divided Legacy: A History of the Schism in Medical Thought.* Vol. 3, *The Conflict between Homeopathy and the American Medical Association.* Berkeley, CA: North Atlantic Books, 1982.

———. *Divided Legacy: A History of the Schism in Medical Thought.* Vol. 4, *Twentieth-Century Medicine: The Bacteriological Era.* Berkeley, CA: North Atlantic Books, 1994.

———. *Vaccination, Social Violence, and Criminality: The Medical Assault on the American Brain.* Berkeley, CA: North Atlantic Books, 1990.

"Doctrine of Signatures." *Io Magazine* 5 (special issue, 1968).

Dudgeon R. E., ed. *The Lesser Writings of Samuel Hahnemann.* New York: William Radde, 1852.

Eisenbud, Jule. "Interview with Jule Eisenbud." January 8, 1972. In Richard Grossinger, ed., *Ecology and Consciousness: Traditional Wisdom on the Environment.* Berkeley, CA: North Atlantic Books, 1992.

Enslin, Theodore. "On Homeopathy." Interview by Richard Grossinger, Cape Elizabeth, Maine, 1969. "Dreams," *Io Magazine* 8 (special issue, 1971): 310–323.

Fasano, Alessio, and Susan Flaherty. *Gut Feelings: The Microbiome and Our Health.* Cambridge, MA: MIT Press, 2021.

Foucault, Michel. *Les Mots et Les Choses.* Paris: Editions Gallimard, 1966; excerpt titled "The Writing of Things," translated by William Christian, in "Doctrine of Signatures," *Io Magazine* 5 (special issue, 1968).

———. *Madness and Civilization: A History of Insanity in the Age of Reason.* Translated by Richard Howard. New York: New American Library, 1967.

Freeland, Christopher. *Other Dimensional Entities: Their Recognition & Release.* Self-published, 2022.

Friedlander, John. *Recentering Seth: Teachings from a Multidimensional Entity on Living Gracefully and Skillfully in a World You Create But Do Not Control.* Rochester, VT: Bear & Company, 2022.

Gorman, James. "Take a Little Deadly Nightshade and You'll Feel Better." *New York Times Magazine,* August 30, 1992.

Grandgeorge, Didier. *The Spirit of Homeopathic Medicines: Essential Insights to 300 Remedies.* Translated by Juliana Barnard. Berkeley, CA: North Atlantic Books, 1998.

Grossinger, Richard. *The Alchemical Tradition in the Late Twentieth Century.* Berkeley, CA: North Atlantic Books, 1991.

———. *The Bardo of Waking Life.* Berkeley, CA: North Atlantic Books, 2008.

———. *Bottoming Out the Universe.* Rochester, VT: Park Street Press, 2020.

———. *Embryogenesis: Species, Gender, and Identity.* Berkeley, CA: North Atlantic Books, 2000.

———. *Embryos, Galaxies, and Sentient Beings: How the Universe Makes Life.* Berkeley, CA: North Atlantic Books, 2003.

———. *Episodes in Disguise of a Marriage*, title tentative, unpublished manuscript.

———. *Migraine Auras: When the Visual World Fails.* Berkeley, CA: North Atlantic Books, 2006.

———. *The Night Sky: Soul and Cosmos.* Berkeley, CA: North Atlantic Books, 2014.

———. *Out of Babylon, Book Two: The James Brothers*, title tentative, unpublished manuscript.

———. *Planet Medicine: Modalities.* Berkeley, CA: North Atlantic Books, 2003.

———. *Planet Medicine: Origins.* Berkeley, CA: North Atlantic Books, 2001.

———. *The Return of the Tower of Babel: Birth Pangs of the Aquarian World.* Published in serial form through *Jovian Bricolage,* Substack (online), 2022–2023.

Haehl, Richard. *Samuel Hahnemann, His Life and Work.* Vol. 1. London: Homeopathic Publishing Company, 1922.

Hahnemann Labs website. "Methods of Preparation of Homeopathic Remedies." Preparation. Accessed December 21, 2023.

Hahnemann, Samuel. *The Chronic Diseases, Their Peculiar Nature, and Their Homoeopathic Cure.* Philadelphia: Boericke & Tafel, 1904.

———. *Materia medica pura*, vol. 1. New York: William Radde, 1846.

Hall, Thomas Steele. *René Descartes: Treatise of Man.* Cambridge, MA: Harvard, 1972.

Handley, Rima. *A Homeopathic Love Story: The Story of Samuel and Mélanie Hahnemann*. Berkeley, CA: North Atlantic Books, 1990.

Hauschka, Rudolf. *The Nature of Substance*. Translated by Mary T. Richards and Marjorie Spock. London: Stuart and Watkins, 1968.

Jung, Carl. *Psychology and Alchemy*. Translated by R. F. C. Hull. London: Routledge & Kegan Paul, 1953.

Kantor, Jerry M. "Donald Trump's Homeopathic Remedy." Hpathy.com, August 17, 2016.

———. "Hillary Clinton's Homeopathic Remedy: Cross Me and You Have Crossed a Rattler." Right Whale Press website, July 26, 2016.

———. *Sane Asylums: The Success of Homeopathy before Psychiatry Lost Its Mind*. Rochester, VT: Healing Arts Press, 2022.

Kent, James Tyler. *Lectures on Homoeopathic Philosophy*. Berkeley, CA: North Atlantic Books, 1979 (orig. 1900).

Lévi-Strauss, Claude. *Totemism*. Translated by Rodney Needham. Boston: Beacon Press, 1963.

Lo, Shui-Yin, "Physical Properties of Water with IE Structures." *Modern Physics Letters B* 10, no. 19 (1996).

Maugh, Thomas H. II. "Journal Probe of Lab Test Results Sparks Furor." *Los Angeles Times*, July 27, 1988.

Nabiar, Chandran. "Nanoparticle Model of Iris Bell and Mary Koithan for Homeopathy—Skyscraper on a Flimsy Foundation." *Redefining Homeopathy* (blog), December 11, 2015.

Pinchbeck, Daniel. "From Vacillation to Vaccination: Why, Despite Uncertainty, I Got the Johnson Shot." *Daniel Pinchbeck's Newsletter*, Substack, August 21, 2021.

Pittman, Robert Allen. *The Chiron Text*, title tentative, unpublished manuscript.

Poole, Robert. "More Squabbling Over Unbelievable Results." *Science* 241 (August 15, 1988): 658.

Remennikova, Ruslana. *Activating Our 12-Stranded DNA*, unpublished manuscript.

Sankaran, Dr. Rajan. *Homeopathy for Today's World: Discovering Your Animal, Mineral, or Plant Nature*. Rochester, VT: Healing Arts Press, 2011.

Shaw, George Bernard. *The Doctor's Dilemma*. New York: Penguin Books, 1965.

Solomon, Andrew. *The Noonday Demon: An Atlas of Depression*. New York: Scribner, 2001.

Specktor, Brandon. "Frozen Tardigrade Becomes First 'Quantum Entangled' Animal in History." *Live Science*, December 20, 2021.

Sperling, Vatsala. *Colubrid Snake Remedies & Their Indications in Homeopathy Practice*. Kandern, Germany: Narayana Verlag, 2023.

Sucher, Willi. "The Zodiac of the Constellations." In *Star Rhythms: Readings in a Living Astrology*, edited by William Lonsdale. Richmond, CA: North Atlantic Books, 1979.

Teilhard de Chardin, Pierre. "The Evolution of Chastity." In *Toward the Future*. Translated by René Hague. San Francisco: HarperOne, 2002.

Tine, Edward P. Sr. "Repertory of the Homoeopathic Materia Medica." *Journal of the American Institute of Homeopathy* 58, no. 1–2 (Jan.–Feb. 1965).

Twain, Mark. "A Majestic Literary Fossil." *Harper's Magazine*, February 1890.

Tyler, M. L. *Homoeopathic Drug Pictures*. Holsworthy Devon, U.K.: Health Science Press, 1942.

Ullman, Dana. *Evidence Based Homeopathic Family Medicine*. Homeopathic Educational Services, 1998.

———. "Extremely Dilute Solutions Create Unique Stable Ice Crystals in Room-Temperature Water: Implications for Medicine, Manufacturing, and Technology." Press release (Berkeley, California: Homeopathic Educational Services), December 29, 1997.

———. "Homeopathic Medicine: A Modern View." *Whole Earth Review* (Fall 1993). Material quoted from prepublication version.

Vithoulkas, George. *The Science of Homeopathy: A Modern Textbook*. Vol. 1. Athens, Greece: A.S.O.H.M., 1978.

Whitmont, Edward. *The Alchemy of Healing: Psyche and Soma*. Berkeley, CA: North Atlantic Books, 1993.

———. *Psyche and Substance: Essays on Homeopathy in the Light of Jungian Psychology*. Berkeley, CA: North Atlantic Books, 1992.

Williams, William Carlos. *Pictures from Brueghel and Other Poems*. New York: New Directions, 1962.

Yates, Frances. *Giordano Bruno and the Hermetic Tradition*. Oxfordshire, U.K.: Routledge and Keegan Paul, 1964.

———. *The Rosicrucian Enlightenment*. Oxfordshire, U.K.: Routledge and Keegan Paul, 1972.

Young, David E. *The Mouse Woman of Gabriola: Brain, Mind, and Icon Interactions in Spontaneous Healing*. Coastal Tides Press, 2013.

Index

Hahnemann Laboratories, 89–90
Hahnemann Medical College, 215
half-homeopathy, 213, 273
Haller, Albrecht von, 160
Handley, Rima, 174, 180
Hauschka, Rudolf, 123
healing. *See also* Contraries;
    homeopathy; Similars
    and energy medicine, xiii
    in esoteric homeopathy, 80
    and life essence, 7–8
    real healing, 155–56
    as theater, 241–42
    transfer of, 237
    via empiricism, rationalism, and
        vitalism, 20–31
healing crisis, 133, 215
health care system, 142–49, 215–16
    why it functions, 153
herbal essences, 251
herbal medicine, compared to
    homeopathy, 266
Hering, Constantine, 195–97
hermeticism, 190
Herophilos of Chalcedon, 28–29
HERV, defined, 84
hexing, medical, 239–42
Hippocrates, 22, 27–28
Holcombe, William, 205
holism, 171, 222, 236–38
    defined, 135–36
homeopathic allopathy, 153–56, 204–6
homeopathic parallels, other Similars
    and microdose effects, 230–65
homeopathic remedies, 62–63, 92–93.
    See also under individual remedy
    names

mirror illness, 6
mystery of, 97–98
names of, 62–63
preparation of, 86–91, 95–97
sales of, 224
why is it noticeable? 10
homeopathic resources, 271–72
homeopathic schools, 14–15
homeopathy. *See also* esoteric
    homeopathy; homeopathic
    remedies; North America,
    homeopathy in
basic rule, 75, 236
benefits of, ix–x
cannot work as substance, 117–18
central principles of, 3, 171
compared to other modalities,
    266–70
critiques of, 11, 176–78, 200–204
defined, 1–3
described, 1–18
as empirical and vitalistic, 1–2
first law of homeopathic pharmacy,
    72–73
function of homeopathic medicine,
    6
the fundamentalist basis of, 157–92
and Hahnemannism, 164–66
how it works, 6–7, 101–10, 116–18
and isopathy, 19–20
key precepts of, 10
as magic, 18
merger with allopathy, 204–6, 211
modern medicine and, 127–56
the mystery of, 166–69
new substances for, 100–101
not a science, 2

OXFORDSHIRE
AT WORK
IN OLD PHOTOGRAPHS

OXFORDSHIRE
AT WORK
IN OLD PHOTOGRAPHS

COMPILED BY
MALCOLM GRAHAM

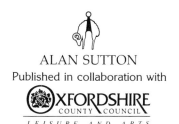

ALAN SUTTON
Published in collaboration with
OXFORDSHIRE
COUNTY COUNCIL
LEISURE AND ARTS

Alan Sutton Publishing Limited
Phoenix Mill · Far Thrupp · Stroud · Gloucestershire

First Published 1991

British Library Cataloguing in Publication Data

Oxfordshire at work in old photographs.
I. Title   II. Graham, Malcolm, *1948–*
942.574

ISBN 0-86299-986-3

Typeset in 9/10 Korinna.
Typesetting and origination by
Alan Sutton Publishing Limited.
Printed in Great Britain by
The Bath Press, Avon.

CONTENTS

INTRODUCTION

Despite all the growth and development of the twentieth century Oxfordshire remains essentially rural in character and farming continues to shape much of the landscape. As late as 1921 agriculture was still the county's largest employer and 234 out of every 1,000 people worked on the land. Before mechanization, farming was highly labour-intensive and much of the community, including women and children, played a part in gathering the harvest. Large numbers of men were also involved in the contract ploughing gangs that were sent out by firms like the Oxfordshire Steam Ploughing Company at Cowley. By contrast, the shepherd's life could be quite isolated, and the ploughman might spend hours with only his horses for company as he plodded to and fro across the fields. For such men the hiring fair or harvest home celebration provided a rare opportunity to let their hair down, especially if something stronger than tea was available (see p. 17). When looking at old photographs of farming scenes it is easy to hanker after a lost Golden Age when agriculture and the environment were in perfect harmony, but the reality was hard work and low pay and Oxfordshire's farm labourers were the worst paid in England in 1911. In addition, the picturesque view of farmwork portrayed by artists and photographers ignored the often dangerous nature of the job (see p. 28).

Oxfordshire was virtually untouched by the Industrial Revolution, and in 1902 the county was felt to be 'prevented, as if by fate, from ever attaining to the position of a great industrial or commercial centre.' Domestic crafts, such as gloving and lace-making, which had helped families eke out low agricultural wages found it difficult to compete with mass-produced, machine-made products. Small scale local trades like stone quarrying and brick making were tending to disappear because non-local building materials could be brought into the county more easily and cheaply, but some local crafts continued to prosper and few villages were without their blacksmith, wheelwright or miller. At the same time, other businesses which had once served a local need now expanded well beyond these confines. The Witney blanket industry, for example, became nationally and internationally known for its products. Frank Cooper's Oxford Marmalade, first made on a virtually domestic scale in 1874, became a household name by the Edwardian period. Local agricultural implement makers, such as Nalder's of Challow and Samuel-

6

son's in Banbury, began to export their products and the size of the Britannia Works at Banbury provided a foretaste of the industry to come in twentieth-century Oxfordshire. The unexpected, unplanned and, at first, unnoticed arrival of the motor industry and other large-scale businesses brought a new prosperity to the county. Oxfordshire people were not, however, entirely immune from the problems of unemployment between the wars.

The local building trade has always been an important employer and accounted for twelve per cent of Oxfordshire's working population in 1901. Photographers were always attracted to major construction projects, commissioned perhaps by building firms or by the originators of particular projects. The demolition of the Cutteslowe Walls in north Oxford was clearly a newsworthy event (see p. 62), but the pictures of men at work on Oxford building sites in the 1920s were snaps taken by their mates (see p. 60). Although the railway lakes in New Hinksey and Wolvercote bear witness to mid-nineteenth-century gravel extraction during the building of the Great Western Railway in Oxford, the massive exploitation of the Thames Valley gravel terraces is a largely twentieth-century phenomenon; the view of gravel workings at Farmoor (see p. 54) shows an early stage in the process which has radically changed much of the county's lowland landscape since the Second World War.

Water and land transport offered a whole range of jobs, both skilled and unskilled. On the River Thames there were, for example, ferrymen, lock- and weir-keepers and maintenance staff; in Oxford Abel Beesley was still using a branch of the river to transport rushes and osiers for basket making. The coming of the railways had taken much commercial traffic off the Thames but, by heavy cost-cutting, the Oxford Canal retained a lot of coal traffic and, as late as 1956, one woman was still heaving coal off a narrow boat in Oxford (see p. 66). The railways, and particularly in Oxfordshire the Great Western Railway, employed 1,298 men in the county in 1901 but railway enthusiasts and company photographers tended generally to photograph locomotives and stations rather than the workforce. The exceptions do, however, emphasise the numbers that were needed to keep the trains running at all times and through all weathers. What railway buff would not give his (or her) eye-teeth for the chance to take the inspection trolley shown on p. 71 down the Witney branch line, or indeed any of the other local lines that are now just memories? The concentration of goods traffic on the railways wrecked the finances of turnpike trusts and, by the end of Victoria's reign, only a few exceptional toll-gates such as those at Swinford and Whitchurch survived. The roads were not entirely peaceful, however, and carriers provided regular links between villages and neighbouring towns; the railways also generated local road traffic as goods were carted to or delivered from the stations. The motor vehicle brought new opportunities for carriers and jobmasters and led to the burgeoning of country bus services in the 1920s. Garages and motoring organizations appeared, to cater for the motorized traveller, and the police took an increasing interest in apprehending the speedy. Road maintenance and improvement assumed a new importance although some of the local experiments proved to be unsuccessful.

A growing number of Oxfordshire men and women found employment in the professions or in public service occupations. There were more students to teach at the University, public education became a greater priority and a County Library

Service was set up in 1923. Communities demanded a better police force and fire brigade and improved standards of health care. The Post Office became a major employer and local authorities, managed of course by unpaid councillors, ran an increasing range of services.

Throughout the county shops existed to cater for local needs and where necessary traders took their products to the customer. The retail trade was very labour-intensive and outlets ranged from sophisticated department stores like Webber's in Oxford through small specialist firms and village shops to the market stall. Commercial advertising stunts could be quite ingenious and delivery vehicles provided opportunities for publicity that were generally taken, though not, apparently, by Mr Crease on his horse-drawn fish and chip van in West Hendred (see p. 122). Country districts could be served by vans from nearby towns and the itinerant tradesman became a rare sight.

Society was underpinned by a veritable army of domestic servants and in Oxfordshire at the turn of the century there were 4,336 males and 13,853 females in service. As Flora Thompson recalled in *Lark Rise to Candleford*, many village girls left their familiar surroundings at an early age to find work in Oxford or other towns. Their initial training depended on the practical skills they had acquired at home or in school, but a few training schools existed to provide quality servants for prosperous households. Domestic service covered a wide range of tasks and there was a huge gulf between the lady's maid or uniformed nursemaid and the humble washerwoman or the Cokethorpe daisy-pickers (see p. 136). Male servants were usually employed as outdoor staff and in higher-status households, but they were common in Oxford, of course, as college servants.

Many other occupations were open to resourceful or necessitous Oxfordshire people. Some public houses offered a good living and, where they did not, the landlord's job could be combined with other employment to generate a decent income. Events such as Henley Royal Regatta and local fairs provided opportunities for gain, although the fairground boxing booth (p. 139) was scarcely a secure occupation. New forms of entertainment, like the cinema or roller skating rink, brought new jobs to the county. One person's deprivation was another's business opportunity, and the absence of a good water supply at Finstock attracted entrepreneurs with buckets of water (p. 143).

At school children learned basic skills although many were already helping to supplement the family income. Old people might have to remain at work, at least until the introduction of Old Age Pensions in 1908, if they were to avoid the dreaded workhouse. The careful or fortunate might have been able to enjoy a rest from their labours, but for the others there was little escape from a life of toil.

Farming

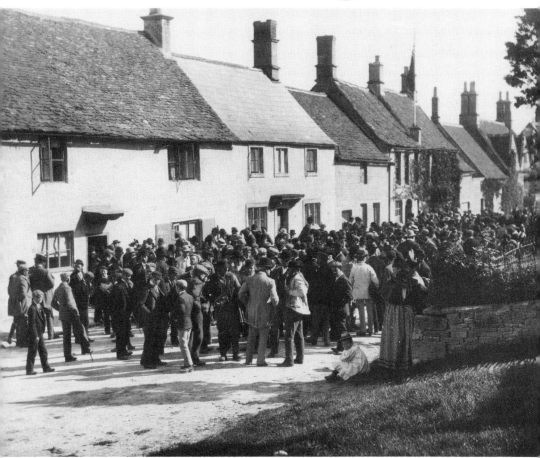

THE ANNUAL HIRING FAIR AT BURFORD in about 1895. At fairs like this farmers took on workers for the ensuing year, and the men and women who wished to be hired carried or wore a symbol of their trade.

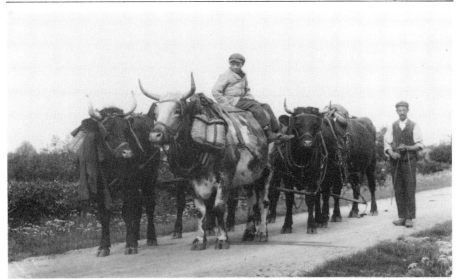

A TEAM OF OXEN ON THE COTSWOLDS.

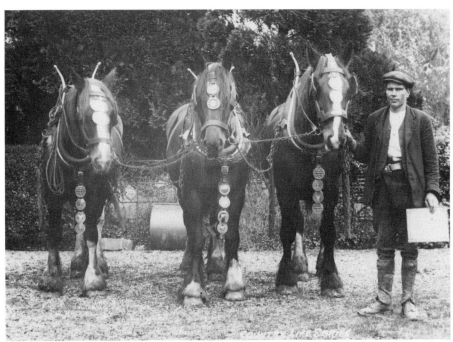

A PROUD PLOUGHMAN with his prize-winning team in June 1910. The horses have been carefully prepared and dressed with brasses on the forehead and four more on the martingale.

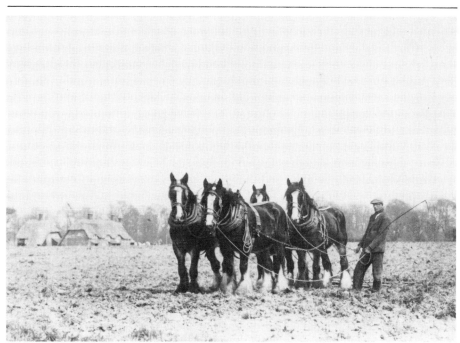

THE PLOUGHMAN WITH HIS TEAM OF HORSES at West Lockinge in about 1930.

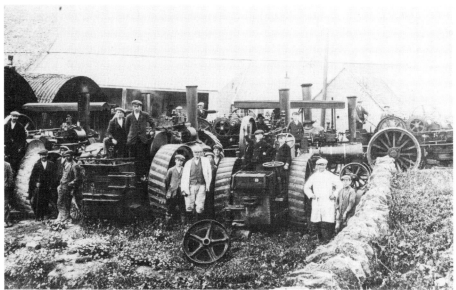

CONTRACT PLOUGHING, perhaps near Woodstock, in about 1900. Gangs like this travelled the countryside for months operating their gargantuan ploughing engines by day and sleeping in vans at night.

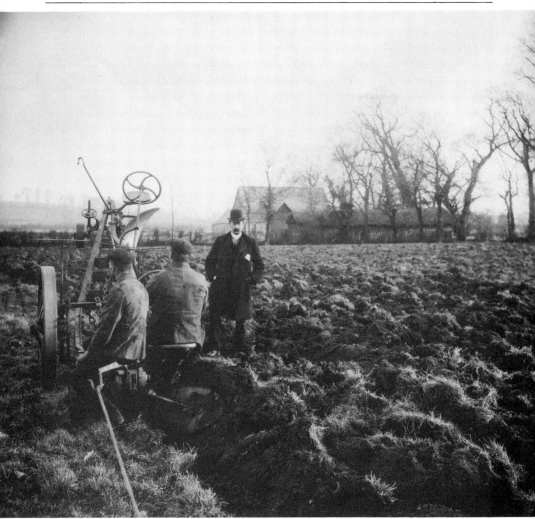

PLOUGHING BY STEAM in about 1898. Ploughing engines out of the picture haul the giant plough backwards and forwards across the field, watched by John Allen, owner of the Oxfordshire Steam Ploughing Company.

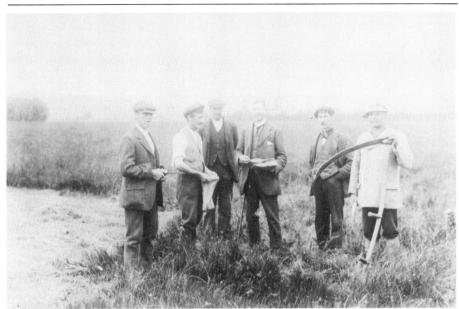

COUNTING THE BALLS prior to drawing lots for strips of land in the Yarnton Lot Meadows in 1917; this ancient custom was last held in 1977.

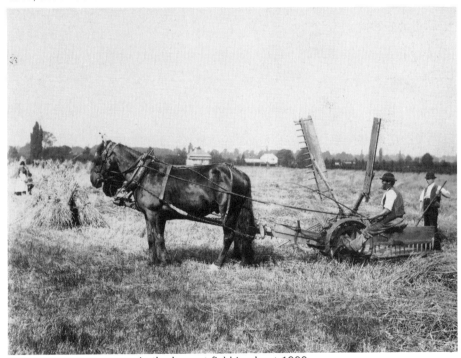

HORSE-DRAWN FLAIL REAPER in the harvest field in about 1900.

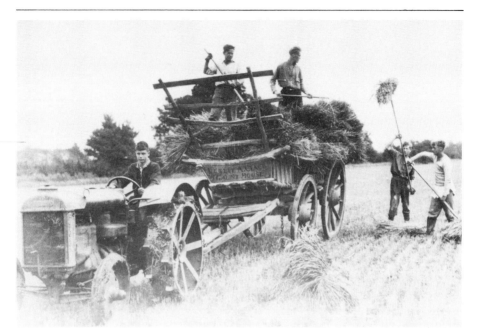

BRINGING IN THE WHEAT by tractor and waggon in about 1941. The boys were evacuees from St Clement Danes Grammar School in London who were taking part in an agricultural camp in Standlake.

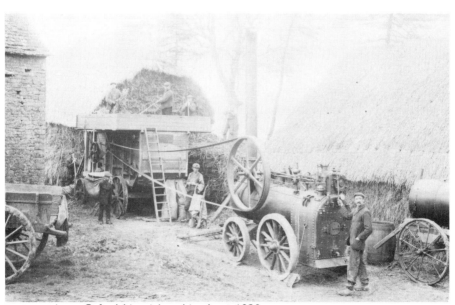

THRESHING in an Oxfordshire rickyard in about 1920.

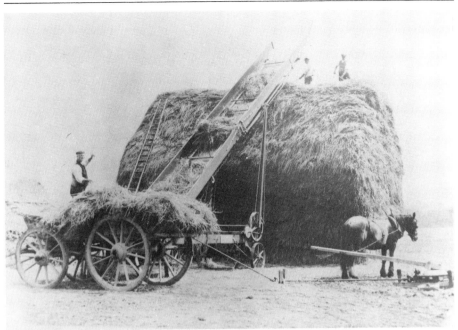

BUILDING A RICK with a conveyor belt at Yarnton in 1911.

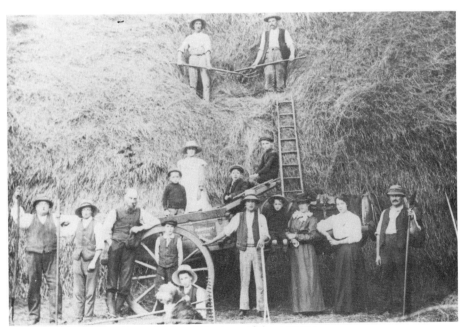

RICK BUILDING at Manor Farm, Hethe at the turn of the century.

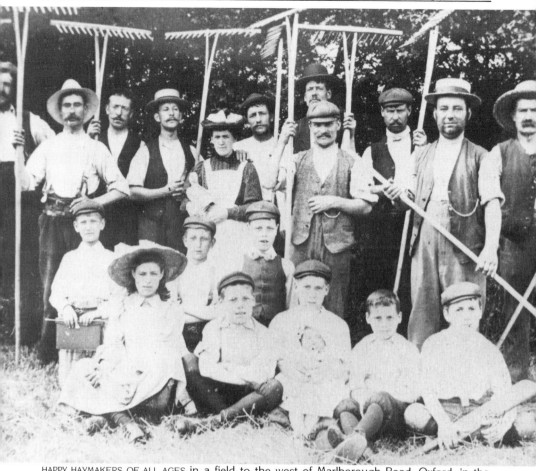

HAPPY HAYMAKERS OF ALL AGES in a field to the west of Marlborough Road, Oxford, in the 1900s.

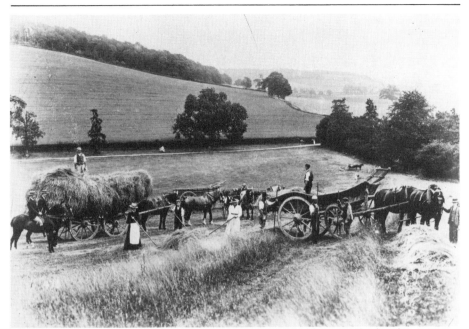

HARD WORK IN A BEAUTIFUL SETTING. Men, women and horses bring in the hay harvest near Henley at the turn of the century.

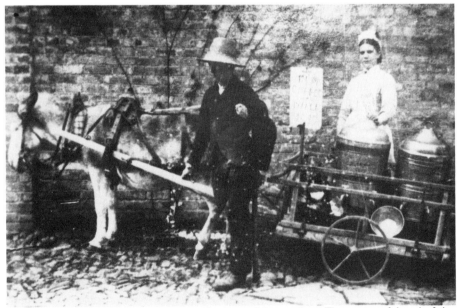

HARVEST TEA-CART AT LETCOMBE REGIS at the turn of the century. The successful end of the harvest was traditionally a time for celebration and some over-indulgence; these beverages were clearly intended to maintain sobriety.

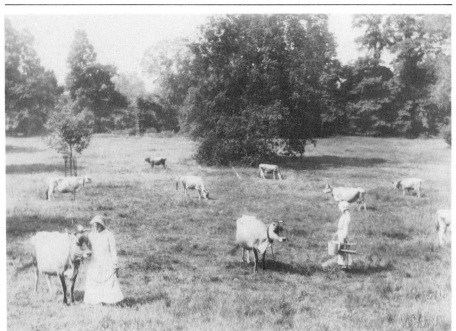

MILKMAIDS AND JERSEY COWS in June 1917; an idyllic scene on the Headington Hill Hall estate of Mrs G.H. Morrell.

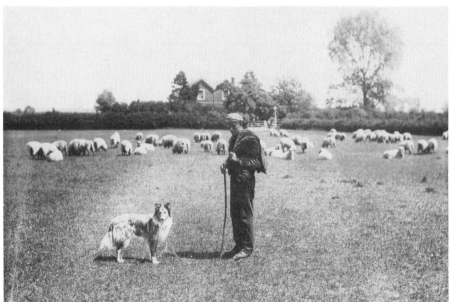

SHEPHERD AND HIS FLOCK in Cowley Road, Oxford in 1901. Rivera, the home of the Oxford photographer Henry Taunt, is visible in the background. Still rural then, it now stands next to the bus garage.

18

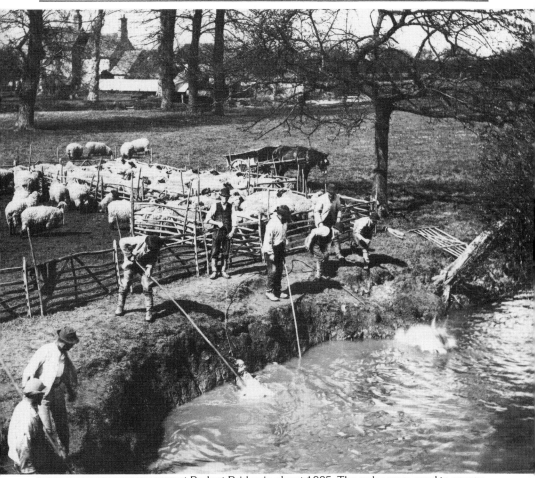

SHEEP WASHING IN THE THAMES at Radcot Bridge in about 1885. The poles were used to ensure complete immersion before the animals were allowed to scramble out of the water.

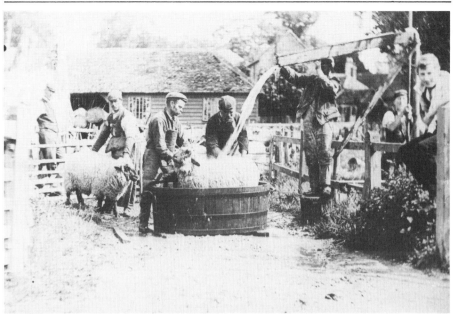

SHEEP WASHING at Sydenham in the 1920s. Where water was not so readily available more ingenious showers were rigged up to wash the fleeces before shearing.

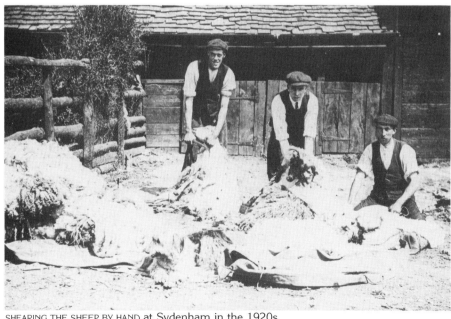

SHEARING THE SHEEP BY HAND at Sydenham in the 1920s.

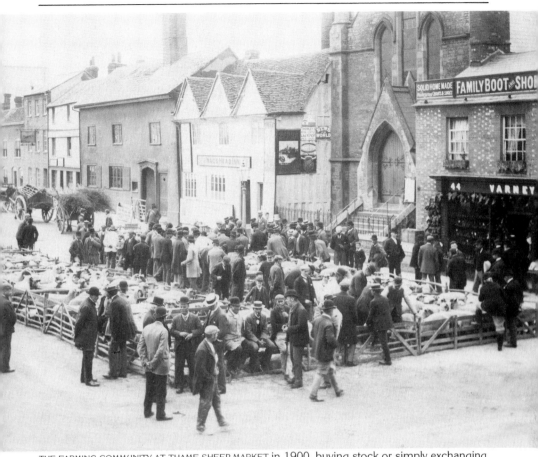

THE FARMING COMMUNITY AT THAME SHEEP MARKET in 1900, buying stock or simply exchanging news and gossip.

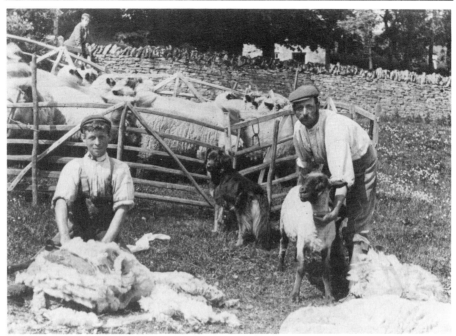

SHEEP SHEARERS BILL GREEN AND ARTHUR LUCKETT at Minster Lovell in about 1910. They took part in a publicity stunt for Early's of Witney in 1906 when sheep's wool was shorn and delivered to the Duke of Marlborough as a blanket in just one day.

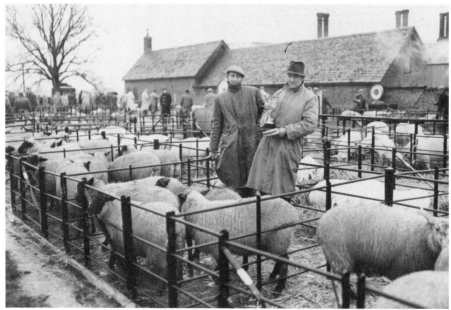

A HAPPY FARMER WITH HIS PRIZE-WINNING SHEEP at Kingham Market in 1957.

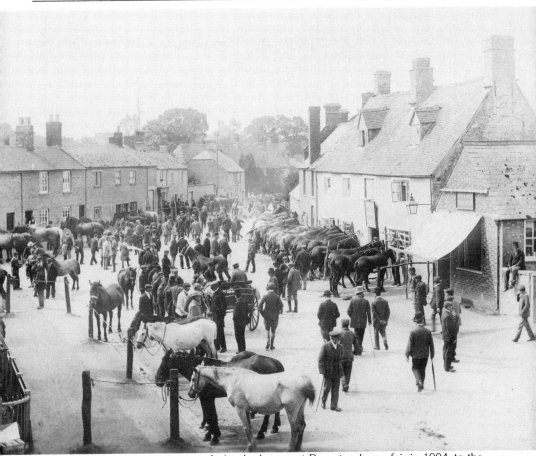

FARMERS, DEALERS AND PASSERS-BY admire the horses at Bampton horse fair in 1904; to the right, hurdles protect the windows of the Horse Shoe pub from the animals just outside.

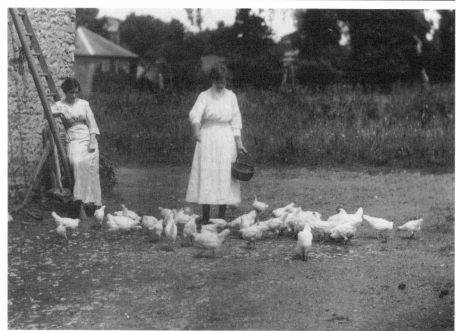

FEEDING FREE-RANGE CHICKENS in about 1920.

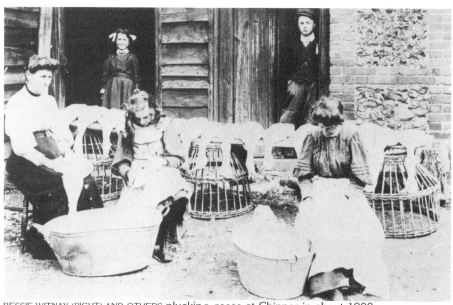

BESSIE WITNAY (RIGHT) AND OTHERS plucking geese at Chinnor in about 1900.

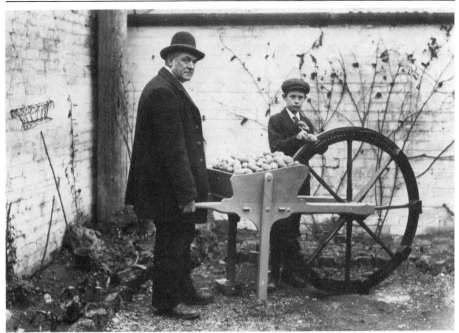

POTATO PLANTING ON A SMALL HOLDING in Cowley in about 1910. This ingenious contraption is being demonstrated by Mr Weston and his son Arthur.

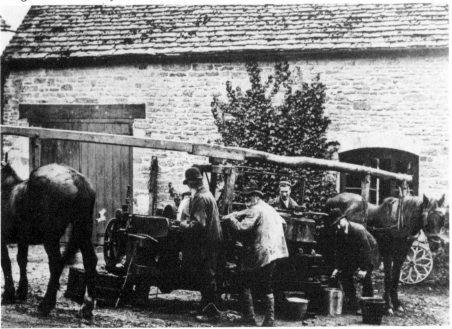

HORSE-DRAWN CIDER PRESS at Shilton in 1900.

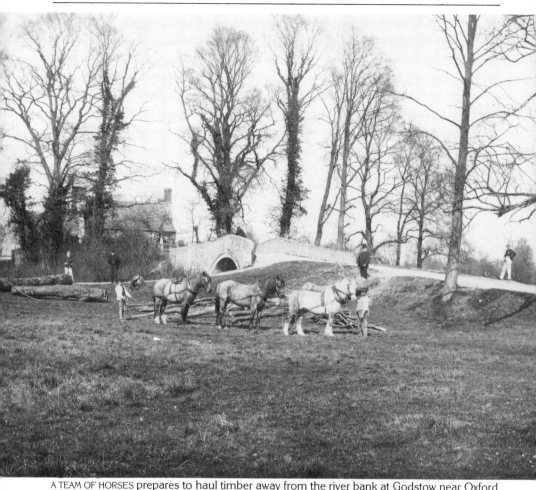

A TEAM OF HORSES prepares to haul timber away from the river bank at Godstow near Oxford in about 1880. The famous Trout Inn is visible beyond the bridge.

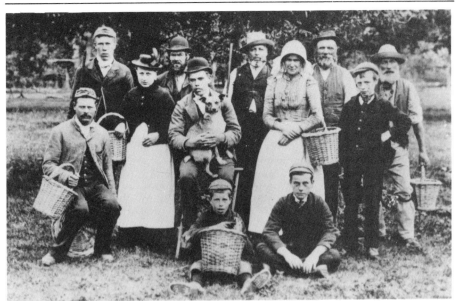

CHERRY PICKERS at Middle Farm, Harwell at the turn of the century.

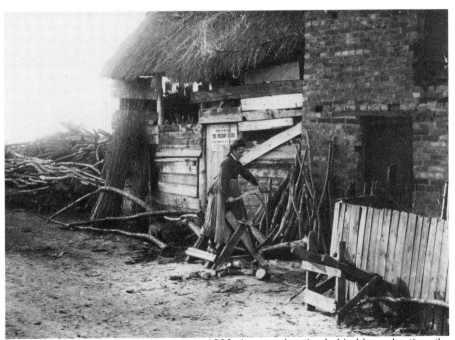

A WOMAN CUTTING WOOD at Wolvercote in 1900. A tattered notice behind her advertises the beginning of a mission at the parish church which had doubtless come and gone.

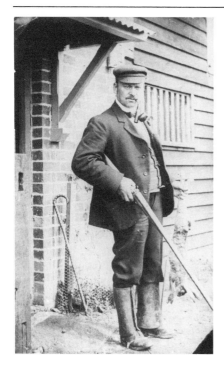

THE GAMEKEEPER and his victim at Sydenham in about 1900.

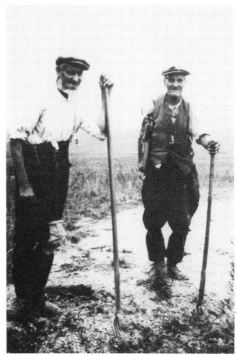

TWO VETERAN FARM LABOURERS at Swinford near Eynsham in the 1920s. Farmwork has always been dangerous and Tom Floyd (right) had lost his arm in a chaff cutter.

Crafts and Industry

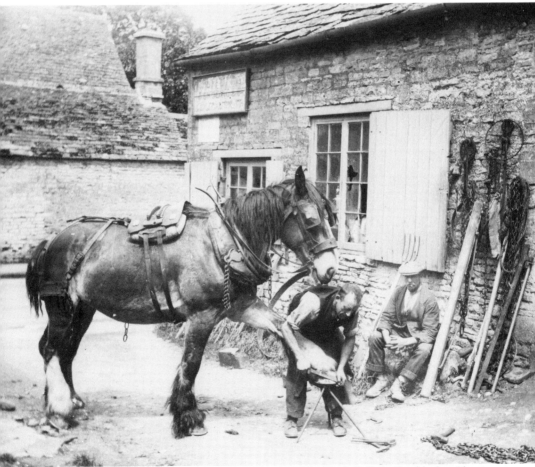

THE GENTLE GIANT. A cart horse stands patiently while Fred Puffett, the blacksmith at Milton-under-Wychwood, fits a new shoe.

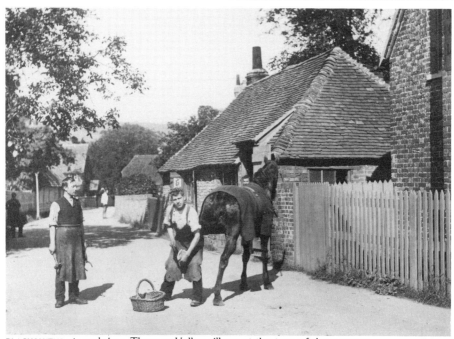

BLACKSMITHS at work in a Thames Valley village at the turn of the century.

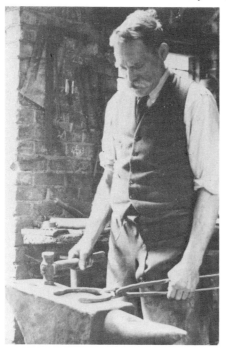

W. STONE, the blacksmith at Harrison's forge in East Hendred, shapes a horseshoe in 1926.

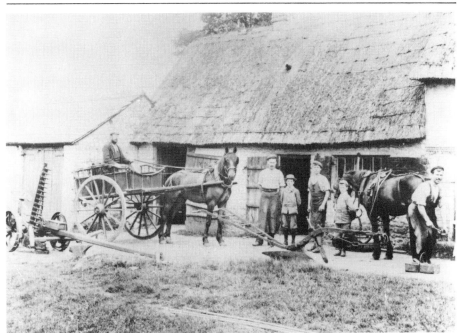

THE FORGE AT FRINGFORD in about 1900. The plough and reaper awaiting repair are a reminder that shoeing horses was only one aspect of the blacksmith's job.

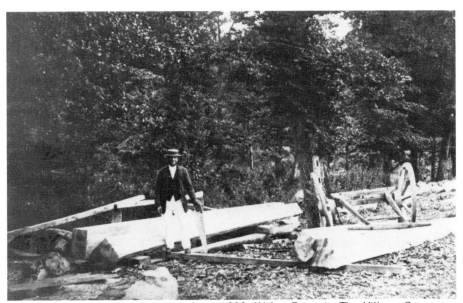

THE SAW-PIT at Letcombe Regis in about 1900. Walter Rose, in *The Village Carpenter*, described the fascination of watching 'the slow creeping forward of the cut' as the two sawyers worked steadily through a large log.

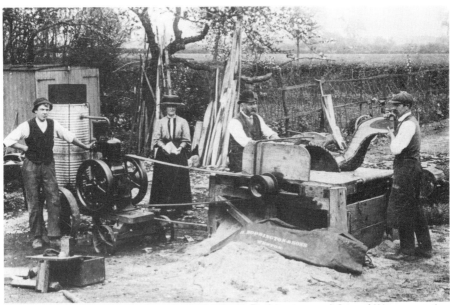

OPERATING A CIRCULAR SAW at the wheelwright's, R. Boddington and Son of Weston-on-the-Green, in 1911. The engine had been bought without the wheels for £36 at the previous year's County Show.

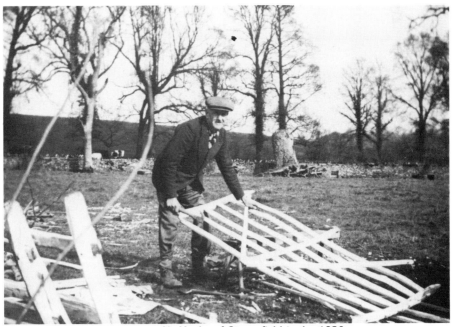

THE CRAFT OF THE HURDLE MAKER: Mr Hanks of Stonesfield in the 1930s.

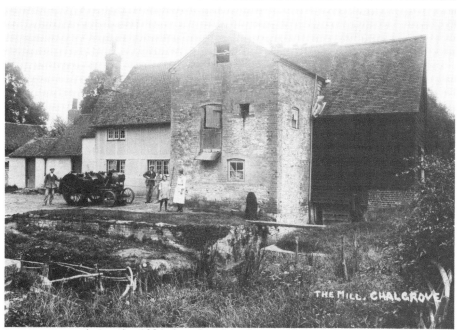

CHALGROVE MILL during the 1921 drought when the machinery had to be driven by a belt attached to a petrol-engined generator.

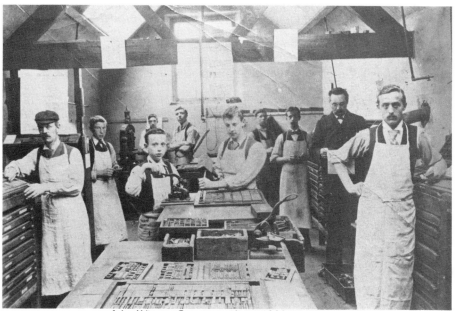

THE COMPOSING ROOM of the *Witney Gazette* in about 1900. In addition to the *Gazette*, which was published weekly from 1882, the firm undertook a variety of jobbing printing.

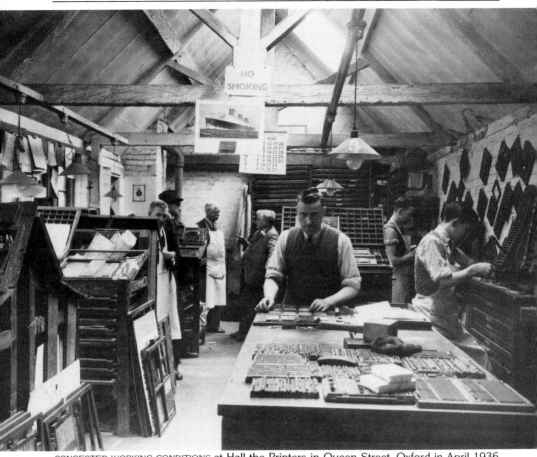

CONGESTED WORKING CONDITIONS at Hall the Printers in Queen Street, Oxford in April 1936.

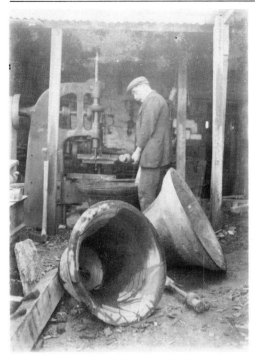

CRAFTSMAN AT BURFORD BELL FOUNDRY in the 1920s. The foundry had been established by Henry Bond in 1861, and was carried on by his sons Henry and Thomas until 1947.

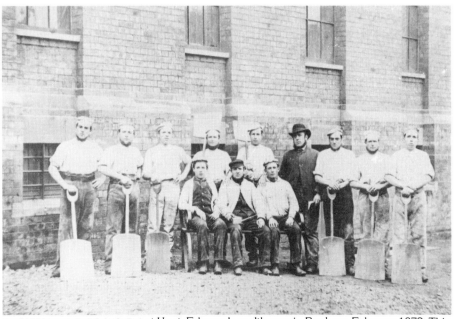

MALTSTERS AND THEIR SHOVELS at Hunt, Edmunds malthouse in Banbury, February 1872. This Banbury brewery was founded in 1807 and ceased brewing in 1967.

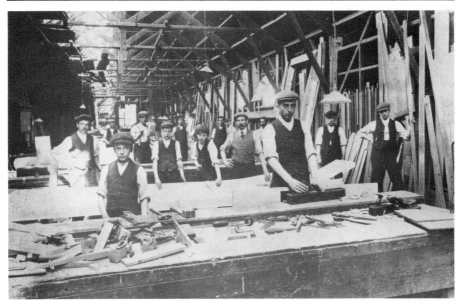

THE FINISHING ROOM at Wrench and Company's plush mill in Shutford in about 1910. Plush, a fabric similar to silk velvet but made mostly of wool or worsted, was hugely popular in the Victorian period.

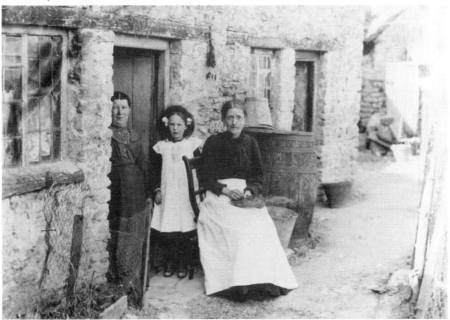

GLOVER MRS BRACKENBOROUGH outside her house in Main Road, Woodstock in about 1900. The gloving industry provided domestic employment for women, enabling them to supplement the earnings of their husbands on the land.

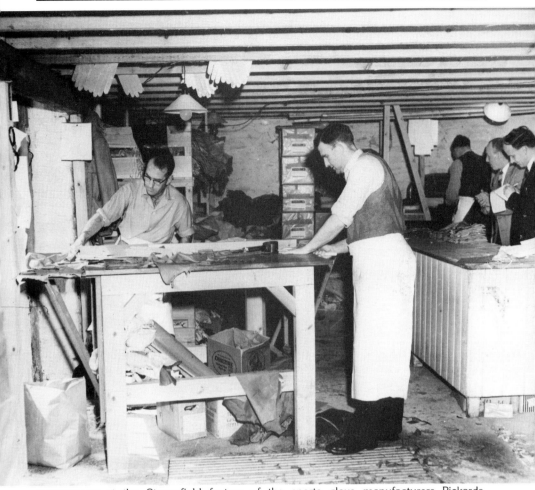

GLOVEMAKERS at the Stonesfield factory of the sports glove manufacturers Pickards (Reading) Limited in 1959.

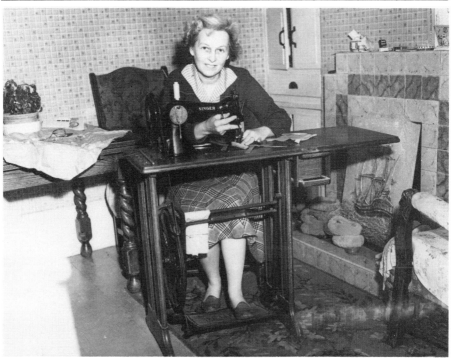

ONE OF PICKARDS' OUTWORKERS photographed in her home at Stonesfield in 1959.

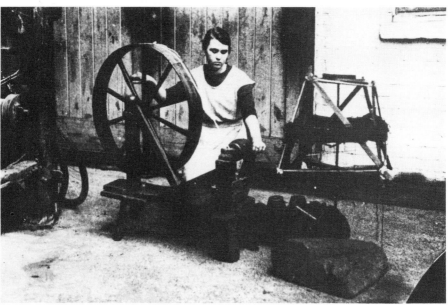

A WOMAN SPINNING JUTE at the Abingdon Carpet Company's Thames-side factory in 1920.

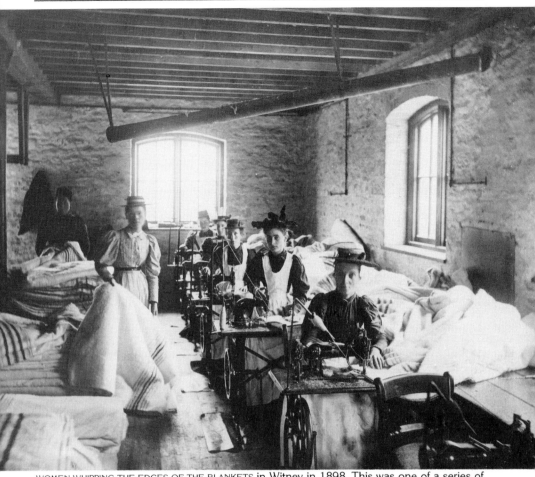

WOMEN WHIPPING THE EDGES OF THE BLANKETS in Witney in 1898. This was one of a series of photographs taken by the Oxford photographer, Henry Taunt, to illustrate a publicity booklet for Early's of Witney.

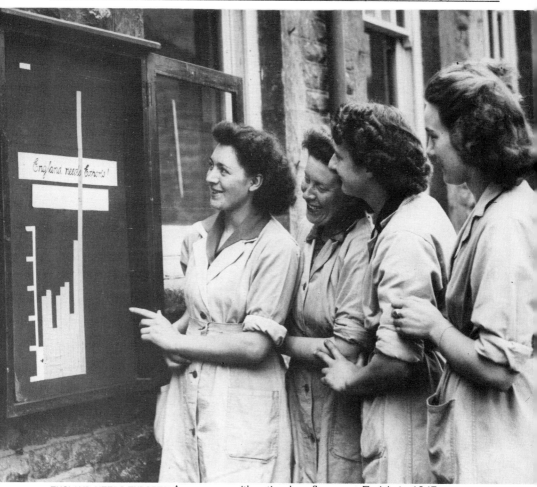

ENGLAND NEEDS EXPORTS! A message with a timeless flavour at Early's in 1947.

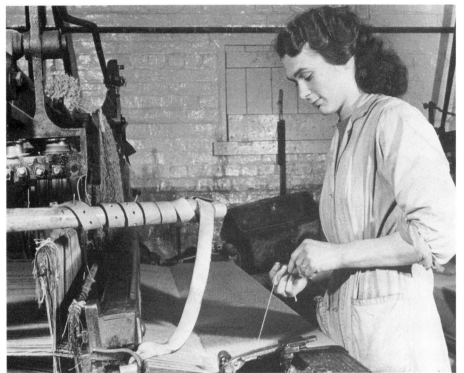

REPAIRING A WARP THREAD at Early's Mill in 1951.

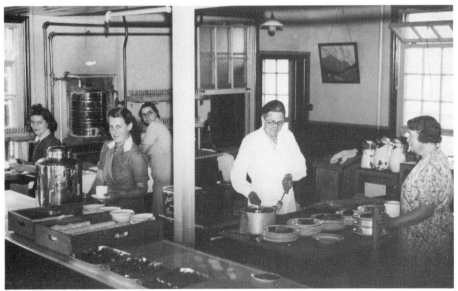

CANTEEN STAFF prepare for the lunch-time rush of hungry blanket makers in the 1940s.

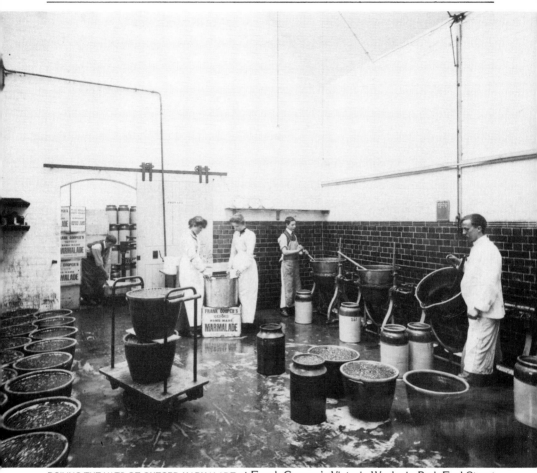

BOILING THE VATS OF OXFORD MARMALADE at Frank Cooper's Victoria Works in Park End Street in about 1905.

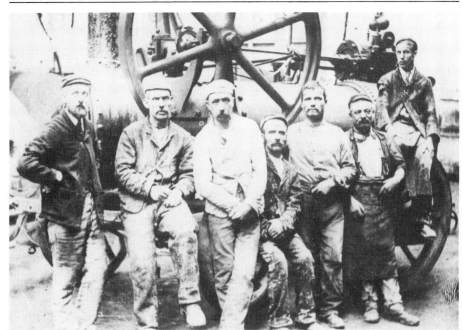

EMPLOYEES AT THE BRITANNIA WORKS in Banbury in about 1900. Bernhard Samuelson took over James Gardner's agricultural engineering business in 1848 and made it Banbury's largest firm, employing 380 people by 1861.

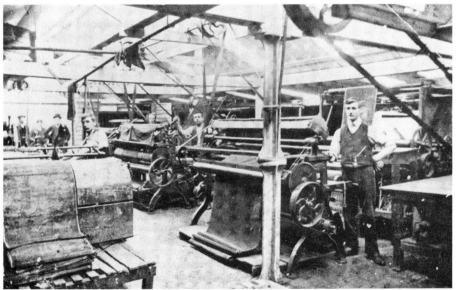

MEN AND BOYS at Nalder and Nalder's Challow Iron Works pose briefly for the camera in about 1900. Founded in 1857, the firm began by making agricultural machinery for the local market but it was exporting huge threshing machines to south-east Europe by 1877.

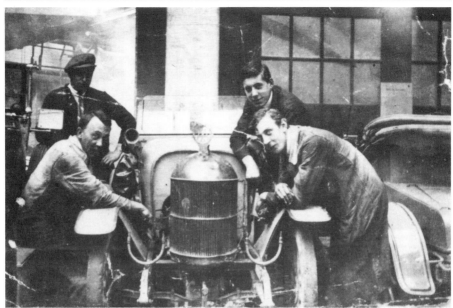

MECHANICS assembling the prototype Bullnose Morris at the Morris Garage in Longwall Street, Oxford in 1912.

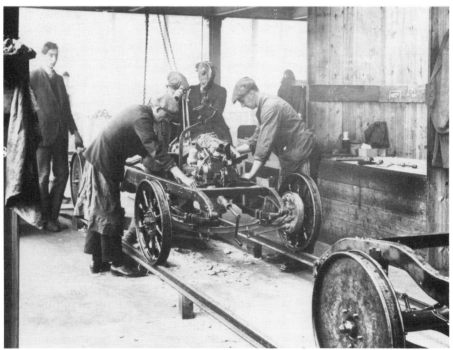

LOWERING THE ENGINE INTO POSITION on the chassis at Morris Motors in Cowley, 1926.

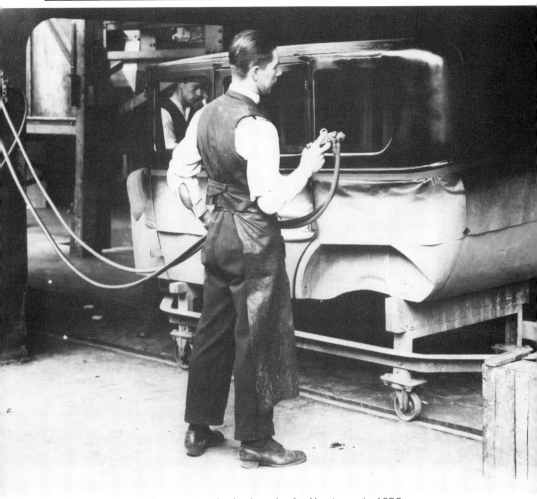

BEFORE THE ROBOT: paint-spraying the bodywork of a Morris car in 1928.

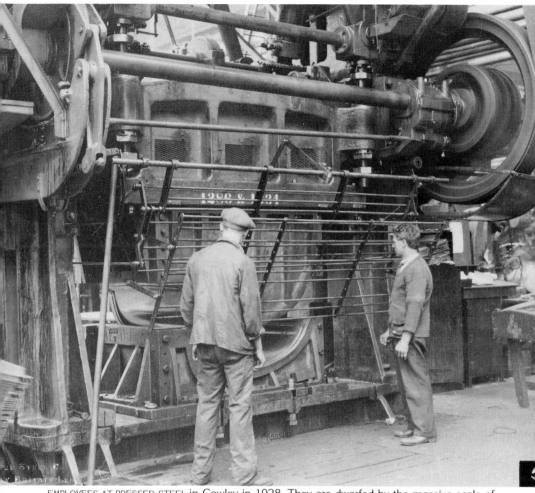

EMPLOYEES AT PRESSED STEEL in Cowley in 1928. They are dwarfed by the massive scale of the press which is delivering the first stike to a roof panel.

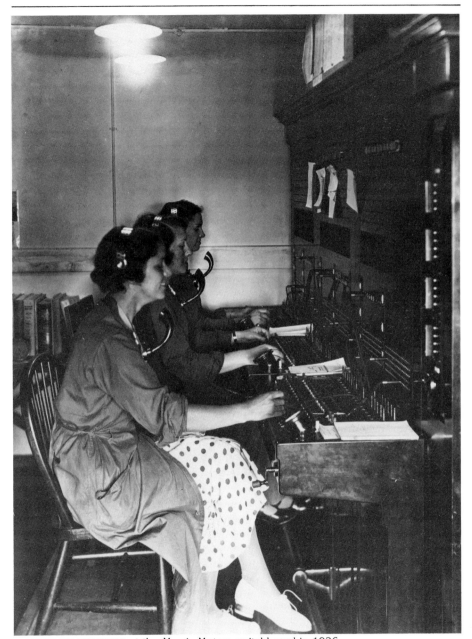

CHEERFUL TELEPHONISTS at the Morris Motors switchboard in 1936.

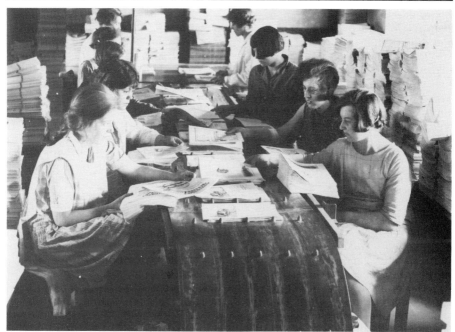

WOMEN AT THE MORRIS OXFORD PRESS in 1929, collating the pages of a house journal on an endless band conveyor.

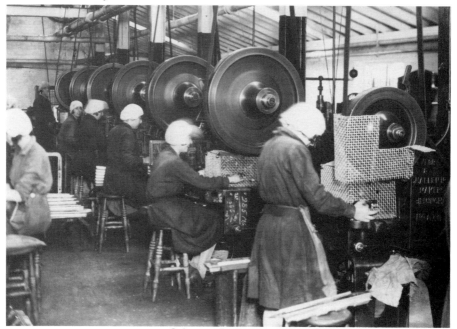

WOMEN OPERATING THE PRESSES at Osberton Radiators in Oxford, 1930.

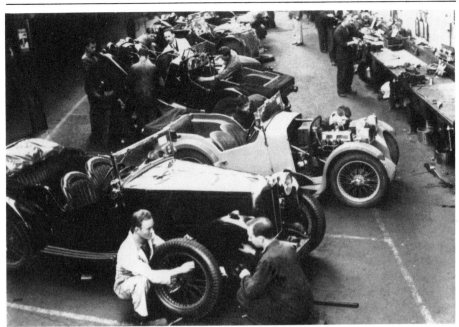

THE MG MIDGET PRODUCTION LINE at Abingdon in about 1934.

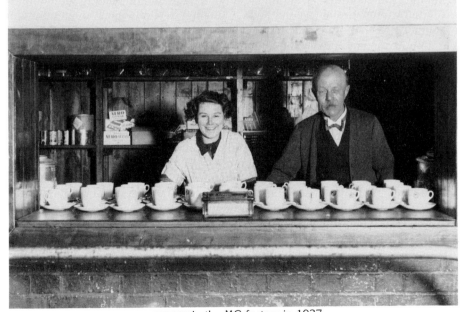

HAPPY FACES AT THE CANTEEN SERVERY in the MG factory in 1937.

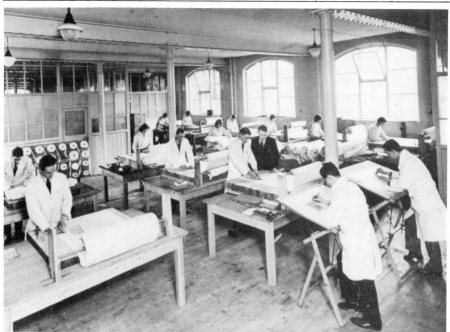

DESIGNING CORSETS at Spencer Corsets Limited in Banbury during the 1930s. As women might have suspected, most of the designers seem to have been men.

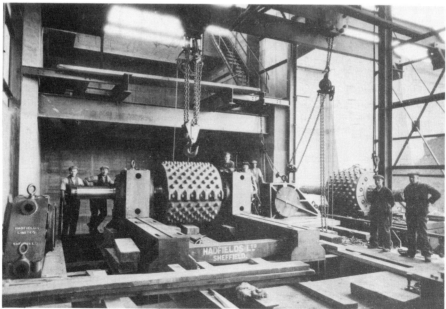

LARGE-SCALE INDUSTRY in rural north Oxfordshire in 1935: workmen installing a crusher and drop bar feeder at the Duffield Ironstone Works in Adderbury.

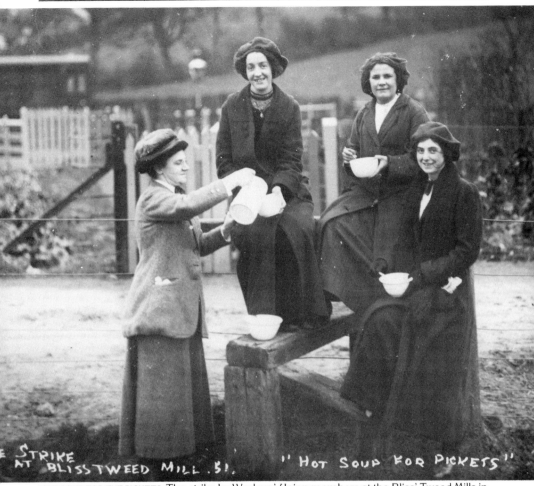

STRIKE AT BLISSTWEED MILL. 51. "HOT SOUP FOR PICKETS"

HOT SOUP FOR THE PICKETS. The strike by Workers' Union members at the Bliss' Tweed Mills in Chipping Norton lasted for seven months from December 1913.

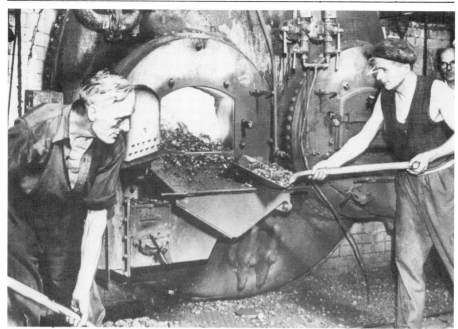

STOKERS feeding coal into the furnace at the Oxford Gasworks in St Ebbe's in August 1955.

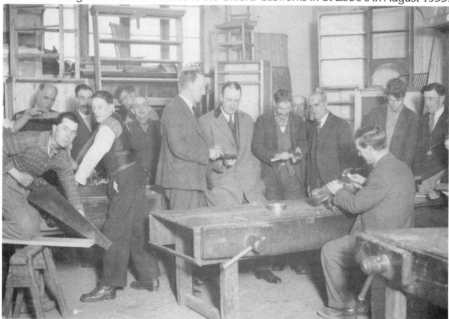

A BOOT REPAIRING AND WOODWORKING CLASS for unemployed men at Eynsham in 1933. The gentleman in their midst was William Goodenough, chairman of the Social Services Group of the Oxfordshire Rural Community Council.

SECTION THREE

Construction

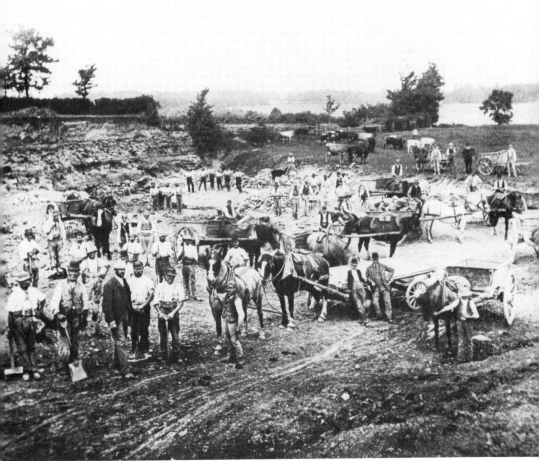

MEN, HORSES AND VEHICLES in Lay's Quarry at Hanborough in about 1890.

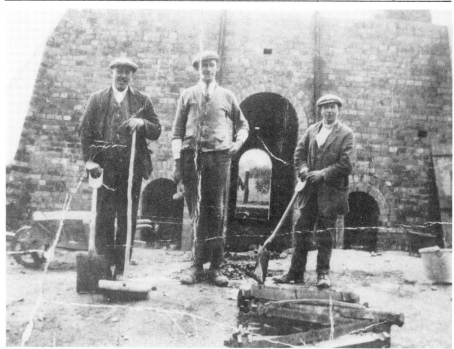

BUILDING THE NEWCASTLE BRICK KILN at Horton-cum-Studley in about 1915. The man in the centre was Harry Green, foreman of the brickyard; Mr Gurl on the right was a brickmaker from Headington.

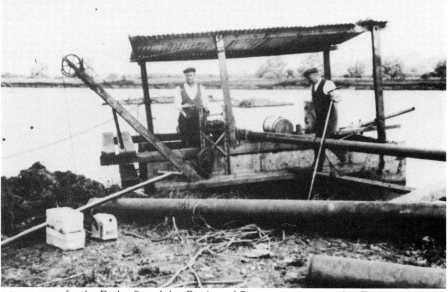

MEN WORKING for the Botley firm John Curtis and Son, extracting gravel at Farmoor in 1930.

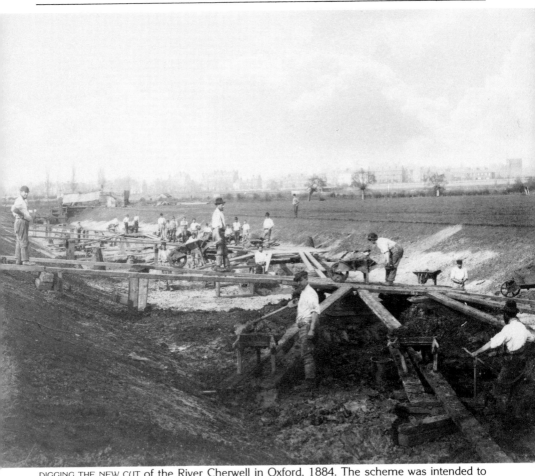

DIGGING THE NEW CUT of the River Cherwell in Oxford, 1884. The scheme was intended to lower river levels and reduce the incidence of flooding in the city.

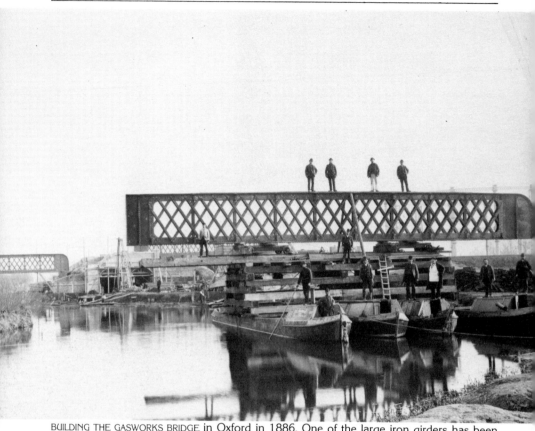

BUILDING THE GASWORKS BRIDGE in Oxford in 1886. One of the large iron girders has been mounted on top of narrow boats and is about to be floated into position.

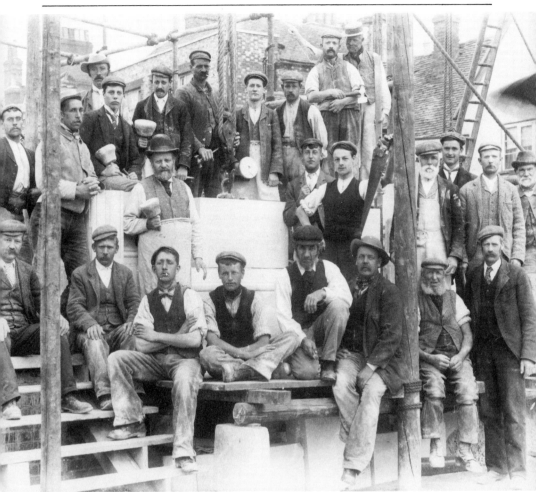

CONSTRUCTION WORKERS at the new Henley Town Hall in 1899. The stone records that the building commemorated sixty years of Queen Victoria's reign.

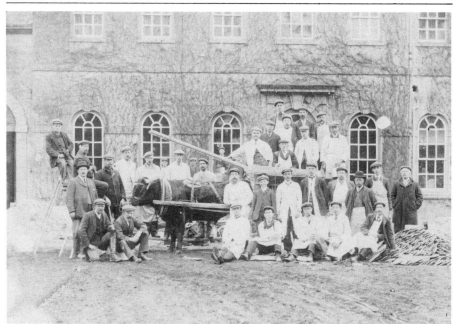

BUILDING EMPLOYEES with their ox cart during construction work at Kingston Lisle House in about 1910.

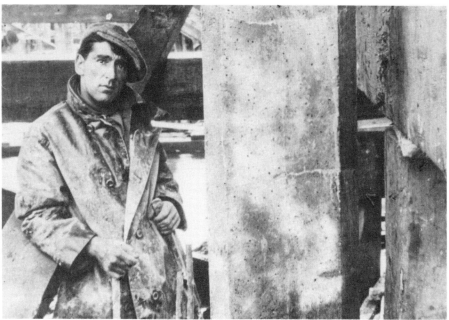

A LABOURER employed on the rebuilding of the Goring and Streatley bridge in September 1922.

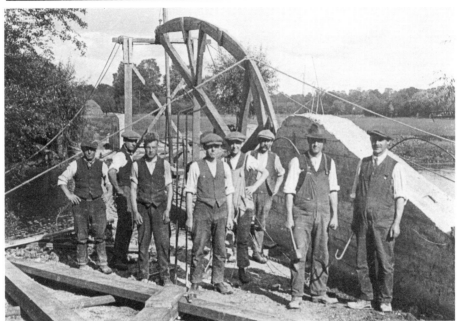

BUILDING THE HIGH BRIDGE in the University Parks in 1923. This link between the Parks and the fields across the river Cherwell was part of a project to relieve local unemployment.

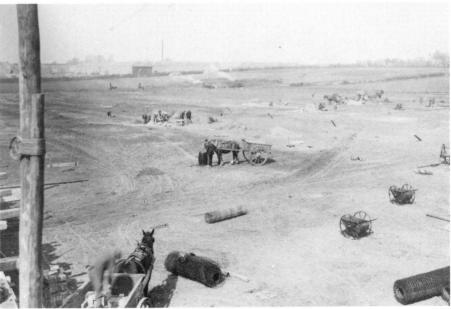

THE EARLY STAGES OF CONSTRUCTION at the Pressed Steel site in Cowley in 1926. Horses and carts and steam ploughing engines pave the way for the giant presses of the new motor industry.

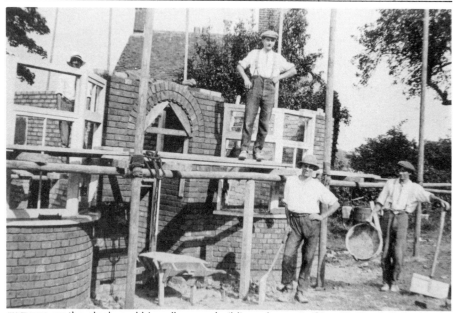

JIM EVANS, on the plank, and his colleagues building a house in Glanville Road, Oxford in the 1920s.

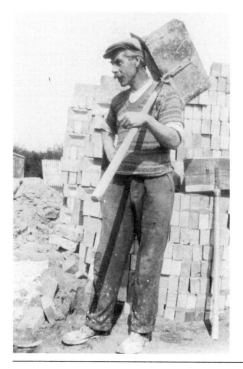

A HOD CARRIER working for the Oxford building firm Organ Bros. in the 1920s.

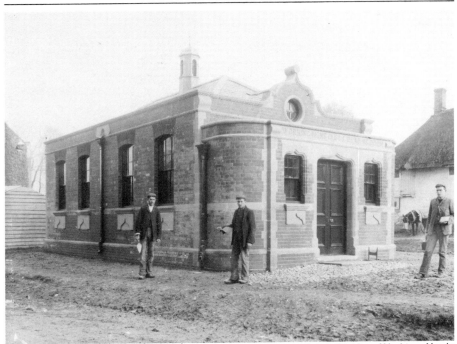

BRICKLAYERS pose with their trowels outside the newly completed Childrey Working Men's Club and Reading Room in about 1910.

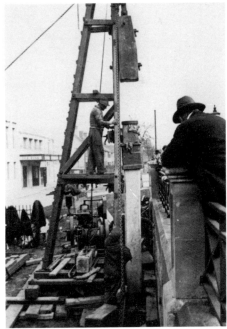

PILE DRIVING near the Ice Rink in Botley Road, Oxford in April 1933. The City Council was laying a 27 in diameter pipeline into Oxford from the new water treatment works at Swinford.

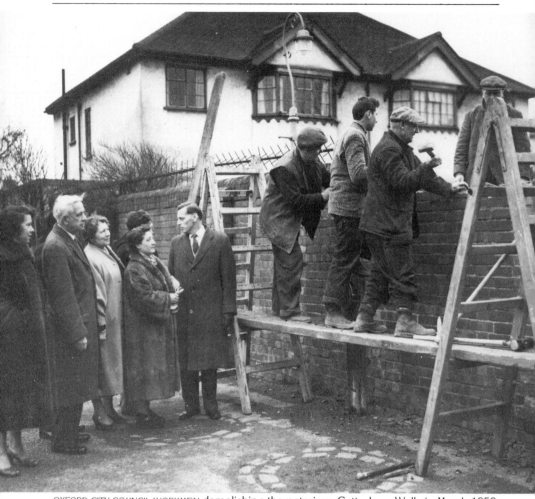

OXFORD CITY COUNCIL WORKMEN demolishing the notorious Cutteslowe Walls in March 1959. Nearest the trestle, Councillors Edmund and Olive Gibbs were particularly enjoying the destruction of this barrier between council and private housing after a battle lasting twenty-five years.

SECTION FOUR

Transport

WATER

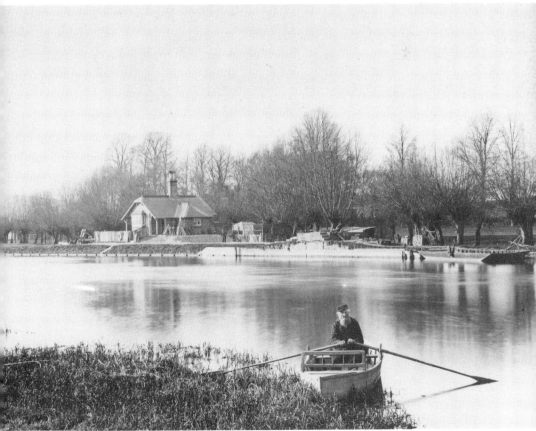

THE FERRYMAN of the Gatehampton to Basildon ferry awaits customers in about 1892. This crossing had been instituted by the Thames Commissioners in 1810.

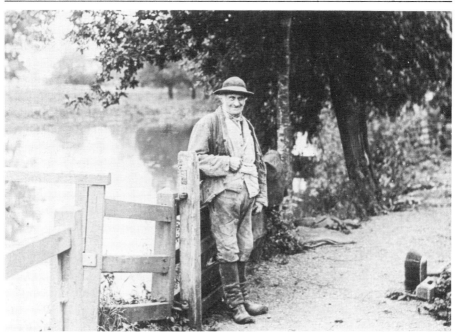

OLD HARPER, the weir-keeper at Old Man's Weir near Radcot, in the 1870s. The Oxford photographer Henry Taunt remarked that he had 'river knowledge enough to teach the best read Oxford Professor that ever lived.'

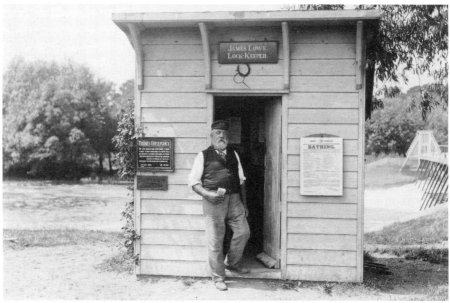

JAMES LOWE, lock-keeper at Day's Lock near Little Wittenham, in 1904. He had worked the lock since 1870 and must have been a well-known Thames character.

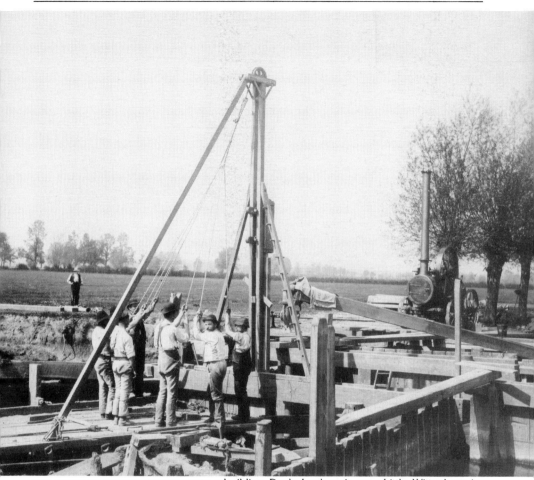

EMPLOYEES OF THAMES CONSERVANCY rebuilding Day's Lock weir near Little Wittenham in about 1885. They were using a 'ringing engine' to drive wooden sheet piles.

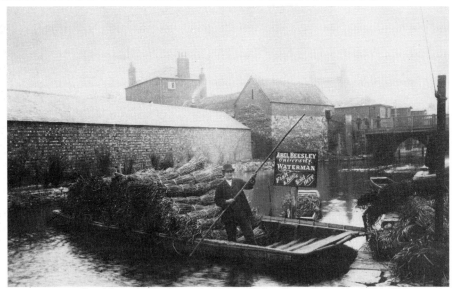

ABEL BEESLEY poling his rush-filled punt in Middle Fisher Row, Oxford in 1901. This was the traditional Oxford working punt, though Beesley was equally adept with racing punts in front of Varsity crowds.

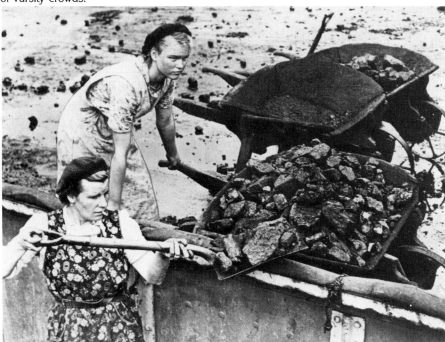

HEAVING COAL at Juxon Street Wharf on the Oxford Canal at Oxford in August 1956: Rose Skinner wields the shovel and Jean Humphries pushes the wheelbarrow.

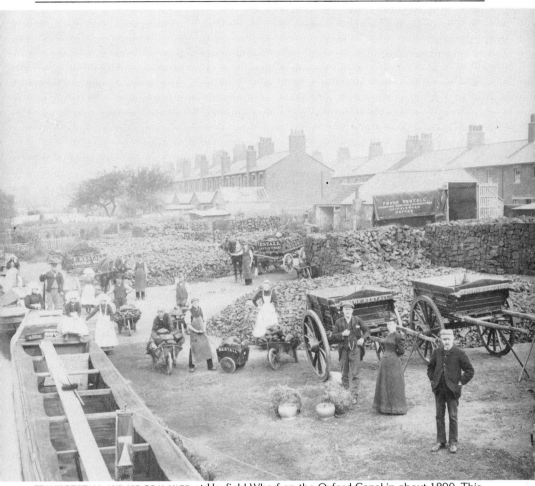

FRANK RESTALL AND HIS COAL YARD at Hayfield Wharf on the Oxford Canal in about 1890. This publicity photograph shows every aspect of the business: employees, the heaps of 'black gold', narrow boats and delivery vehicles.

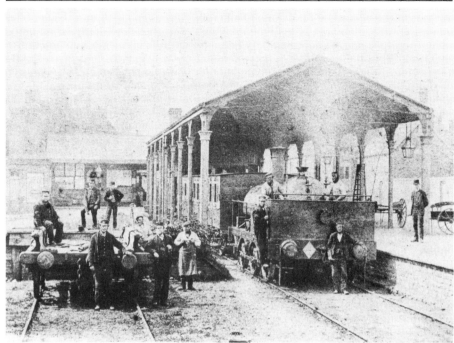

RAILWAY EMPLOYEES at Abingdon station in about 1860. The short branch line from Radley opened in 1856 and, as this photograph shows, was originally built to Brunel's broad gauge.

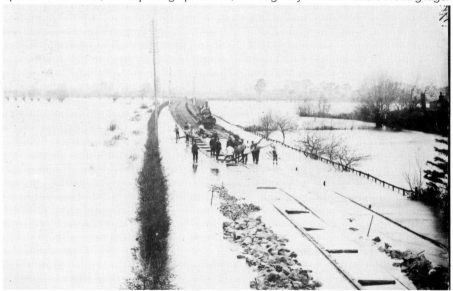

GREAT WESTERN RAILWAY EMPLOYEES working to reinstate the line south of Oxford during the floods of November 1875. The photograph was taken from Red Bridge on the Abingdon road.

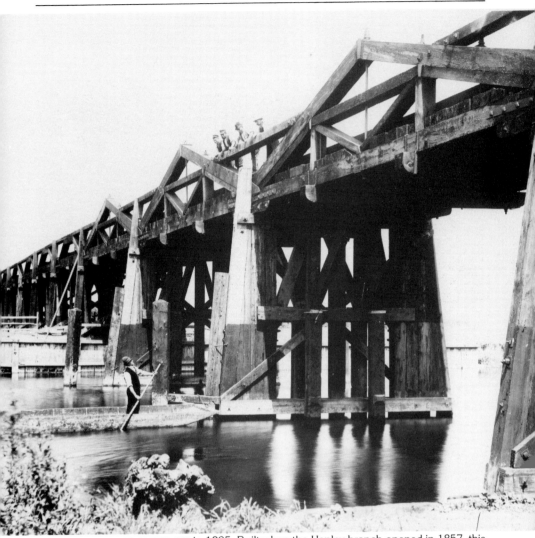

THE RAILWAY VIADUCT AT SHIPLAKE in 1895. Built when the Henley branch opened in 1857, this wooden structure was replaced in 1896, and it seems likely that these men were discussing its poor condition rather than idly passing the time of day.

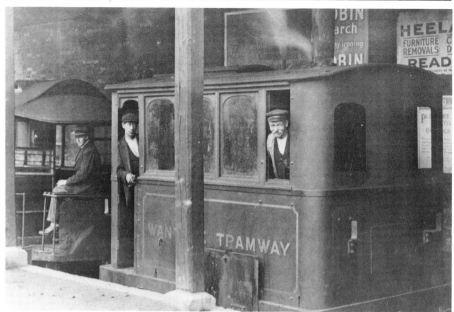

WANTAGE TRAMWAY ENGINE NO.6 at Wantage Town station in about 1925. Driver, fireman and a smart passenger pose at the terminus of this tramway which linked Wantage to the Great Western main line at Wantage Road.

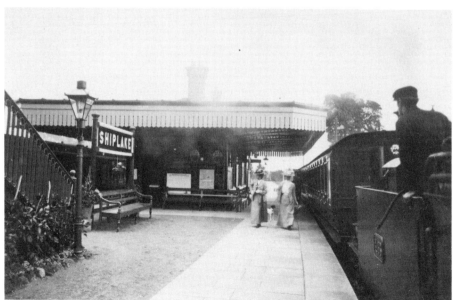

HENLEY BRANCH TRAIN AT SHIPLAKE STATION in the 1900s. Awaiting the 'right away' signal, perhaps the driver finds time to admire the trim ankles of the two lady passengers?

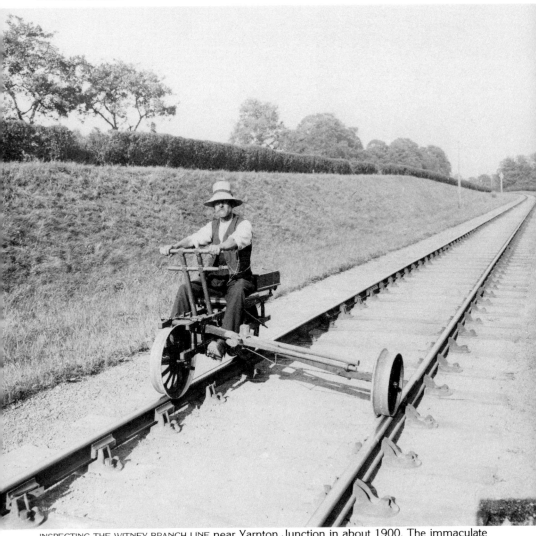

INSPECTING THE WITNEY BRANCH LINE near Yarnton Junction in about 1900. The immaculate condition of the track and the well-trimmed embankment and hedge are a tribute to the men who maintained this line.

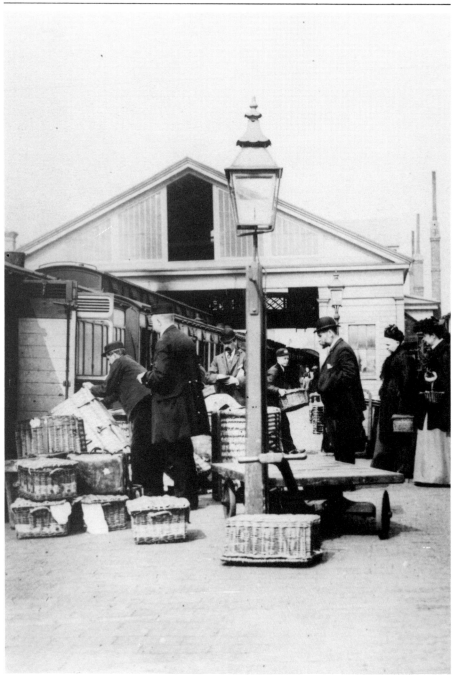

A PORTER wrestles a large basket into the luggage van at Banbury's Great Western Railway station in 1905.

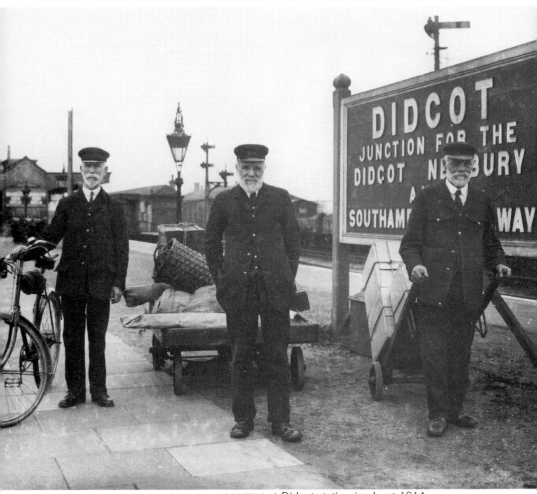

LONG-SERVING GREAT WESTERN RAILWAY PORTERS at Didcot station in about 1914.

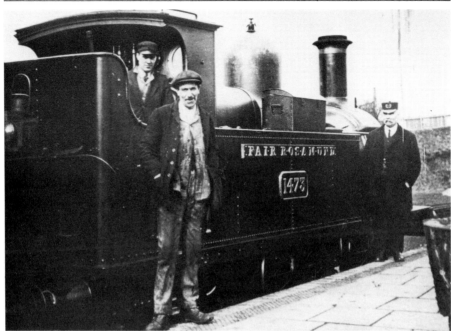

DRIVER BILL POMEROY AND STATION MASTER WILLIAM COOKE pose beside *Fair Rosamund* at Kidlington station in 1925. This loco worked on the Woodstock branch line from 1890 to 1935.

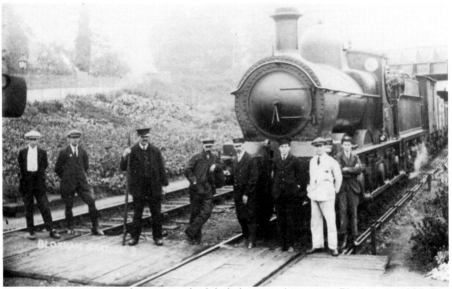

THE LOCAL GOODS TRAIN makes an unscheduled photographic stop at Bloxham in 1925. The group in front of the locomotive includes the guard W. Clarke (with the shunter's pole), the station master Herbert Lloyd and, on the right, the photographer's son Basil Packer.

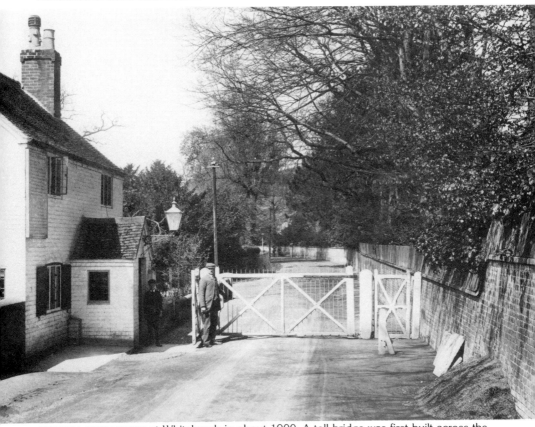

THE TOLL-GATE KEEPER at Whitchurch in about 1900. A toll-bridge was first built across the Thames between Pangbourne and Whitchurch following an Act of Parliament in 1792.

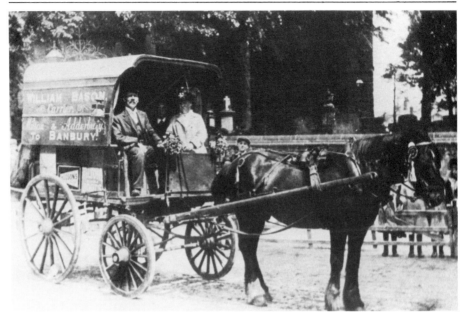

WILLIAM BASON'S CARRIER'S CART at Banbury in 1908. Bason travelled from Milton and Adderbury three days a week taking people and produce into Banbury and returning with shopping orders for those who stayed behind.

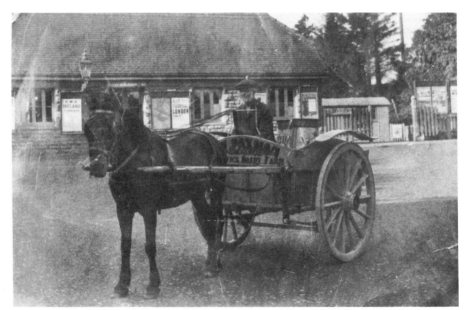

CHARLES FOSTER, a cowman at Mr Paxman's farm at Hardwick, delivering milk churns to Witney station in the late 1900s. They were then sent on to London by the 7.40 a.m. milk train.

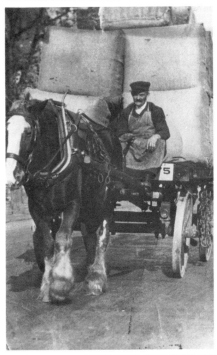

HARRY LOWE, a Great Western Railway drayman, guides another load of blankets from
Witney Mills to the railway station in 1936.

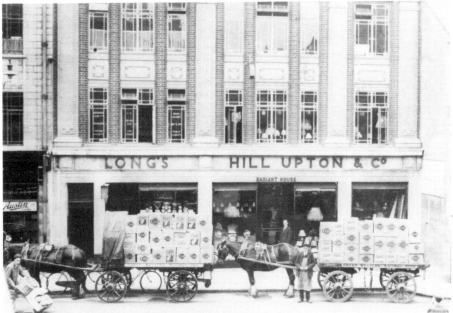

RAILWAY WORKERS delivering Osram light bulbs to Hill, Upton and Company in George Street,
Oxford in October 1931.

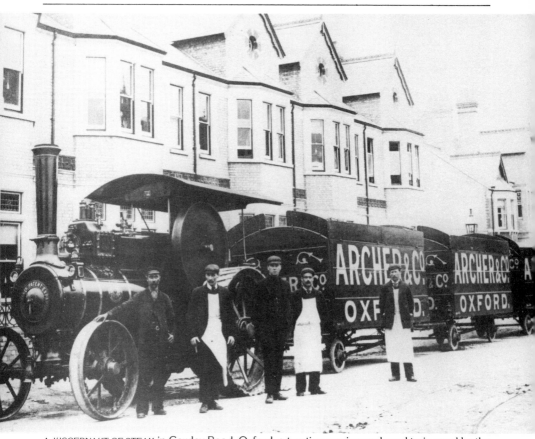

A JUGGERNAUT OF STEAM in Cowley Road, Oxford: a traction engine and road train used by the Oxford removal firm Archer & Co. in about 1900.

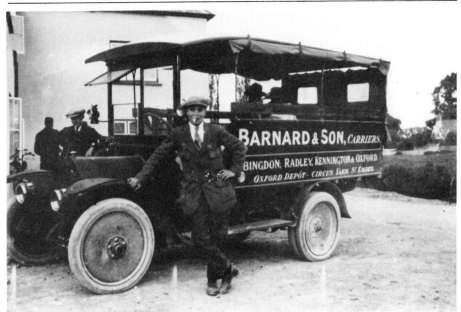

BARNARD & SON'S CARRIER'S VAN in Abingdon in about 1922. Barnard's were clearly proud of their new van, which made the journey to Oxford five days a week, stopping at Circus Yard near St Ebbe's church.

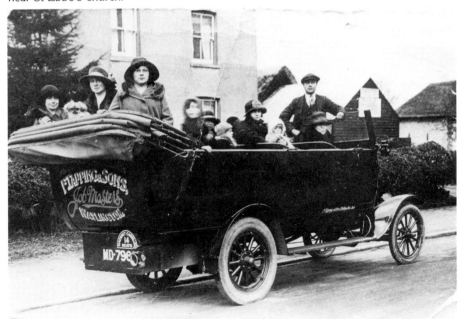

FRANCIS TAPPING'S CHARABANC in Watlington in the early 1920s. Jobmasters who had dealt with horse-drawn vehicles adapted easily to the new technology.

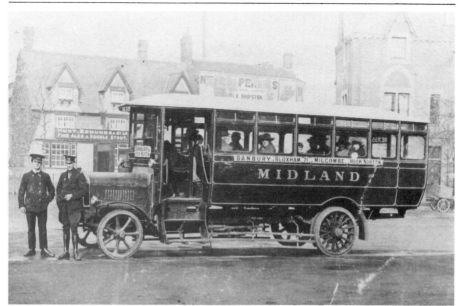

DRIVER AND CONDUCTOR beside their Midland Red bus in Bridge Street, Banbury in the early 1920s. Were the passengers perhaps a little impatient with this delay to the Hooky bus?

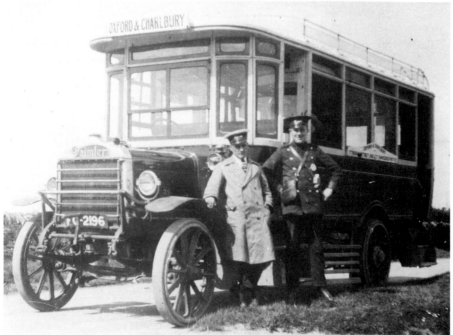

THE DRIVER AND CONDUCTOR of the Oxford and Charlbury service enjoy a spot of sunshine besides their bus in the early 1920s.

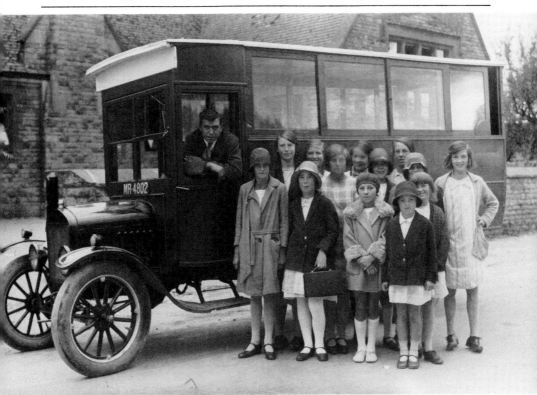

JONES OF CARTERTON'S BUS in 1929. He was employed to take the children from Brize Norton School to their cookery class.

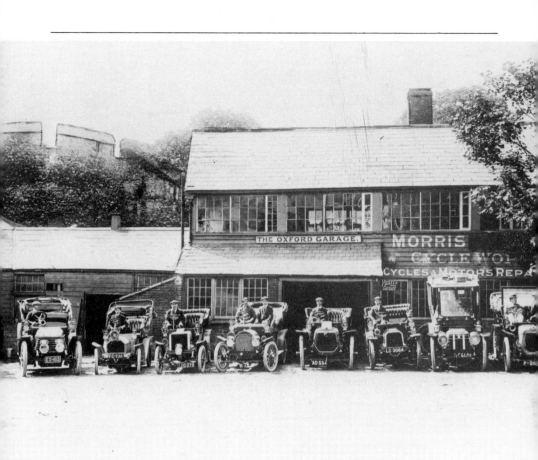

DRIVERS WITH A VARIED COLLECTION OF HIRE CARS at the Morris Garage and Cycle Works in Holywell Street, Oxford in 1907 or 1908. William Morris, later Lord Nuffield, is seated in the passenger seat of P2198 to the right of the picture.

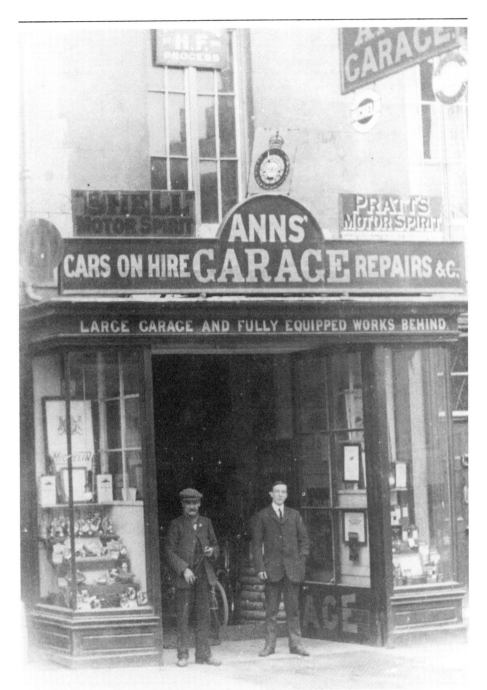

ANNS' GARAGE in Market Place, Faringdon in 1912. Henry Robins (left) and Edgar Argant stand ready to welcome motorists on the main road between Oxford and Swindon.

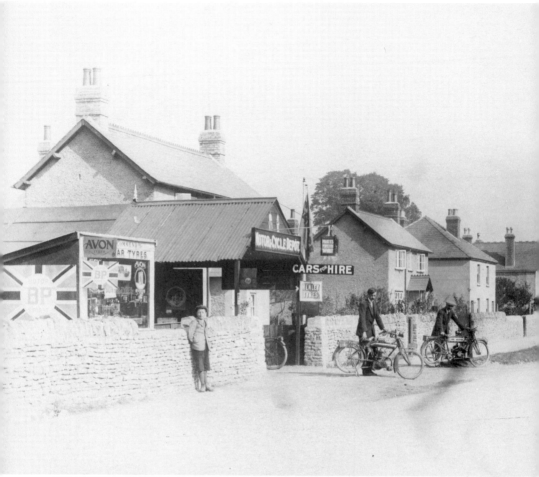

EMPLOYEES HAVE WHEELED OUT TWO MOTOR BIKES to promote the Motor & Cycle Depot at Long Hanborough in the early 1920s. The Pratts Perfection Spirit advertised above 'Cars for Hire' changed its name to Esso in the '30s.

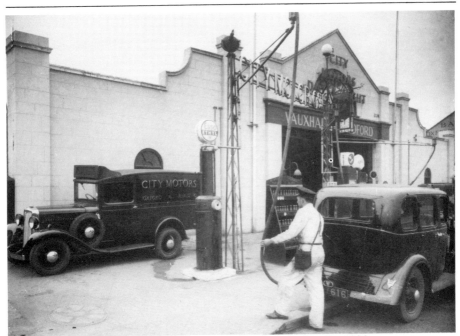

FILLING HER UP at City Motors Garage in Botley Road, Oxford in the 1930s.

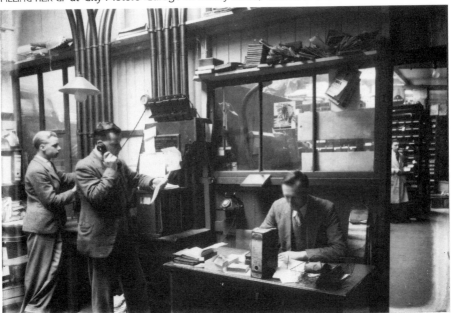

THE WORKADAY OFFICE at City Motors' Gloucester Street premises in Oxford during the 1930s. The pneumatic tubes shot your money to a central cash point and returned your change with a whoosh – much more exciting than an electronic till.

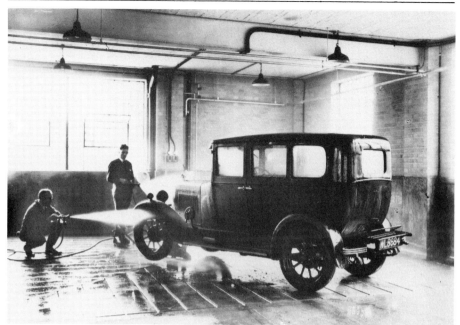

THE CAR WASH at Morris Garages in St Aldate's, Oxford in 1932. This huge motor palace designed by Henry Smith comprised showroom, offices, forecourt, service area and a large public car park.

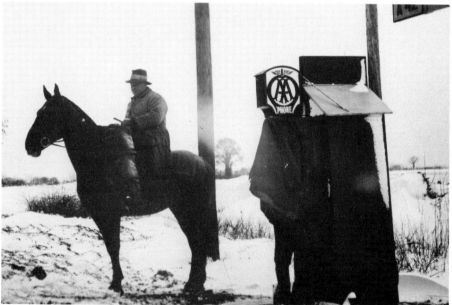

THE AA WILL GET THROUGH! A stranded motorist uses a call-box near Chipping Norton during the hard winter of 1947.

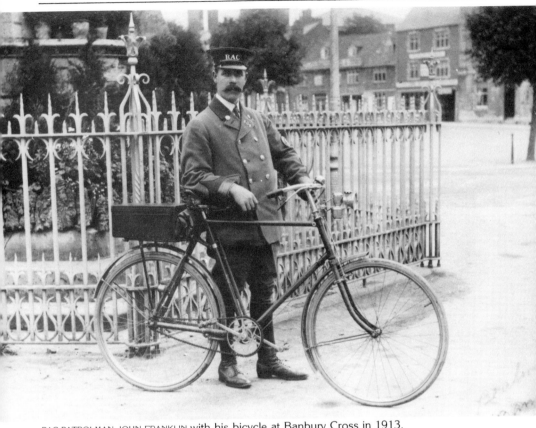

RAC PATROLMAN JOHN FRANKLIN with his bicycle at Banbury Cross in 1913.

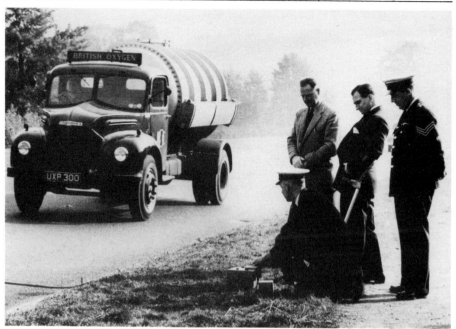

A RATHER CONSPICUOUS SPEED TRAP mounted by the Oxfordshire Constabulary in October 1959.

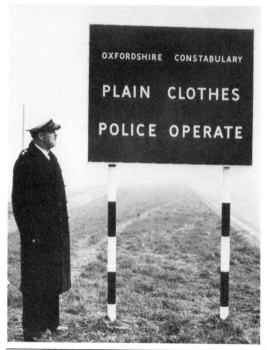

OXFORDSHIRE   CONSTABULARY

PLAIN CLOTHES

POLICE OPERATE

A CAMPAIGN AGAINST SPEEDING on the outskirts of Oxford in 1959. The plain clothes traffic policemen were seen as rather unsporting.

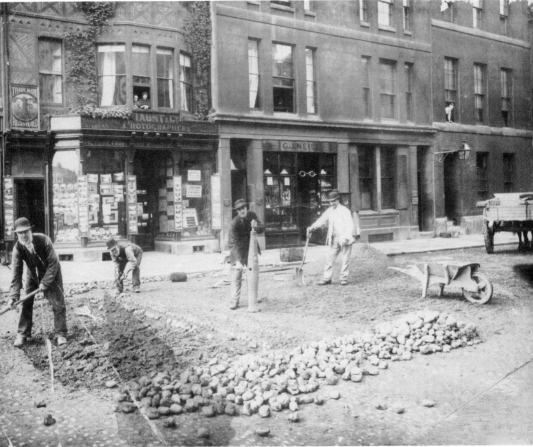

WORKMEN RE-LAYING THE COBBLES in Broad Street, Oxford in about 1875. The group is carefully posed outside the shop of Henry Taunt, the famous Oxford photographer.

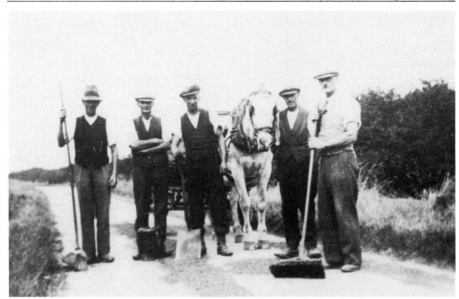

OXFORDSHIRE COUNTY COUNCIL ROAD GANG at Clanfield in the 1920s. The three central figures are, from left to right: Bill Garner, George Cross and Ernest Yeatman.

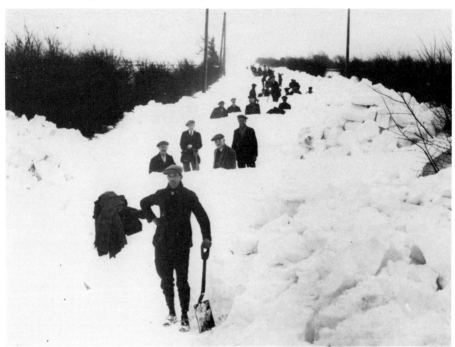

CLEARING THE SNOW near Chipping Norton in 1929. This sort of job often provided the unemployed with welcome cash during the difficult winter months.

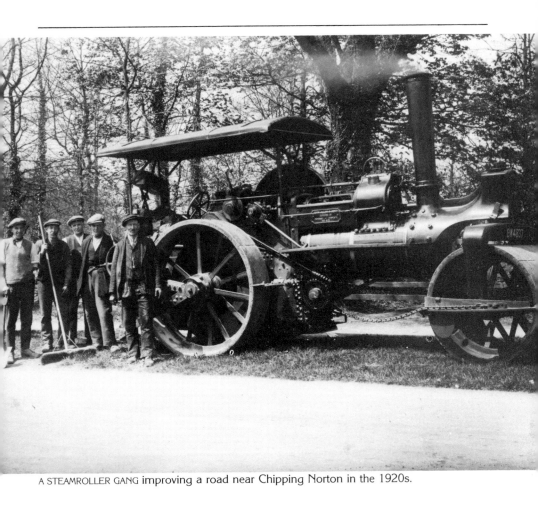

A STEAMROLLER GANG improving a road near Chipping Norton in the 1920s.

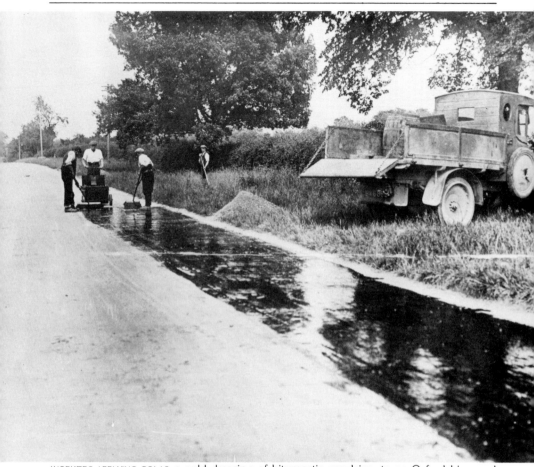

WORKERS APPLYING COLAS, a cold dressing of bitumastic emulsion, to an Oxfordshire road. Between the wars country roads that had been alternately dusty or muddy were transformed into smooth highways for motor vehicles.

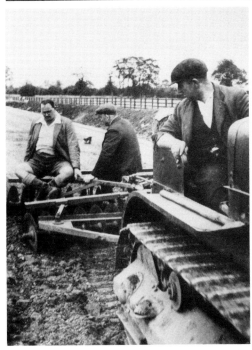

BUILDING THE NEW BICESTER ROAD in 1938. This soil stabilization experiment needed Senior Assistant Divisional Surveyor Bill Sewell to provide extra weight on the back. Even with his help the result was 'mud pies'.

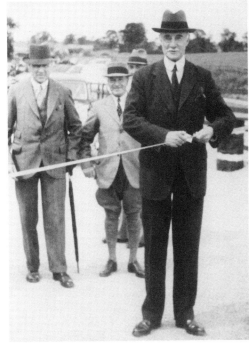

OPENING THE NEW BANBURY ROAD CANAL BRIDGE north of Kidlington in June 1938. The cutter of the ribbon was the chairman of the County Council's Highways Committee, Lt.-Col. H.E. Du Cane Norris.

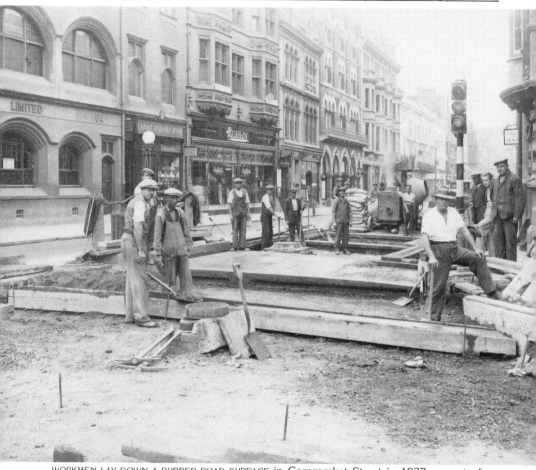

WORKMEN LAY DOWN A RUBBER ROAD SURFACE in Cornmarket Street in 1937 as part of an experiment to reduce vibration to Oxford's historic buildings. The rubber blocks proved to be very slippery in wet weather and were removed in 1955.

Professions and Public Service

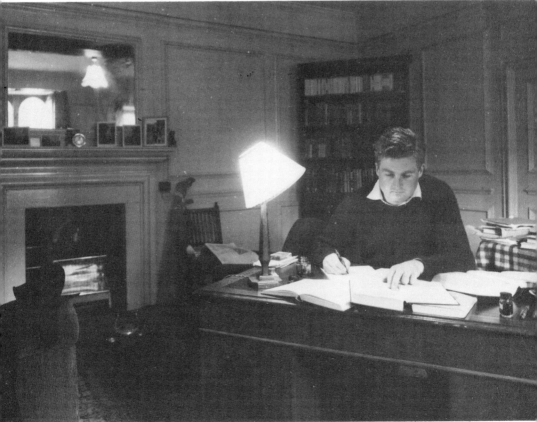

BURNING THE MIDNIGHT OIL at Brasenose College in 1958: an undergraduate struggles to complete his work.

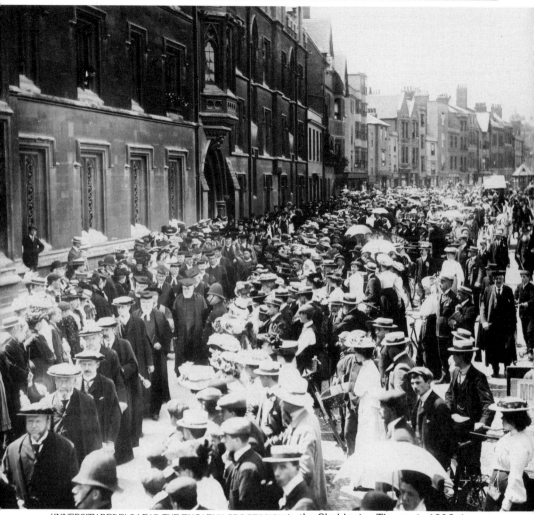

UNIVERSITY BEDELS LEAD THE ENCAENIA PROCESSION to the Sheldonian Theatre in 1906. Away to the right a sandwich-board man advertises John Collier and Sons, a former cycle business which had come to terms with the motor car.

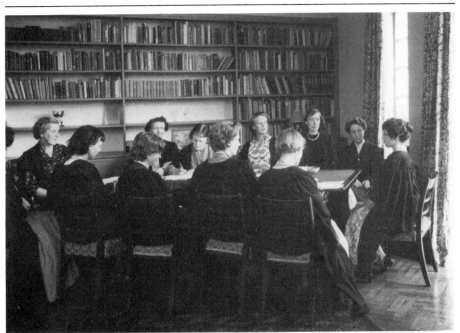

'DID YOU REALLY MEAN THAT?' An undergraduate at St Anne's College in the 1950s listens uncomfortably to the Principal's end of term report in the presence of College tutors.

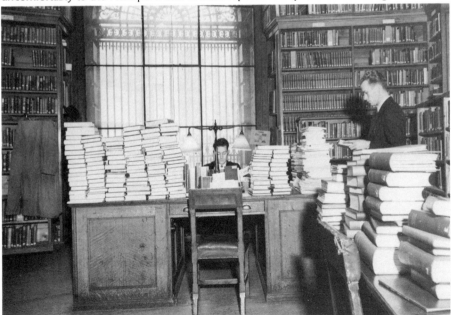

LIBRARIANS AT THE BODLEIAN LIBRARY in the 1950s, when the library received this daunting quantity of new books every four or five days.

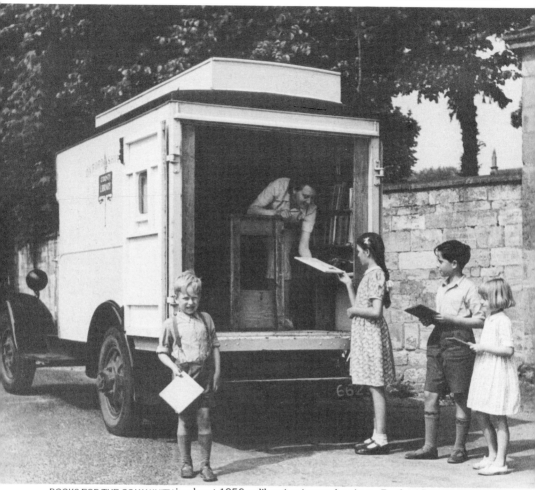

BOOKS FOR THE COMMUNITY in about 1950: a librarian issues books to Burford Primary School children from the dark recesses of the Children's Book Van.

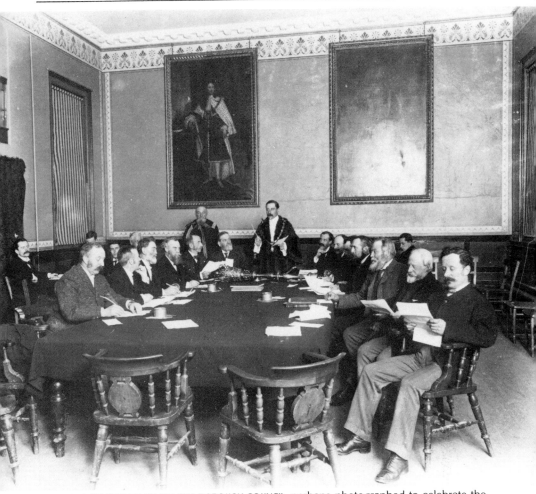

A MEETING OF HENLEY-ON-THAMES BOROUGH COUNCIL, perhaps photographed to celebrate the opening of the new Town Hall in 1900.

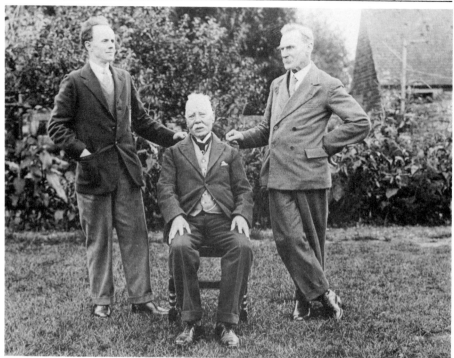

THREE GENERATIONS OF HEADMASTER at Brize Norton School in 1931. From left to right: Mr Jones (1925–32), Mr Hawkins (1876–96) and Mr Williams (1896–1925).

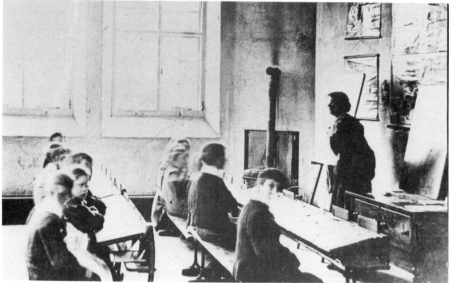

ALONE AT THE CHALK FACE: a school teacher seeks to retain the attention of her class at Stratton Audley School in 1905.

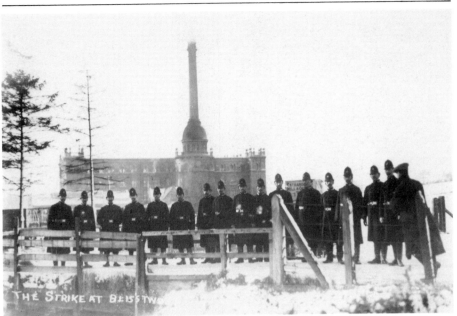

A STRONG POLICE PRESENCE guards the approach to Bliss' Tweed Mill at Chipping Norton during the strike of 1913/14.

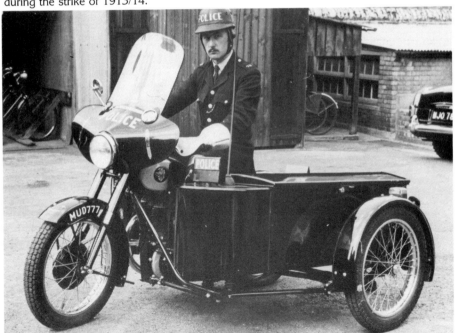

A PROUD POLICE OFFICER with one of the radio-equipped motor cycles which the Oxfordshire Constabulary introduced in 1958.

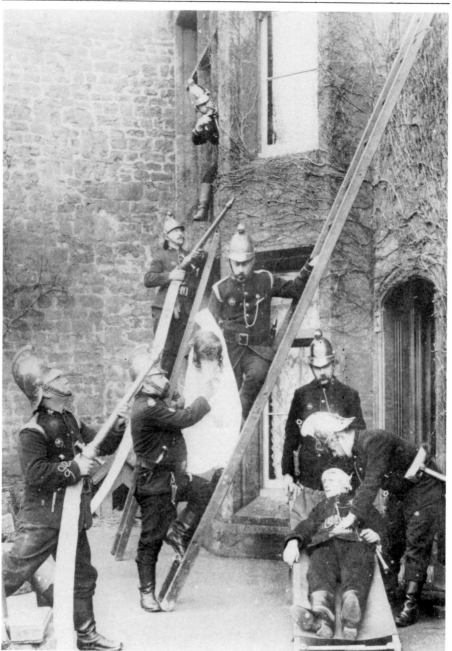

A POSED RESCUE at Calthorpe Manor by members of the Banbury Volunteer Fire Brigade in the 1890s.

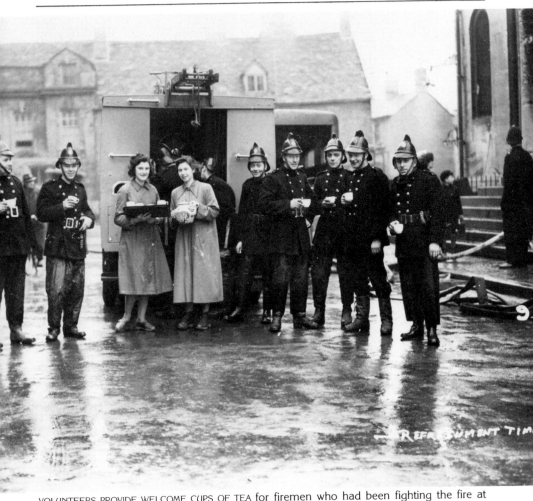

VOLUNTEERS PROVIDE WELCOME CUPS OF TEA for firemen who had been fighting the fire at Chipping Norton Town Hall in March 1950.

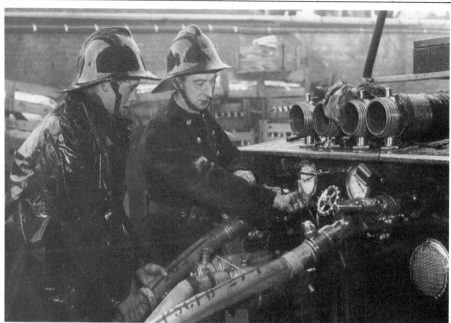

FIREMEN from the Pressed Steel fire brigade fighting a fire in Q Building in 1958.

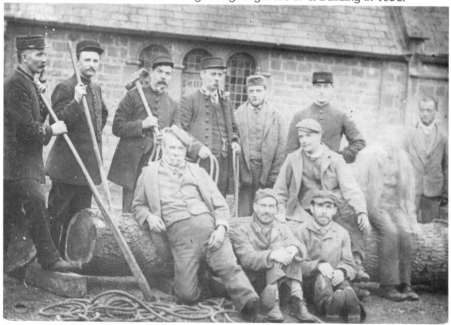

NURSING STAFF AND PATIENTS at Littlemore Hospital in about 1910. They formed the 'Scratch Gang' which did work around the site and are posing proudly beside the tree they had just felled.

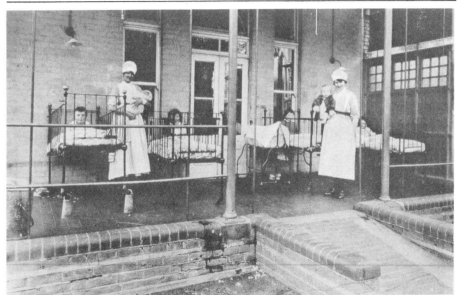

NURSES AND PATIENTS at the children's ward of the Radcliffe Infirmary, Oxford in about 1910.

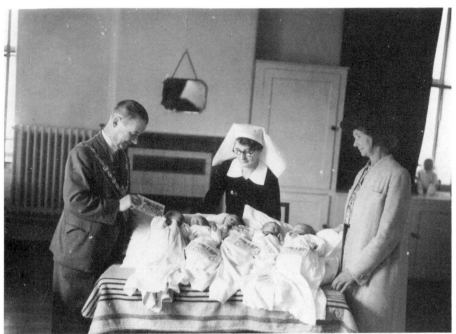

MATRON SHOWS OFF five Christmas or New Year babies at Chipping Norton Hospital in the 1940s.

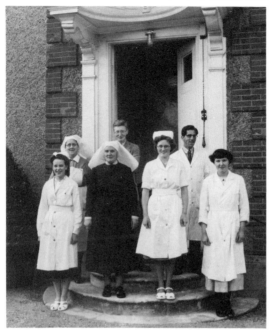

DOCTORS AND NURSES at Longworth Hospital in 1946.

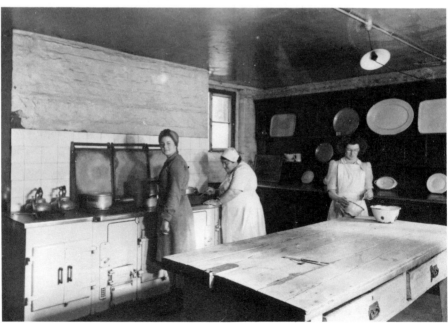

STAFF WORKING IN THE KITCHENS of the Downs Hospital, the former Wantage Union workhouse, in 1946. The building was eventually demolished in the 1960s.

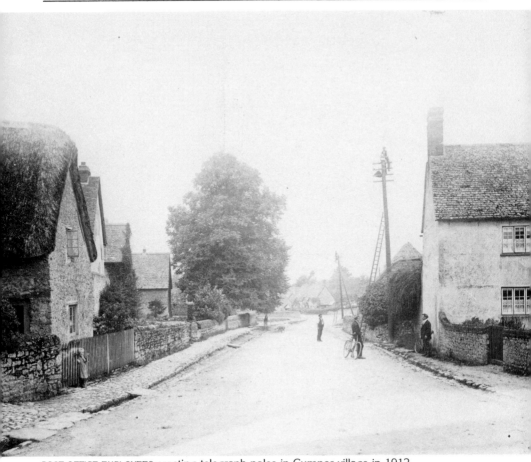

POST OFFICE EMPLOYEES erecting telegraph poles in Cumnor village in 1912.

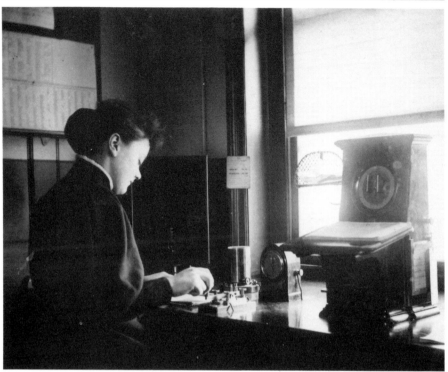
MISS JONES, the telegraphist at Banbury post office, in the 1890s.

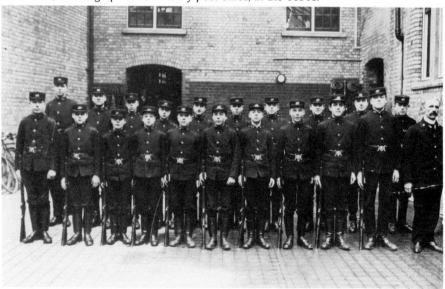
OXFORD POST OFFICE MESSENGER BOYS attend morning parade in 1912, before going to drill in Christ Church Meadow.

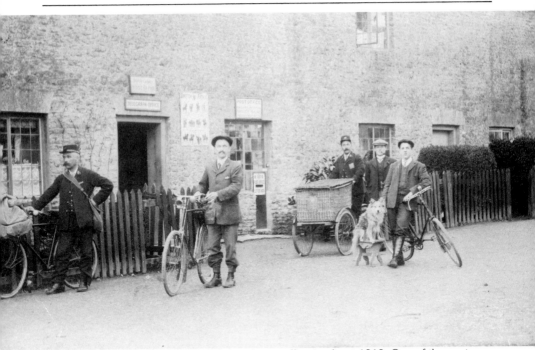

POSTMEN AND CUSTOMERS outside Buckland post office in about 1910. One of the postmen has a tricycle with a huge basket for delivering parcels. It is tempting to see the dog as the defender of postmen on their rounds.

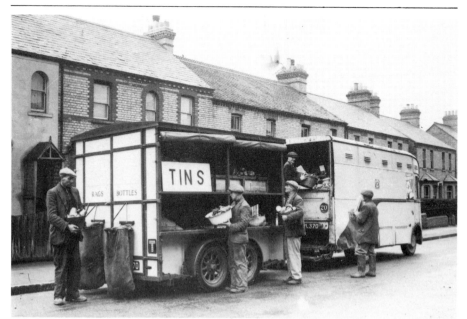

RECYCLING in Oxford during the Second World War: City Council workmen sort the refuse into categories as part of the war effort.

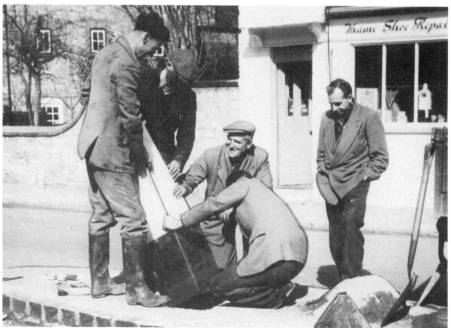

MANY HANDS MAKE LIGHT WORK in Thame in 1956. Council workmen struggle to erect a bollard at the junction of Upper High Street and East Street.

Shops

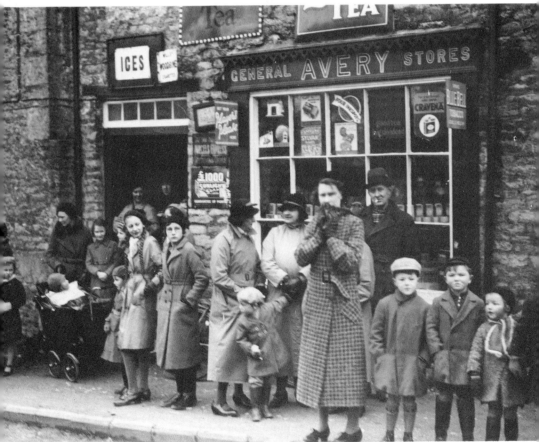

SHOPPERS OF ALL AGES outside Avery's general stores in Chipping Norton in about 1950.

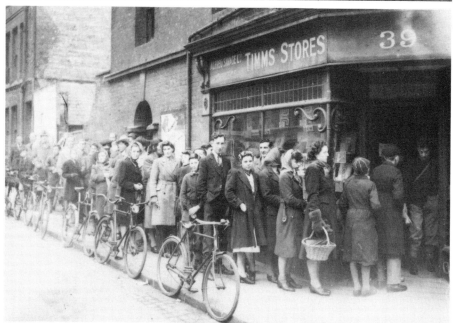

QUEUEING FOR BARGAINS at Timms' toy shop in George Street, Oxford in the years of austerity following the Second World War.

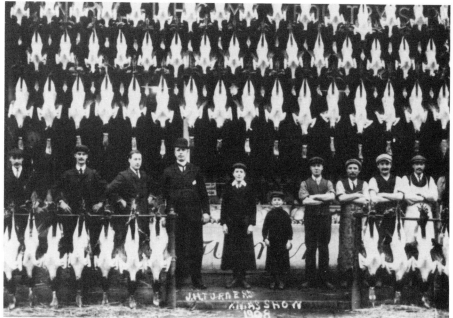

CHRISTMAS DISPLAY at J.H. Turner's fish, game and poultry shop in Broad Street, Banbury in 1908.

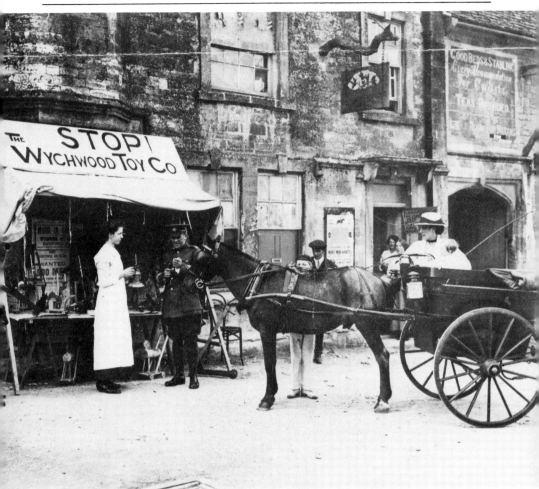

A SOLDIER considers buying a toy for his child at a Burford toy shop in 1914. Posters behind him urge Oxfordshire men to join the struggle against the Kaiser's Germany.

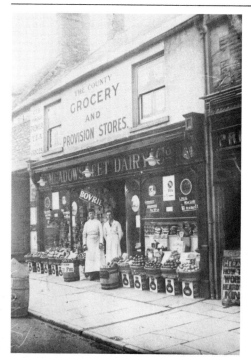

A BOVRIL SPECIAL PROMOTION at the Meadowsweet Dairy in High Street, Witney, possibly in 1932. The *Daily Herald* placard to the right is probably referring to King George V's first Christmas broadcast which took place in that year.

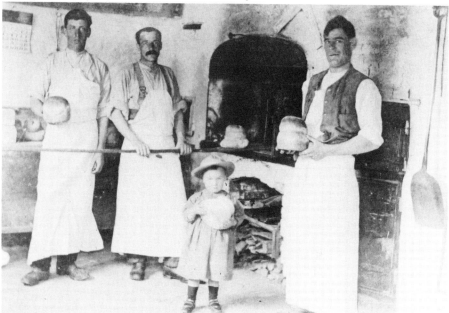

BAKERS AND A VERY YOUNG HELPER at the old Co-operative Society bakery in Heyford Road, Steeple Aston in 1895.

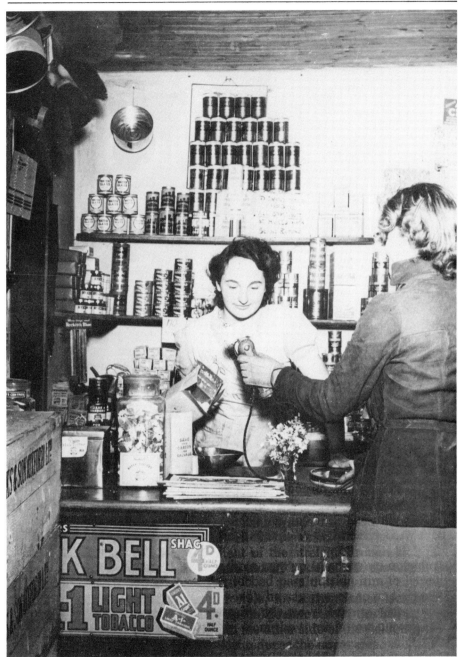

INSIDE THE POST OFFICE at Cassington in 1946. The assistant is being interviewed for the BBC programme *Portrait of a Village*.

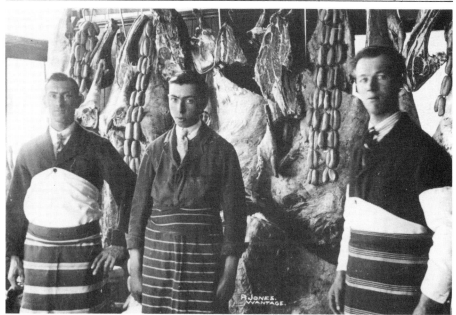

THE BRITISH ARGENTINE MEAT COMPANY SHOP in Market Place, Wantage in 1930. The staff were, from left to right: Mr Moore, Charles Crook and George Taylor.

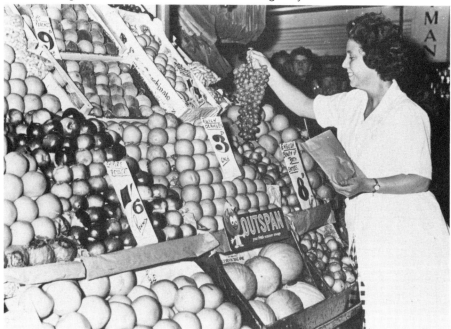

EMPIRE DESSERT APPLES for 1s. 6d. a pound, and oranges at 3d. each. Service with a smile in Oxford's Covered Market in August 1960.

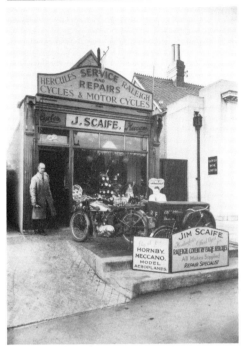

PARADISE FOR BOYS OF ALL AGES. Jim Scaife poses briefly outside his cycle and toy shop at 83 London Road, Headington in October 1936.

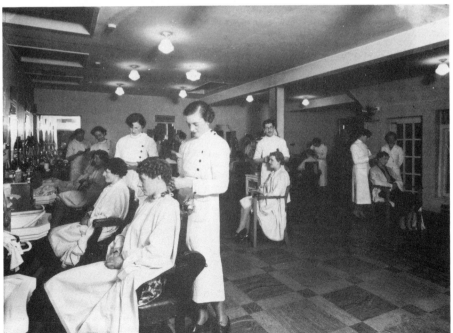

HAIRDRESSERS at Strange's Salon in Market Street, Oxford in March 1937.

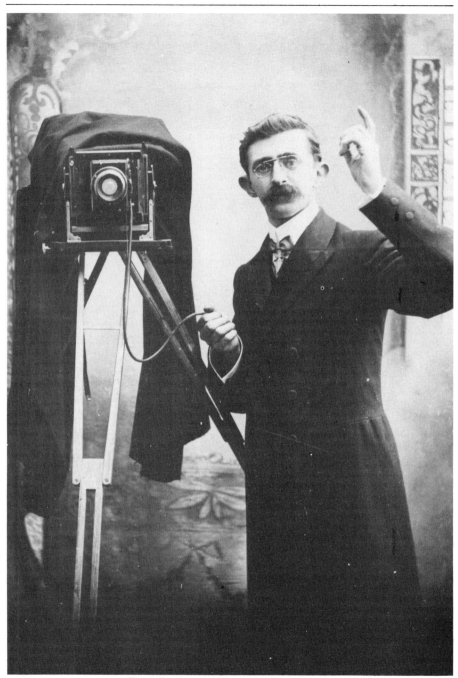

WATCH THE BIRDIE, PLEASE! Frank Packer, the Chipping Norton photographer, prepares to add another face to his hall of fame.

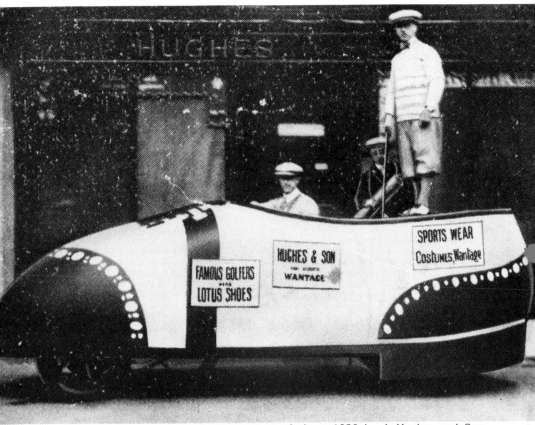

THE MOBILE SHOE: an original advertising stunt of about 1930 by J. Hughes and Son, shoemakers in the Market Place, Wantage.

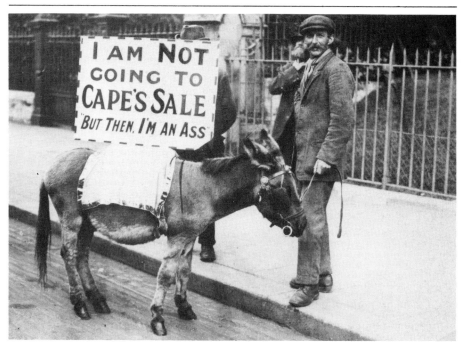

USING A DONKEY to publicize the sale held by Oxford drapers, F. Cape and Company. The photograph was taken outside the New Road Baptist church in about 1929.

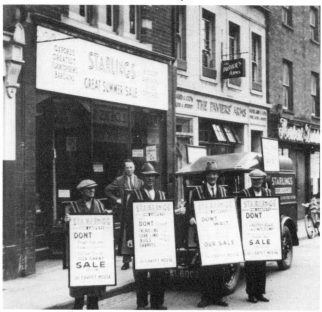

SANDWICH-BOARD MEN set off to proclaim the news of Starling's carpet sale in Castle Street, Oxford in about 1930.

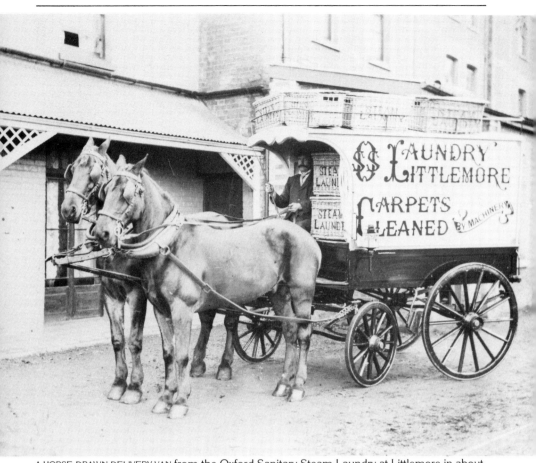

A HORSE-DRAWN DELIVERY VAN from the Oxford Sanitary Steam Laundry at Littlemore in about 1900.

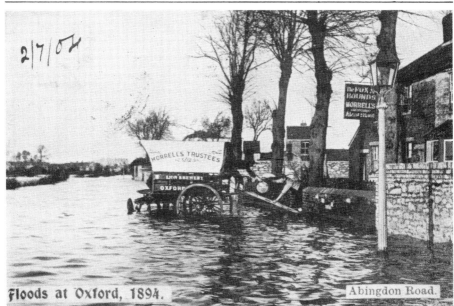

UNDAUNTED BY THE FLOODS, a Morrell's drayman delivers the beer to the Fox and Hounds pub in Abingdon Road, Oxford in 1894.

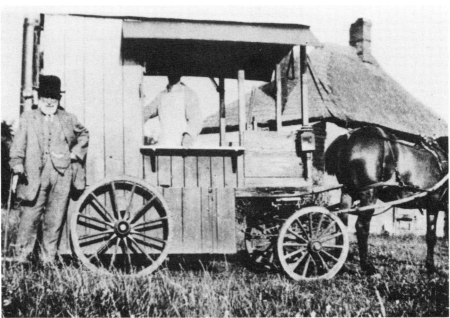

FISH AND CHIPS by horse-drawn van at West Hendred in about 1910. Mr Crease is standing by the rear wheel and Larry Roberts is in the van.

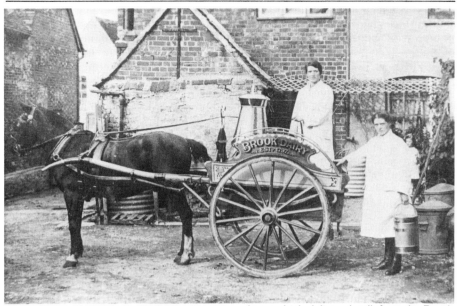

MILK-O! Two women pose with the smart pony and trap which delivered milk from the Brook Dairy at Watlington. This was possibly taken during the First World War.

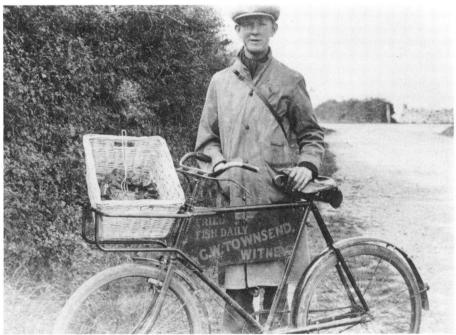

FISH AND CHIPS by bicycle around Witney in the 1920s. G.W. Townsend ran this enterprising, if improbable service.

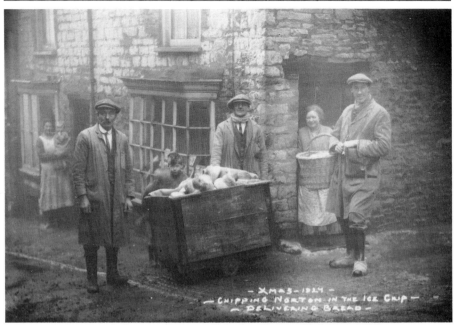

DELIVERING THE BREAD in icy conditions at Chipping Norton, Christmas 1927.

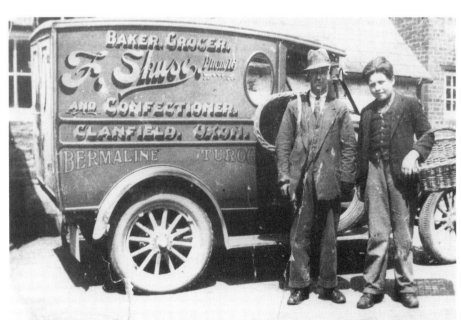

FRED SKUSE with his delivery van and baker's boy, Bob Blake, at Clanfield in the 1920s.

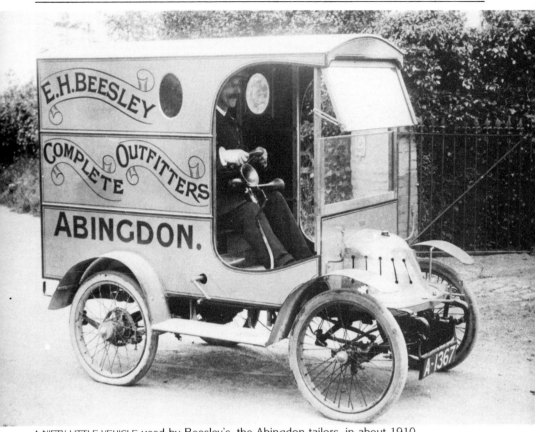

A NIFTY LITTLE VEHICLE used by Beesley's, the Abingdon tailors, in about 1910.

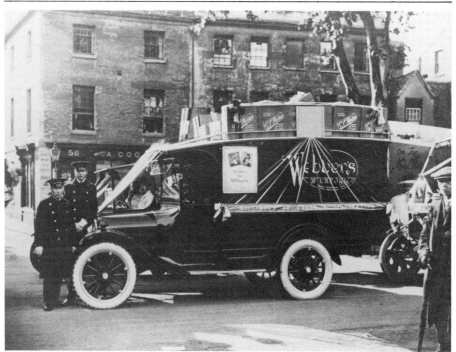

WEBBER'S OF OXFORD DELIVERY VAN in St Giles' in 1923. Dressed overall for the Oxford Shopping Carnival, the van formed a splendid advertisement for the High Street department store.

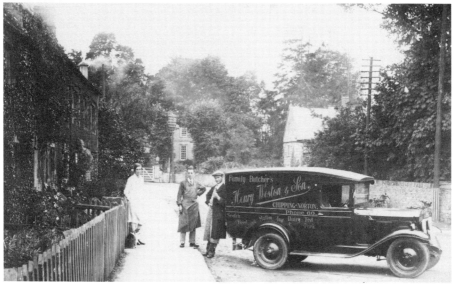

HENRY WESTON & SON'S BUTCHERS chat to a customer in Kingham in the 1930s; the cat stares hopefully at the delivery van.

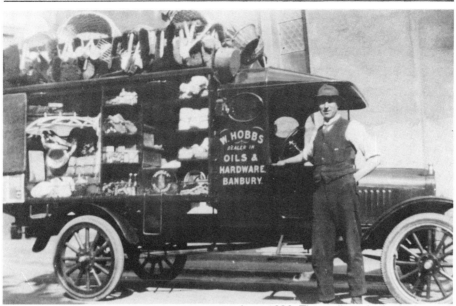

W. HOBBS WITH HIS TRAVELLING HARDWARE SHOP in about 1930. This well-stocked vehicle must have been a welcome sight in Banburyshire between the wars.

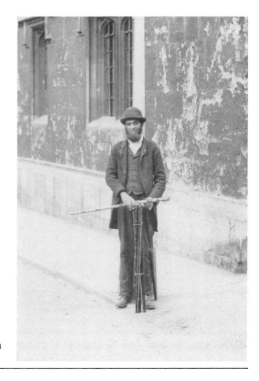

AN ITINERANT VENDOR OF WALKING STICKS in Radcliffe Square, Oxford in the 1870s.

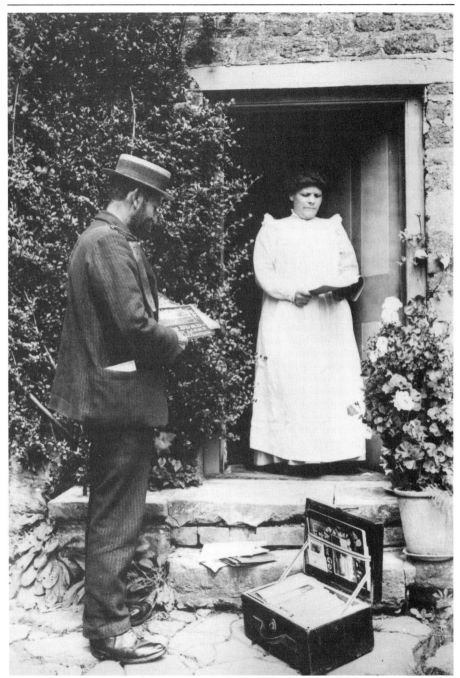

NOT TODAY, THANK YOU! A colporteur, or travelling salesman with religious tracts, receives a frosty welcome from a woman in the Banbury area.

SECTION SEVEN

Servants

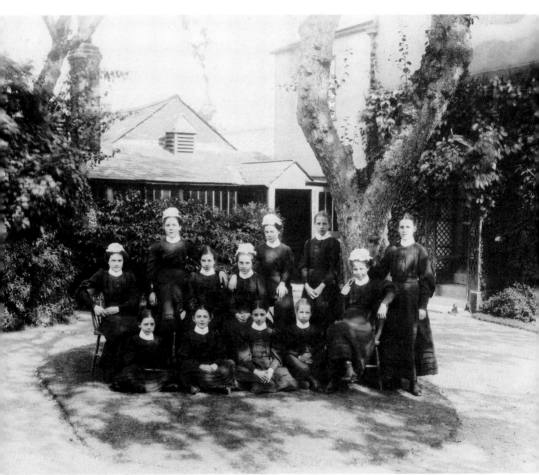

YOUNG GIRLS at the domestic servants' training school in Headington Hill Hall, 1913. This school had been started in 1858 by Mrs Morrell, wife of the Oxford brewer.

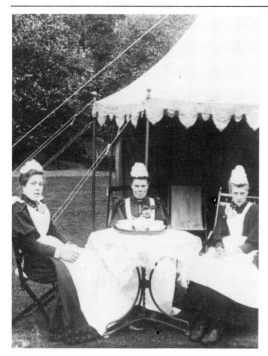

SERVANTS taking a well-earned rest during a tea party at Garsington Rectory in the 1890s.

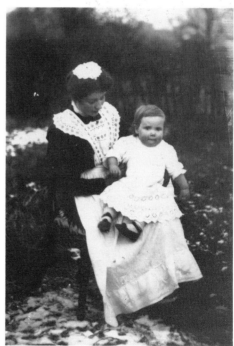

AN UNKNOWN NURSEMAID AND HER CHARGE, photographed for a family album by B.R. Morland of Banbury in about 1910.

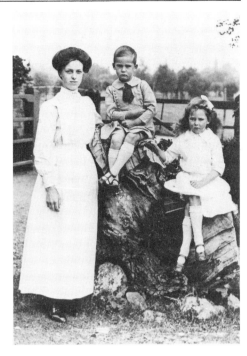

NURSEMAID KATE WITH STELLA AND JOSEPH MAWLE at Manor Farm, Cogges in the 1900s.

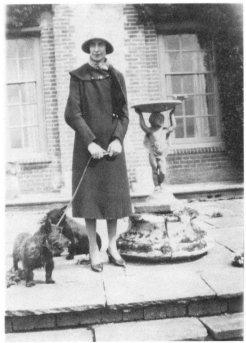

LORD NUFFIELD'S MAID, KATHLEEN FRANCIS, with the family's scotties at Nuffield Place in the 1930s.

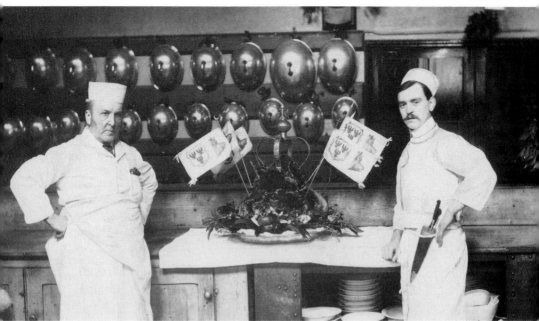

QUEEN'S COLLEGE CHEFS WITH THE BOAR'S HEAD in about 1900. The Boar's Head ceremony is an annual Christmas custom at the College and is said to commemorate a student's lucky escape from a wild boar on Shotover Hill.

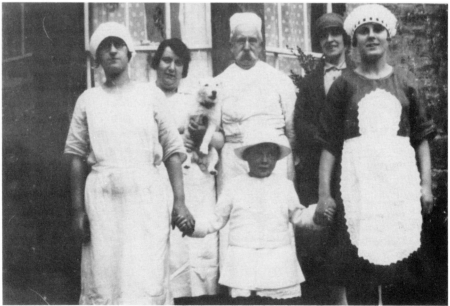

DOMESTIC STAFF at the Bear Hotel, Woodstock in about 1930. They were, from left to right: the kitchen maid, the waitress, the chef, the chambermaid and the between maid.

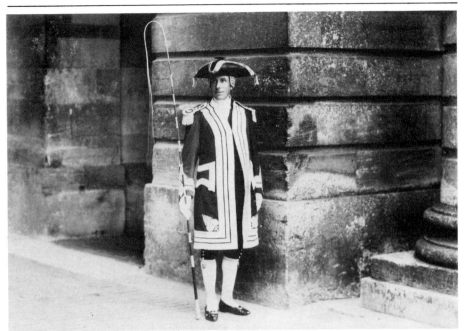

THE DUKE OF MARLBOROUGH'S COACHMAN at Blenheim Palace, photographed outside the massive East Gate in about 1900.

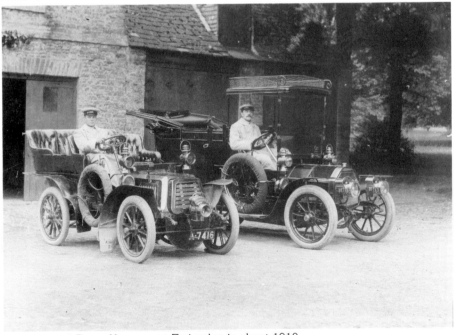

CHAUFFEURS at Pusey House near Faringdon in about 1910.

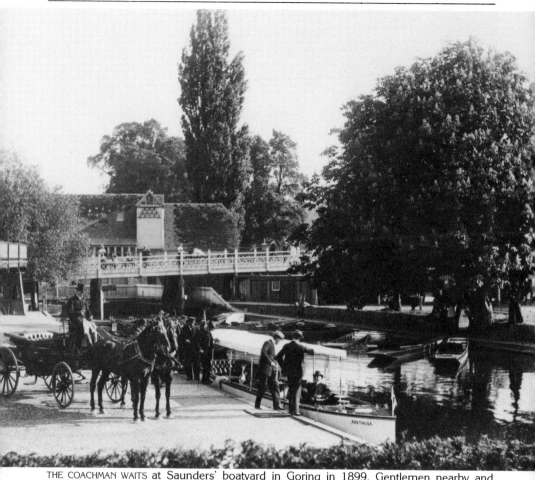

THE COACHMAN WAITS at Saunders' boatyard in Goring in 1899. Gentlemen nearby and spectators on the bridge admire the steam launch *Arethusa*.

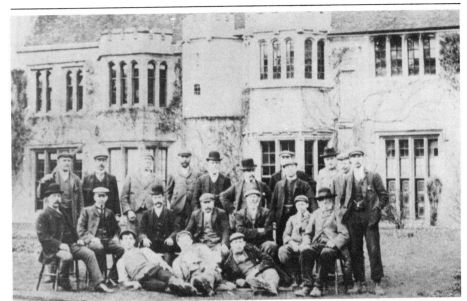

THE ESTATE STAFF of Thame Park in about 1900. This large group of gardeners, grooms, bricklayers and other outdoor servants is posed outside the picturesque early sixteenth-century range.

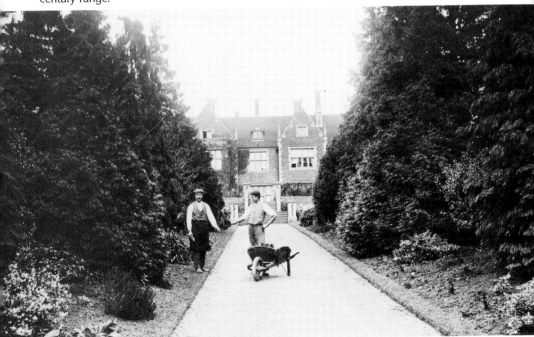

TWO GARDENERS discuss their work at Barcote Manor near Faringdon in about 1910. The house was built for a director of the Great Western Railway Company in 1875.

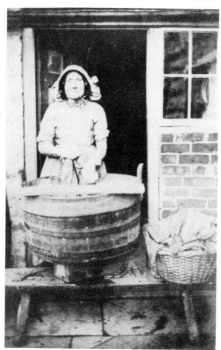

WASHDAY BLUES for a washerwoman, possibly at Gaunt House in Standlake, in about 1900.

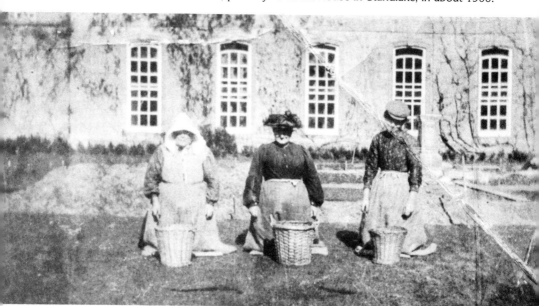

DAISY PICKING at Cokethorpe House near Witney in about 1908. This group, with Elizabeth Foster in the centre, graphically illustrates that a servant's work was never done.

SECTION EIGHT

Miscellany

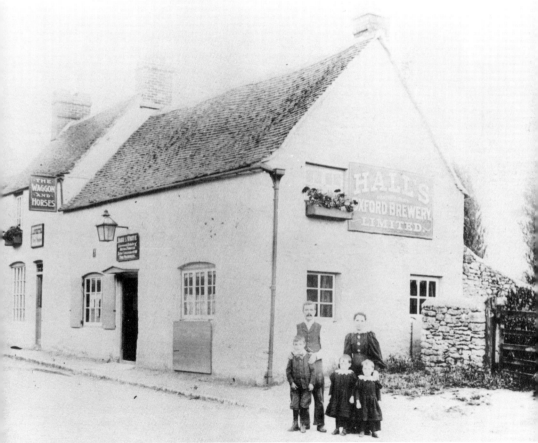

JIM AND SARAH WHITE with their three children, Tom, Flo and Win, outside the Waggon and Horses in Cowley in about 1900. As well as being landlord of the pub, Jim kept the adjoining butcher's shop.

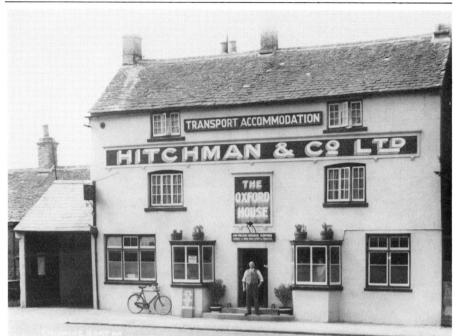

LANDLORD JOHN SCRIVENER outside the Oxford House in Chipping Norton in the 1930s. His comfortable proportions were, perhaps, a promising advertisement for the establishment's food.

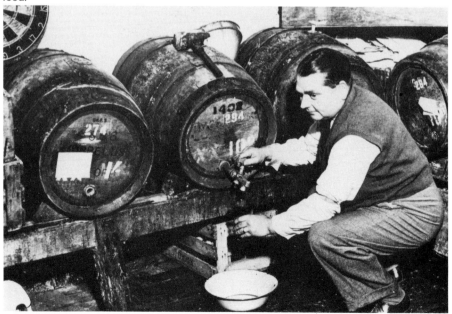

BILL LONG drawing the first pint at The Chequers in Cassington in 1946.

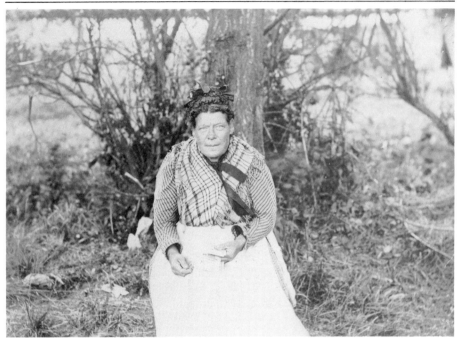

PROGRAMME BETTY at Henley Royal Regatta in July 1902.

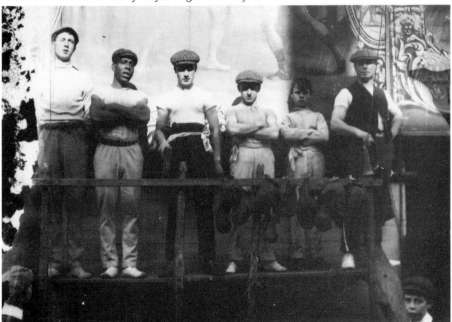

TAKING ON ALL COMERS. Pugilists of varying sizes, weights and ages stand ready to fight local lads at Banbury Fair.

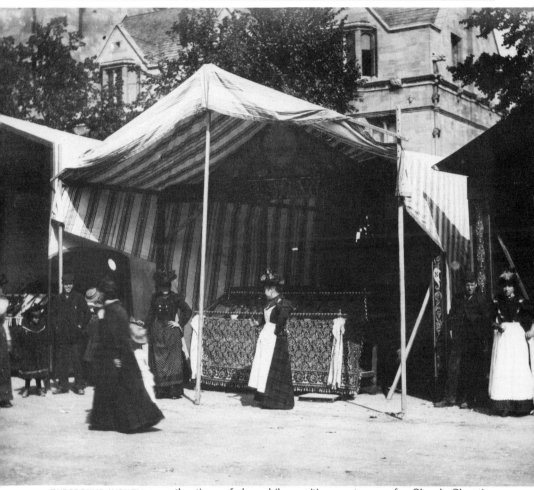

FAIRGROUND WOMEN pass the time of day while awaiting customers for Shaw's Shooting Gallery at St Giles' Fair in 1895.

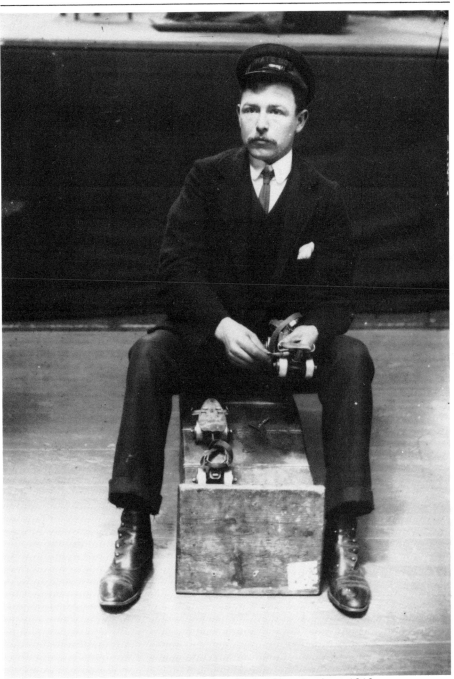

SKATEBOY at the Banbury roller skating rink in Market Place in about 1910.

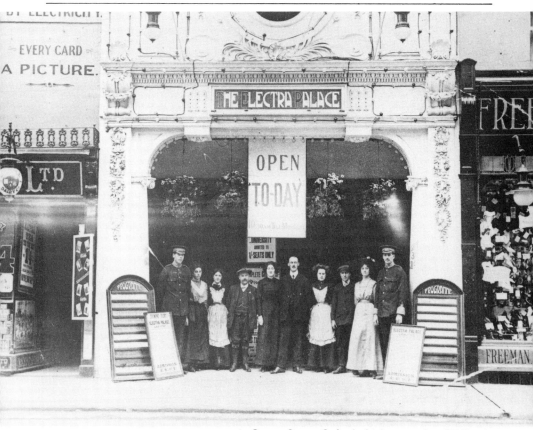

THE STAFF OF THE ELECTRA PALACE CINEMA in Queen Street, Oxford which opened on 25 March 1911. The tall commissionaires were doubtless needed to deal with University rowdies who were only admitted to the expensive 1s. seats.

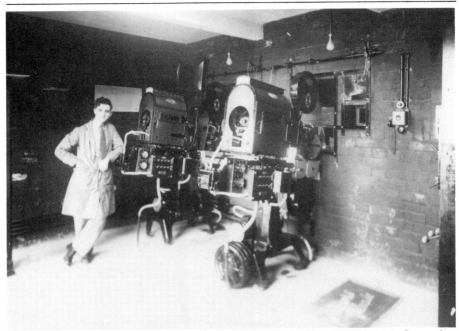

THE PROJECTIONIST at the New Cinema, later the Regent, in Chipping Norton in December 1934. The first feature film was *Roman Scandals*, starring Eddie Cantor.

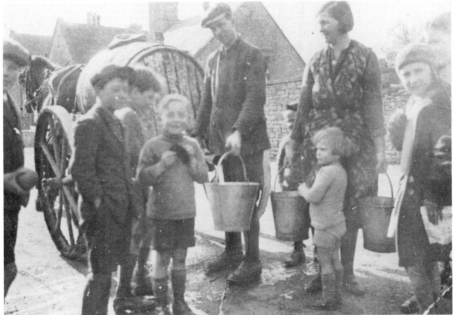

DELIVERING WATER to the villagers of Finstock in the 1920s. The cart came from Fawler and the water cost ½d. a bucket.

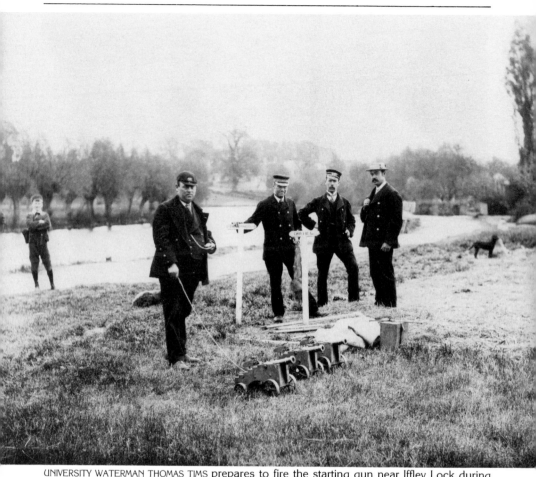

UNIVERSITY WATERMAN THOMAS TIMS prepares to fire the starting gun near Iffley Lock during Eights Week in May 1908.

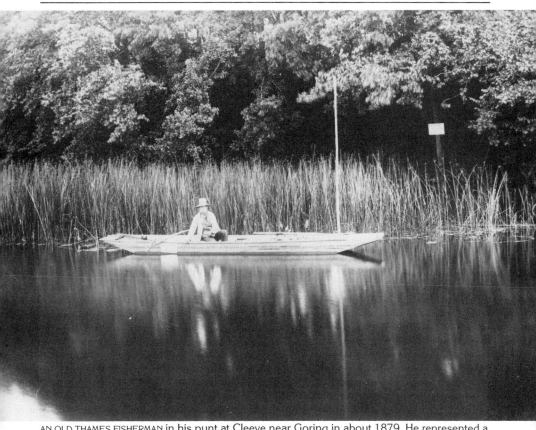

AN OLD THAMES FISHERMAN in his punt at Cleeve near Goring in about 1879. He represented a dying breed as amateur anglers and pleasure seekers began to take over the river.

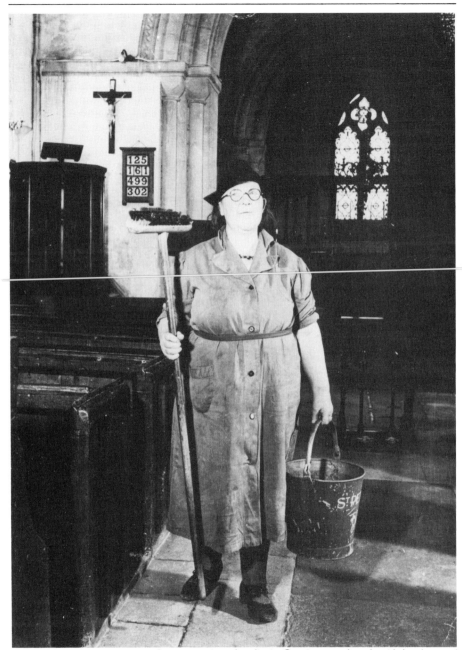

HESTER NEWMAN prepares to advance against the dirt in Cassington church with bucket and brush in 1946.

SECTION NINE

Children

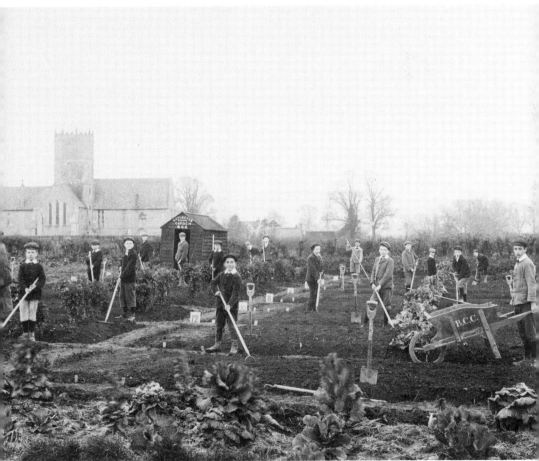

GARDENING CLASS for the boys of Uffington School in 1910.

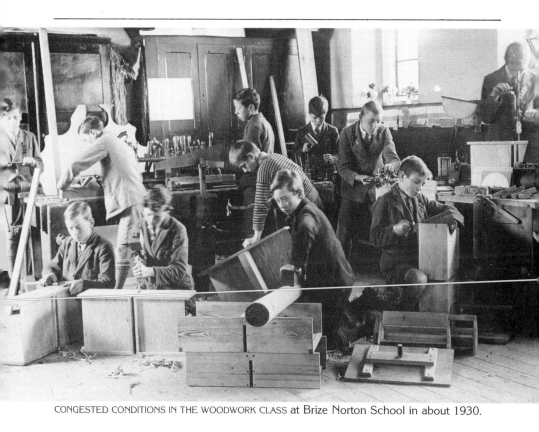

CONGESTED CONDITIONS IN THE WOODWORK CLASS at Brize Norton School in about 1930.

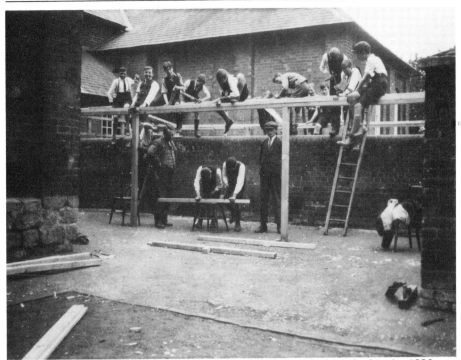

SAFETY AT WORK? Boys of Thame Church of England School build a shed in the 1920s.

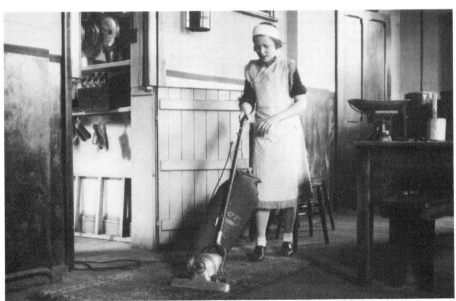

PRACTISING WITH THE HOOVER at Thame Church of England School in 1937.

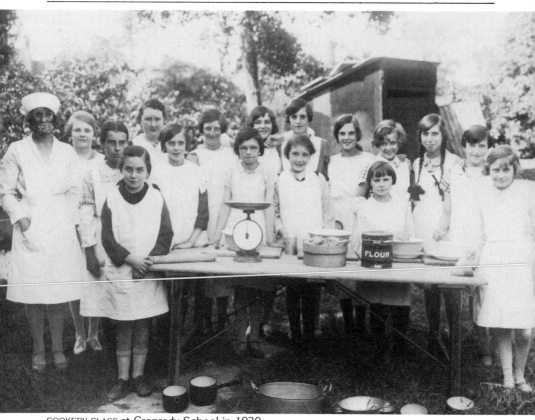

COOKERY CLASS at Cropredy School in 1930.

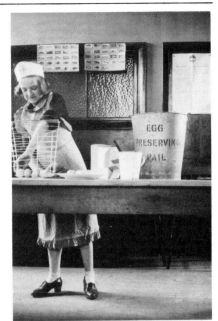

DOMESTIC SCIENCE WORK at Thame Church of England School in 1937. A girl prepares to lay down eggs in the preserving pail.

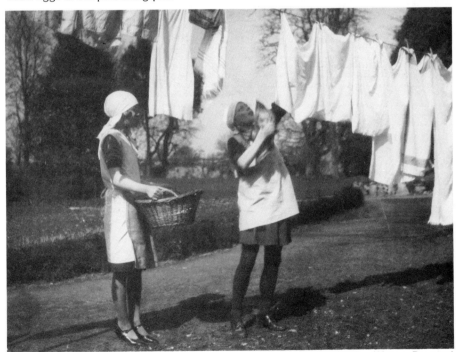

HANGING OUT THE WASHING: part of the domestic science lesson at the Witney Practical Subjects Centre in 1932.

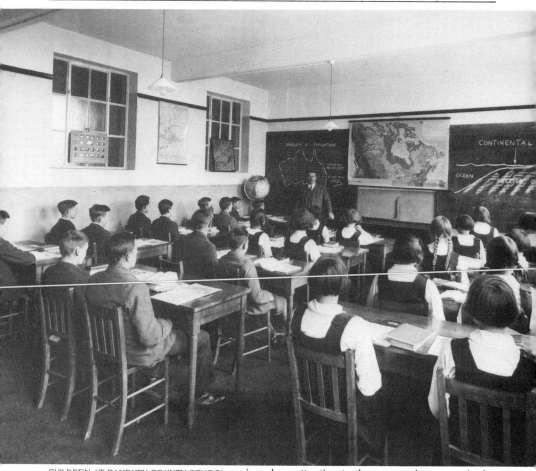

CHILDREN AT BANBURY COUNTY SCHOOL paying close attention to the geography master in the 1930s.

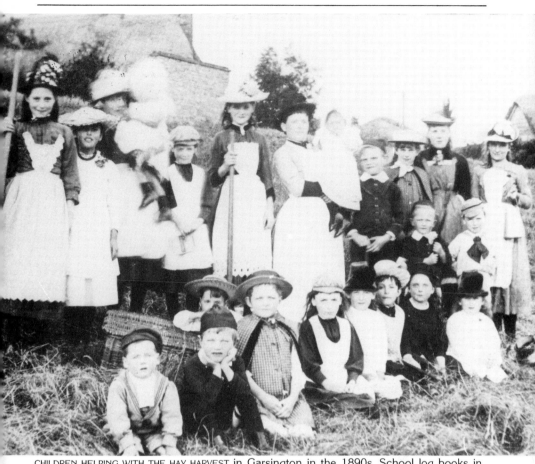

CHILDREN HELPING WITH THE HAY HARVEST in Garsington in the 1890s. School log books in country areas frequently recorded the absence of children doing farmwork.

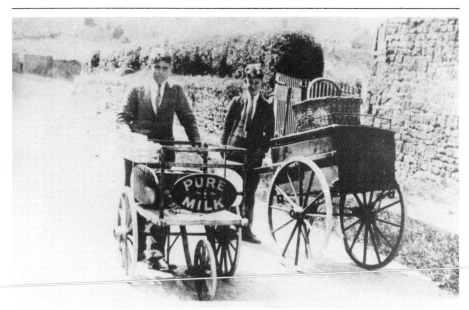

CO-OPERATIVE SOCIETY DELIVERY BOYS Vic Lynes (left) and Len West in Round Close Road, Adderbury in the early 1930s.

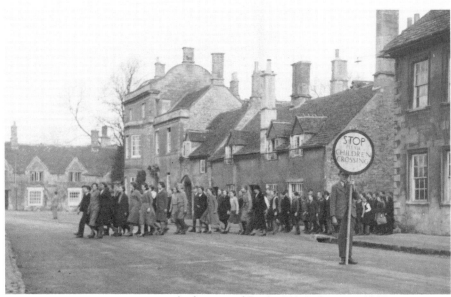

PUPILS ON TRAFFIC CONTROL CUTY at the bottom of Burford High Street in 1935.

SECTION TEN

Old Age

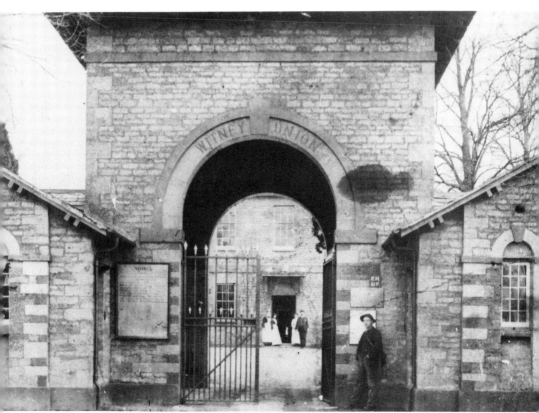

THE ENTRANCE TO WITNEY WORKHOUSE in about 1900. After a life of toil, ending your days in the workhouse or 'spike' was a very real fear for the less fortunate.

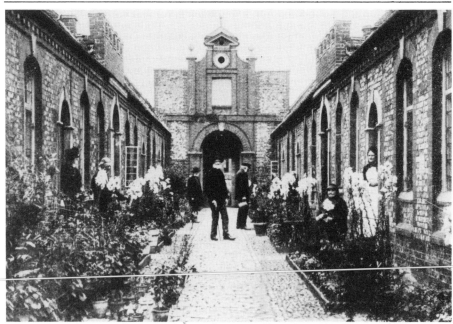

ALMSMEN AND WOMEN at the early eighteenth-century Tompkins Almshouses in Abingdon in 1907.

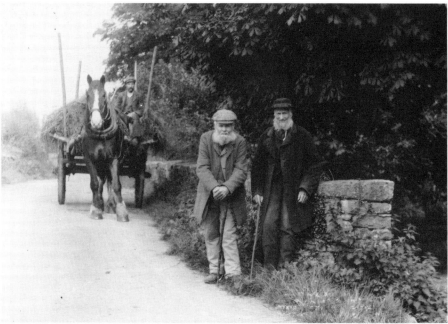

'GAFFERS' BY THE ROADSIDE in an unknown village in the early 1900s: an attractive study by the Chipping Norton photographer, Frank Packer.

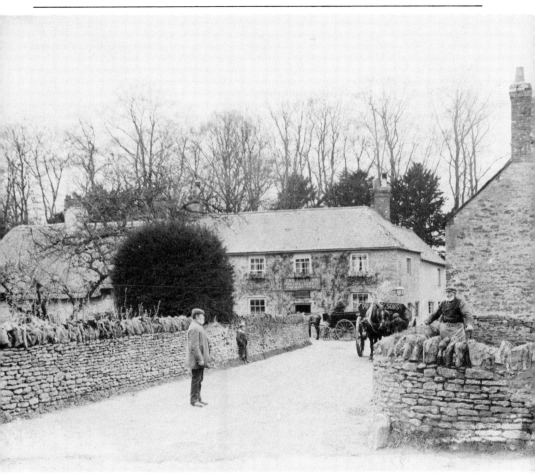

TWO OLD MEN EXCHANGE PLEASANTRIES in Buckland in about 1910. Behind them, Phillips & Son's dray has replenished the Lamb Inn's supplies of fine ales and stouts.

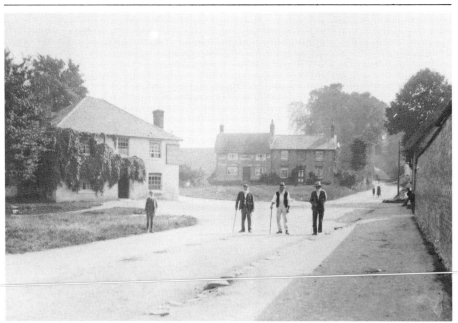

COMING FROM THE HATCHET PUB in Childrey in about 1910. Three veterans make their slow way home with no need to worry about traffic.

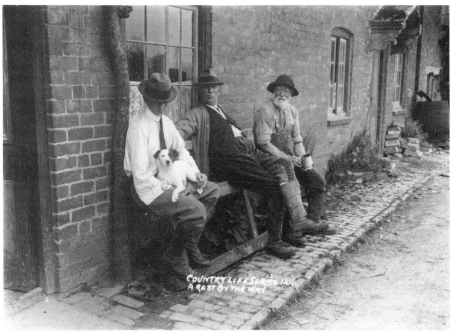

A REST AND A POT OF ALE outside a wayside pub, one of Packer's Country Life photographs.

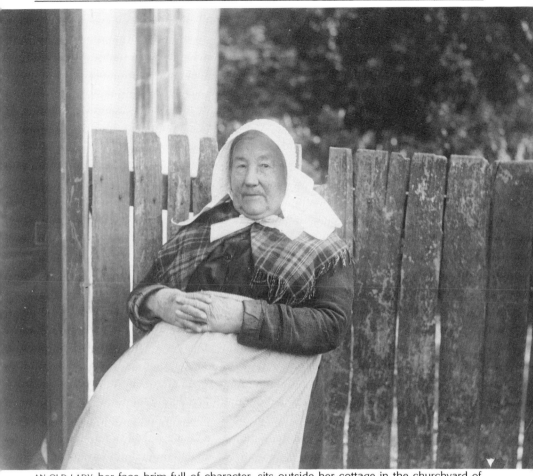

AN OLD LADY, her face brim-full of character, sits outside her cottage in the churchyard of Dorchester Abbey in 1907.

OXFORDSHIRE PHOTOGRAPHIC ARCHIVE

The photographs in this book are selected from the Oxfordshire Photographic Archive, a superb resource of over 150,000 images, which is housed in the Centre for Oxfordshire Studies at the Central Library, Westgate, Oxford. The creation of the Archive in 1990 was the brainchild of the County Council's Department of Leisure and Arts and has brought together the formerly separate collections of the Local Studies Library and the County Museum Service.

The Archive provides free public access to pictures of local places, people, events and activities and has been built up over many years by purchase, by donation and by copying borrowed photographs. It is perhaps best known for the work of Henry Taunt (1842–1922), the Oxford photographer, and for the Packer Collection from Chipping Norton. Both collections range beyond Oxfordshire, but the Archive concentrates upon building up a visual record of the county past and present and welcomes the opportunity to acquire interesting or unusual images. It also aims to widen access to the photographs through improved documentation and the use of new technology.